ADAMS'
Coding and
Reimbursement
A Simplified Approach

Fourth Edition

Wanda L. Adams

Wanda L. Adams and Associates, Inc.
Troy, Tennessee

ELSEVIER

3251 Riverport Lane
St. Louis, Missouri 63043

ADAMS' CODING AND REIMBURSEMENT: A SIMPLIFIED APPROACH, FOURTH EDITION   978-0-323-08434-5

Notice

Knowledge and best practice in this field are constantly changing. As new research and experience broaden our understanding, changes in research methods, professional practices, or medical treatment may become necessary.

Practitioners and researchers must always rely on their own experience and knowledge in evaluating and using any information, methods, compounds, or experiments described herein. In using such information or methods they should be mindful of their own safety and the safety of others, including parties for whom they have a professional responsibility.

With respect to any drug or pharmaceutical products identified, readers are advised to check the most current information provided (i) on procedures featured or (ii) by the manufacturer of each product to be administered, to verify the recommended dose or formula, the method and duration of administration, and contraindications. It is the responsibility of practitioners, relying on their own experience and knowledge of their patients, to make diagnoses, to determine dosages and the best treatment for each individual patient, and to take all appropriate safety precautions.

To the fullest extent of the law, neither the Publisher nor the authors, contributors, or editors, assume any liability for any injury and/or damage to persons or property as a matter of products liability, negligence or otherwise, or from any use or operation of any methods, products, instructions, or ideas contained in the material herein.

ISBN: 978-0-323-08434-5

Acquisitions Editor: Jeanne R Olson
Developmental Editor: Luke Held
Publishing Services Manager: July Eddie/Hemamalini Rajendrababu
Project Manager: Andrea Campbell/Srividhya Vidhyashankar
Designer: Jonarth Nill

Printed in the United States
Last digit is the print number: 9 8 7 6 5 4 3 2

On a personal note, I would like to dedicate this edition to my late husband, John, who always told me to reach for the highest star. Without his support, encouragement, and patience, I would not have had the courage or strength to reach for a star.

Reviewers

Renii Modisette, MHA, RHIT, CCS
AHIMA-approved ICD 10 Trainer and Ambassador
Systems Program Director, HIT/MBC
Pinnacle Career Institute
Kansas City, Missouri

Dee Mollenbernd
California Credentialed Instructor
Martinez Adult Education
Business Training Center
Martinez, California

Janet Roberts-Andersen, EdD, MT (ASCP)
Associate Professor, Medical Assisting Program
  Chair
Mercy College of Health Sciences
Des Moines, IA

Preface

Here's the concise, friendly textbook that makes coding, insurance, and claims easy for you to understand and so you can succeed on the job!

Adams' Coding and Reimbursement: A Simplified Approach, Fourth Edition, gives you the big picture so that you understand how each step in the coding and claims process affects reimbursement. It begins with coding rules and applications as its foundation and then moves into insurance carrier specifics, helping you understand the impact of carrier rules on claims submission. Then it helps you through the maze of the reimbursement system, all with plenty of real-world practice along the way!

NEW TO THIS EDITION

Chapter 2: Working with ICD-10-CM

This chapter provides the student with the opportunity to learn the new diagnostic coding system that goes into effect in October, 2013. By having this advanced knowledge of the changing face of diagnostic coding, the student will be better prepared for the exciting challenges that await the future of coding. This chapter provides a detailed look at the system, as well as case studies and coding exercises to develop the required skills to code using this new system.

Chapter 4: HCPCS Coding

To provide students with a better understanding of the purpose and uses of HCPCS coding, this section has been deleted from the Medicare chapter. By creating a new chapter devoted to the complexities of HCPCS coding, the student is able to visualize the greater potential of this code set. This chapter further demonstrates that HCPCS coding is not just for Medicare claims but that these codes are also accepted by most insurance companies. This chapter contains exercises and scenarios to provide the student with practical coding experience. Also included are:

- Updated content, tips, notes, and reminders
- Updates on industry and governmental changes, along with special notes and tips to keep students on the right track.

SUPPLEMENTAL RESOURCES

1. Enhanced TEACH Instructor's Resource, which includes:
   - PowerPoint Slides
   - ExamView test bank files—generate test questions at the click of a mouse
   - Curriculum information—effortlessly prepare for your course with sample syllabi, teaching tips, course outlines, course calendar, and lesson plans
2. An online program on Evolve, called *Code It & Claim It*, provides students with the opportunity to practice and hone their coding skills in an interactive environment.

Acknowledgments

I would like to say a special thank you to all of the people who took the time to review and comment on my book. I appreciate the kind comments and the assistance that this service provided.

I would like to send a very special thank you to the editorial staff at Elsevier who worked long hours in making this project happen and for their belief in this book.

To the entire marketing staff: Thank you for your hard work in presenting this material to your clients.

Contents

4   HCPCS Coding System, *140*

5   Understanding Insurance Policies, *149*

Diagnostic Coding: International Classification of Diseases, Ninth Revision, Clinical Modification (ICD-9-CM)

1

CHAPTER OUTLINE

KEY TERMS

Term	Definition
APG	Ambulatory patient group: A payment system similar to DRG but designed for the ambulatory care facility.
CMS	Centers for Medicare and Medicaid Services: The federal agency responsible for maintaining and monitoring the Medicare program, beneficiary services, and Medicaid and state operations.
Comorbidity	An ongoing condition that exists with another condition for which the patient is receiving treatment.
Compliance Plan	A structured format stating office policies and procedures for identifying and correcting inaccurate documentation and billing criteria.
Complication	A disease or condition that arises during the course of or as a result of another disease and that modifies medical treatment requirements.
Conventions	Terms and symbols used to provide instructions for using diagnostic codes.
CPT	Current Procedure Terminology
Cross References	Directions to look in another area for the correct code.
DRG	Diagnosis-related group: A patient classification system to categorize patients who are medically related with respect to diagnosis or treatment or who are statistically similar with regard to length of hospital stay.
DRG Rate	A fixed dollar amount payable to hospitals for patient care.
DSM-V	*Diagnostic and Statistical Manual of Mental Disorders, Fifth Edition:* A reference for coding psychiatric disorders or conditions.
E Codes	Codes for the external cause of injury or disease.

Eponym	A condition or procedure named after a person or place.
Etiology	The cause of a disease.
ICD-9-CM	*International Classification of Diseases, Ninth Revision, Clinical Modification:* The source of diagnosis coding required by insurance carriers and government agencies.
Index	Another term for ICD-9-CM, Volume 2, the alphabetical listing of terms to describe injuries or diseases.
Manifestation	Signs or symptoms of a disease.
NEC	Not elsewhere classified: A category of codes to be used only when the coder lacks the information required to code the term to a more specific category.
Nonessential Modifiers	Terms listed in parentheses that provide supplemental information but do not affect the code selection.
NOS	Not otherwise specified: This abbreviation is equivalent to "unspecified."
Rubric	Three-digit root code for the classification of illness, disease, or injury.
Specificity	Coding a diagnostic statement to the highest degree reportable within the ICD-9-CM manual, using fourth and fifth digits when available, while avoiding overuse of unspecified codes.
Tabular List	Another name for ICD-9-CM, Volume 1, the numerical listing of disease and injury.
V Codes	Supplemental codes that are used when a patient presents for something other than illness or disease.

OBJECTIVES

After completing this chapter, readers should be able to:

- Identify the specific volumes of *International Classification of Diseases, Ninth Revision, Clinical Modification* (ICD-9-CM) as they pertain to medical practices.
- Apply the five basic steps used to code diagnoses.
- Recognize and use ICD-9-CM conventions and guidelines.
- Recognize the various applications of numerical codes, V codes, and E codes.
- Understand and use the tables in the ICD-9-CM Index.
- Recognize and correct coding problems and errors.
- Correctly enter ICD-9-CM codes on a claim form.

This chapter is designed to introduce the reader to the ICD-9-CM coding system. It provides an overview of the coding system based on instructions and exercises for the practical application of ICD-9-CM coding principles. The ICD-9-CM is important because it is the national standard for reporting diagnoses, conditions, and signs and symptoms on insurance claim forms.

The Health Insurance Portability and Accountability Act of 1996 (HIPAA) was passed by the U.S. Congress to set standards (similar to those used in the financial field for transactions such as ATM use) for electronic health care transactions. A number of HIPAA regulations now set consistent standards and protect the privacy and security of a patient's health information.

The ICD-9-CM coding system is a part of HIPAA regulations called the HIPAA Electronic Health Care Transactions and Code Sets (TCS). Using these standards, physicians can prepare and transmit electronic claims in the same format, regardless of the insurance carrier. Every health plan must accept the standard format and standard codes and must send electronic messages back to the provider, also in standard formats, advising the provider of claim status, payment, and other key information.

Although ICD-9-CM coding is not easy, it will be easier for coders who have a good working knowledge of medical terminology and of basic anatomy and physiology, as well as a fundamental understanding of ICD-9-CM conventions and applications.

HISTORY

The statistical study of disease began as early as the seventeenth century with the work of John Graunt. In 1837 William Farr urged the adoption of a uniform classification of causes of death. In 1893 a French physician, Jacques Bertillon, developed the *Bertillon Classification of Causes of Death*. The United States began using Bertillon's classification system in approximately 1898. In 1938 the name was changed to *International Classification of Diseases* (ICD). With the publication of the ninth revision of the ICD in 1978, the words "Clinical Modification" (CM) were added to the title. This new title, *International Classification of Diseases, Ninth Revision, Clinical Modification (ICD-9-CM)*, is the one most recognized and used by coders today.

When it was published in 1978, the ICD-9-CM was a three-volume set compiled from the classifications that the World Health Organization (WHO) had established in 1977. However, since then, publishers have condensed the volumes into one book that contains either two or three of the volumes. Medical offices have the option of buying one book containing only the volumes that pertain to their particular practices or buying the complete three-volume set.

PURPOSE

The original purpose of the ICD system was to provide morbidity statistics for the WHO. Today medical offices use ICD-9-CM codes to provide information to substantiate the need for patient care or treatment and to provide statistics for analyzing the appropriateness of health care costs.

ICD coding translates written medical terminology or descriptions into codes that provide a universal language. Standard codes prevent the problems that arise when different terms are used for the same disease or condition. These standard codes are reported to insurance carriers with descriptions of the care or treatments patients received.

CODING COMPLIANCE

For many years, physicians were not required to give more than a simple descriptive phrase or perhaps the first three digits of the diagnosis code. Today, in order to have a profitable practice, a physician needs to understand the importance of coding and coding relationships. Federal agencies and most other insurance carriers require correct diagnosis coding. Coding has a direct impact on reimbursement to the practice.

Compliance with the rules for reporting codes is also important to correct coding. As you will see in this chapter, there are many guidelines (e.g., correct sequencing of codes) that must be followed for correct diagnostic coding. In most medical offices, a **compliance plan** covers the policies and procedures that must be followed. The compliance plan monitors the fulfillment of government regulations, especially in coding and billing.

Payers check the linkage between the condition and the care to determine if the services were medically necessary and should be reimbursed. Given the patient's condition, a payer or insurance company will seek answers to such questions as the following:

- Does the treatment match the diagnosis?
- Was the treatment elective or experimental? (Insurance companies do not pay for unnecessary or unapproved procedures.)
- Was the care furnished at an appropriate level?

> ## E X A M P L E
>
> A patient received a complete physical examination after visiting the physician with symptoms of a common cold. The diagnosis of only a cold does not support billing for a complete physical examination. The office would need to provide another diagnosis to support this type of service, because a payer is unlikely to reimburse this level of care for just a common cold.

In a medical office the chief source of ICD-9-CM codes should be the physician. The physician is the individual with the in-depth knowledge of the patient's condition and appropriate medical terminology. Although it is the physician's responsibility to advise staff concerning the patient's diagnosis, office staff should have a working knowledge of the coding systems, diagnoses (ICD-9-CM), and procedures (CPT) to assist the physician in coding patient services.

One recommendation is to confer with the physician on an annual basis and review the diagnosis codes most often used in the practice. By having a complete list of these codes, the office staff can prevent costly delays and questions on future claims.

CONTENTS OF ICD-9-CM

Let's begin our study by examining the design of ICD-9-CM and each of its three volumes to obtain a better understanding of the contents of each and how to apply them.

In the ICD-9-CM the way the text is printed is an important clue to the use of a particular code. In the introduction to each book, the publisher provides important facts and information to help the coder understand the basic uses of the ICD-9-CM. Each person involved in coding for the practice should read the introduction before beginning to code from that volume.

Tabular (Volume 1)

The Tabular List is a numerical listing of diseases and injuries. It contains 17 chapters for the classification of diseases and injuries, grouping problems by **etiology** (cause) or anatomical (body) site.

Composition of the Tabular List (Volume 1)

Main Classifications

1. 001-139   Infectious and Parasitic Diseases
2. 140-239   Neoplasm
3. 240-279   Endocrine, Nutritional, and Metabolic Diseases and Immunity Disorders
4. 280-289   Diseases of the Blood and Blood-Forming Organs
5. 290-319   Mental Disorders
6. 320-389   Diseases of the Nervous System and Sense Organs
7. 390-459   Diseases of the Circulatory System
8. 460-519   Diseases of the Respiratory System
9. 520-579   Diseases of the Digestive System
10. 580-629   Diseases of the Genitourinary System
11. 630-679   Complications of Pregnancy, Childbirth, and the Puerperium
12. 680-709   Diseases of the Skin and Subcutaneous Tissue
13. 710-739   Diseases of the Musculoskeletal System and Connective Tissue

14. 740-759   Congenital Anomalies
15. 760-779   Certain Conditions Originating in the Perinatal Period
16. 780-799   Symptoms, Signs, and Ill-Defined Conditions
17. 800-999   Injury and Poisoning

Supplementary Classifications

1. V01-V90   V Codes: Factors Influencing Health Status and Contact with Health Services
2. E000-E999   E Codes: External Causes of Injury and Poisoning

Appendices

A. Morphology of Neoplasm
B. This appendix, Glossary of Mental Disorders, was deleted October 1, 2004.
C. Classification of drugs by American Hospital Formulary Service List Number and ICD-9-CM Equivalents
D. Classification of Industrial Accidents According to Agency
E. List of Three-Digit Categories
    Table A: Table of Bacterial Food Poisons (May not appear in all publisher editions)

Index (Volume 2)

The Alphabetic Index is a listing of codes used as a guide to assist in locating the complete code in Volume 1.

Contents of Index (Volume 2)

- Index to Diseases
- Tables
  - Hypertension
  - Neoplasms
- Table of Drugs and Chemicals
- Index to External Cause of Injury and Poisoning

Volume 3

Volume 3 is a tabular alphabetical and numerical listing used primary by hospitals to report inpatient care. It includes a tabular list of procedures by anatomical sites, miscellaneous diagnostic and therapeutic procedures, and an alphabetical index. This volume is not intended for use by physician practices. Because the primary focus of this volume is on the medical office and outpatient services, it will not be discussed further.

TEST YOUR KNOWLEDGE   Exploring Volume Contents

1.   There are _____ chapters in Volume 1.

2.   Another name for Volume 1 is _____

3.   List the three tables in Volume 2, also called the Index.

    a. _____

    b. _____

    c. _____

4.   Which codes are used to describe the cause of injury or poisoning?

    _____

5.   Name the organization responsible for maintaining ICD-9-CM coding.

    _____

ICD-9-CM CODE FORMAT

In the diagnostic coding system, codes are broken down into a three-digit code category, or **Rubric**. Most of these three-digit codes are further broken down into a fourth-digit subcategory and a fifth-digit subclassification based on the descriptive terms needed to complete the diagnosis and achieve the highest degree of description, or **specificity**, for coding. However, not every code will require a fourth or fifth digit to be at its highest level of coding. There are a few codes that are at the highest level possible with only the three-digit number.

    To understand how a code is built based on three, four, or five digits, let's examine the code for diabetes mellitus (250).

Three-Digit Codes

The first three digits of a code classify a disease or a group of similar diseases within a particular category.

> EXAMPLE
>
> Code 250: Diabetes mellitus
>   The three digits *250* inform the coder that anything beginning with these three numbers will pertain to diabetes mellitus.

Fourth-Digit Subcategory

The addition of a fourth digit provides information about the cause, site, or description for the diagnosis. Its purpose is to add clinical detail.

> ### E X A M P L E
>
> Code 250.0: Diabetes mellitus without mention of complication
> The addition of the .0 has provided the coder with more information about the patient's condition or problem.

Fifth-Digit Subclassification

The fifth digit is provided to add even greater definition or to isolate terms for accuracy in clinical study.

> ### E X A M P L E
>
> Code 250.01: Diabetes mellitus without mention of complication, type 1 [juvenile type] or unspecified type, not stated as uncontrolled.
> The fifth digit tells the coder that the patient is insulin dependent and has a controlled case of diabetes.

 CODING TIP

To code diabetes, select the code based on whether the diabetes is juvenile onset versus type 2 or unspecified type or adult onset, not whether the patient is insulin dependent or noninsulin dependent. For example, "diabetes mellitus without complication, insulin dependent" would be coded as 250.00.

CONVENTIONS OF ICD-9-CM

To correctly apply the coding system, coders need to understand the various symbols, abbreviations, and other **conventions** that are used in ICD-9-CM. These descriptions and explanations are usually found in the introduction of the ICD-9-CM volume. With each new edition, publishers have deleted important definitions for some conventions. Let's review some of the conventions pertinent to diagnostic coding.

Use of Print Types

Bold Face

Volume 1, the Tabular List

All titles and codes are printed in bold type—for example, **876, Open wound of back.**

Volume 2, the Alphabetic List

The main term is printed in bold face—for example, **Emphysema.**

 CODING TIP

A main term represents a disease (e.g., pneumonia), condition (e.g., open wound), noun (e.g., syndrome), or adjective (e.g., large) that allows the coder to find the correct information and code number for a particular problem or condition.

Italics

In both volumes, italics are used to highlight all exclusion notes and to identify Rubrics (category codes) that ***should not*** be used as the primary code for a condition or problem. For example, in the Tabular List, look up the following:

Code 359.5, Myopathy in endocrine diseases classified elsewhere

You will see that the given code is written in italics with the instruction to code first the underlying disease, such as Addison's disease, 255.4. Because Addison's disease is the primary problem or condition of the patient, it should be listed first on the claim form as the primary diagnosis (Dx) and followed by the **manifestation** (359.5), or secondary diagnosis.

EXAMPLE
Primary Dx: 255.41, Addison's disease (code requires fifth digit)
Secondary Dx: 359.5, Myopathy in endocrine diseases classified elsewhere

LOCATING AN ICD-9-CM CODE

Table 1-1 contains the format and conventions used in the ICD-9-CM. Once we have reviewed these conventions, the next step is to learn how to locate a code. Coders must understand how each of the volumes (1 and 2) relates to the coding process.

Volume 1, often referred to as the Tabular List, is used as the final resource to apply the diagnosis, symptom, or condition. Because the Tabular List is in numerical order based on etiology instead of anatomy, it is difficult to find the correct code using this volume. When one is using the tabular listing, it is important to remember to *always* code to the highest level of the description. Use fourth and fifth digits only when they are applicable and are given in the coding sequence.

To solve the problem of finding the correct code, Volume 2, the Index, lists signs, symptoms, conditions, and so forth, in alphabetical order. The Index gives the coder an easy method of locating the correct code. It is important that you remember ***never*** to code directly from the Index. The Index is a reference tool to help locate the correct code in Volume 1. The Index might not list all the pertinent information for selecting the correct code.

Steps to Locating a Code

Developing good research habits is the key to correct coding. There are five basic steps to locating the correct diagnosis code. When these steps are followed, the coder will be successful in locating even the most elusive codes.

1. Correctly identify the main term or condition to be coded.
2. Use the Index to locate the condition or problem.
3. Refer to all notes, and review the information given while following all instructions or cross references.
4. Locate and confirm the correct code in the Tabular List and review all notes and information to select the correct code.
5. Place codes in correct sequence when using multiple diagnoses. The main or primary diagnosis should always be coded as the condition or reason that caused a patient to seek medical care.

EXAMPLE
A patient with a history of peptic ulcers (533.9) was seen in the office for acute pharyngitis (462). The ulcer code would not be listed unless it affected the patient's care or was addressed during the office visit.

TABLE 1-1   ICD-9-CM Conventions and Terms

Convention or Term	Explanation
{ } Brace	Used to enclose a series of terms, each of which is modified by the statement to the right of the brace (e.g., code 385.3).*
[ ] Brackets	Used to enclose synonyms, alternative wordings, or explanatory phrases (e.g., code 460).
Code First Underlying Disease	Used in categories not intended for primary tabulation of disease. These codes are also written in italics with a note. The note requires that the underlying disease or cause be recorded first and the particular manifestation be recorded second (this note will appear only in the Tabular List) (e.g., code 365.44).
: Colon	Used after an incomplete term that needs one or more of the modifiers that follow (usually indented) to make it assignable to a given category (e.g., code 366.12).
Eponym	Disease or syndrome named after the person who discovered it or the person who first developed the condition (e.g., 331.11, Pick's disease).
Excludes	Terms following this word indicate you must look to a different code series (e.g., code 333.3).
Includes	This note appears immediately under a three-digit code to further define or give an example of the contents of the category (e.g., code 007).
NEC	Not elsewhere classified. Used with ill-defined terms to alert the coder that specified terms for a condition may be classified differently or with terms when a more specific category is not provided in the code lists (e.g., code 519.1).
NOS	Not otherwise specified. Equivalent to unspecified. Used when the physician has insufficient data to code a specific condition (e.g., code 295.9).
Notes	Used to define terms and provide coding instructions (e.g., code 139).
( ) Parentheses	Used to enclose supplementary words that might or might not be present in a statement without affecting the code assignment (e.g., code 134.9).
Section markers	The section mark or indicator is provided to advise the coder that a footnote appears at the bottom at the page (e.g., code 852.1). Based on the publication it may appear as a circled number, a flag with arrows, or curved marks (§).†
See	A cross reference used primarily in the Index. It is an explicit direction for the coder to look elsewhere for the correct code. This term must always be followed to obtain the correct code (e.g., Volume 2, Rupture, oviduct).
See also	A cross reference to direct the coder to look elsewhere when the main term or subterm is not sufficient to code the condition or problem (e.g., Volume 2, Sinus—*see also* Fistula).
Use additional code	An explicit command that the selected code needs more information to provide an accurate clinical picture of the patient's problem or condition (e.g., code 250.4).

*Some publishers may not use this convention in their publications.
†Some publishers may use color-coded bars or symbols to provide coding assistance.

In addition to correctly sequencing codes, it is important to list all codes that affect patient care or for conditions that cause a patient to seek medical attention.

EXAMPLE

Situation

A patient is seen in a follow-up office visit for hypertension (401.1). During the examination, the patient complains of problems of frequent urination and a burning sensation. The physician orders a urinalysis for the patient and a complete blood count (CBC). The diagnosis listed on the encounter form only indicates the diagnosis of high blood pressure (401.1).

Problem

The claim is sent to the insurance company and lists the office visit, a urinalysis, and a CBC with a diagnosis of hypertension (401.1). The insurance company denies payment for the CBC and the urinalysis as being medically unnecessary.

Solution

To correct this problem, the office would have to file an appeal, accompanied by additional information, with the insurance company. This process could delay payment for the laboratory work for another 4 to 8 weeks.

   To have prevented this problem, the office should have submitted a secondary diagnosis of a urinary tract problem in addition to the primary diagnosis of the hypertension. The hypertension diagnosis should only have been associated with the office visit—not the laboratory services on the claim form.

The following pages contain coding exercises to assist you in checking your understanding of the conventions used in the ICD-9-CM manuals.

ICD-9-CM CODING EXERCISE 1   Using ICD-9-CM Conventions

Directions: Answer the following questions by giving the specified information. You might wish to list the ICD-9-CM page number for easy reference.

Example: Code 491 is assigned to chronic bronchitis. The complete code number for simple chronic bronchitis is as follows:

Page *131*, _____ Volume 1, _____ Answer: *491.0*

1.   Identify the site that is *excluded* from code 011.3, Tuberculosis of bronchus.

Page _____ Volume _____ Answer: _____

_____

_____

2. Identify the fifth digit(s) used with category 250.

   Page _____   Volume _____   Answer: _____

   _____

   _____

3. Rheumatism excluding the back is classified under codes 725 to 729. Which other categories are included in these codes?

   Page _____   Volume _____   Answer: _____

   _____

   _____

4. In some editions of ICD-9-CM, a brace is located under entry 560.9. What does a brace signify?

   Page _____   Volume _____   Answer: _____

   _____

   _____

5. Code 321.0 appears in italics. What is the significance of italics?

   Page _____   Volume _____   Answer: _____

   _____

   _____

6. Code 017 is preceded by a section mark. What does this indicate?

   Page _____   Volume _____   Answer: _____

   _____

   _____

7. Code 473 includes several words in parentheses. Is it necessary for these words to appear in the written definition of the diagnosis? Why or why not?

    Page _____   Volume _____   Answer: _____

    _____

    _____

8. Code 041 includes a note. What is the purpose of the note?

    Page _____   Volume _____   Answer: _____

    _____

    _____

9. Code 292 contains the instruction "Use additional code for any associated drug dependence (304.0-304.9)." Which code(s) would you use to completely code a diagnosis of drug-related hallucination due to cocaine dependence?

    Page _____   Volume _____   Answer: _____

    _____

    _____

10. Locate the following entries in the Alphabetic Index and list any cross reference entry.

    1. Patellar; 2. Backflow (pyelovenous); 3. Compression with injury

    Answers:

    1. _____   Page _____

    2. _____   Page _____

    3. _____   Page _____

ICD-9-CM CODING EXERCISE 2   Basic ICD-9-CM Coding

Directions: Underline the main term in each coding problem. Locate the term in the Alphabetic Index. Record the page number and code.

Example: Irritable colon, Code 564.1, Page 430

TERM	CODE	PAGE
1. Diabetes insipidus	_____	_____
2. Yellow jaundice	_____	_____
3. Diverticulitis of colon	_____	_____
4. Major depression, single, mild	_____	_____
5. Tobacco dependence, continuous	_____	_____
6. Myocardial infarction with hypertension, initial episode of care	_____	_____
7. Bleeding peptic ulcer without obstruction	_____	_____
8. Actinic keratosis	_____	_____
9. Common migraine with blurred vision	_____	_____
10. Urinary tract infection with vaginitis NOS	_____	_____
11. Food poisoning NOS with vomiting	_____	_____
12. Colles' fracture	_____	_____

ICD-9-CM CODING SPECIFICS

Now that you have been introduced into the world of diagnosis coding and have a basic understanding of ICD-9-CM formats and conventions, it is time to take a closer look at coding as it relates to a medical practice. We will examine issues dealing with coding chronic conditions, surgery, neoplasms, and suspected conditions. We will explore the tables in Volume 2 to determine just how beneficial they are to the coder. Also, you will learn about **V codes** and **E codes**.

A key factor in accurate coding is the importance of reading the notes and other instructions provided with a code. Most coding questions can be answered simply by returning to the beginning of the chapter or code series and reviewing the instructions given for that code.

Hypertension Table

In the Index, you will find the Hypertension Table (Table 1-2) by looking up the word *Hypertension*. This table contains a complete listing of all conditions that are due to or associated with hypertension.

TABLE 1-2 Hypertension Table

Hypertension	Malignant	Benign	Unspecified
Hypertension, hypertensive (arterial) (arteriolar) (disease) (essential) (fluctuating) (idiopathic) (intermittent) (labile) (low renin) (orthostatic) (paroxysmal) (primary) (systemic) (uncontrolled) (vascular)	401.0	401.1	401.9
with			
heart involvement (conditions classifiable to 428, 429.0-429.3, 429.8, 429.9 due to hypertension) (*see also* Hypertension, heart) with kidney involvement—*see* Hypertension, cardiorenal	402.00	402.10	401.90
renal involvement (only conditions classifiable to 585, 586, 587) (excludes conditions classifiable as 584) (*see also* Hypertension, kidney)	403.00	403.10	403.90
with heart involvement—*see* Hypertension, cardiorenal			
failure (and sclerosis) (*see also* Hypertension, kidney)	403.01	403.11	403.91
sclerosis without failure (*see also* Hypertension, kidney)	403.00	403.10	403.90
accelerated (*see also* Hypertension, by type, malignant)	401.0	—	—
antepartum—*see* Hypertension, complicating pregnancy, childbirth, or the puerperium			
cardiorenal (disease)	404.00	404.10	404.90
with			
heart failure	404.01	404.11	404.91
and renal failure	404.03	404.13	404.93
renal failure	404.02	404.12	404.92
and heart failure	404.03	404.13	404.93

Source: International Classification of Diseases, Ninth Revision, Clinical Modification (ICD-9-CM).

Note that some descriptions have a code listed under each category and other descriptions have only one code listed under just one column. This information is found only in the hypertension table. By initially looking for a code in the table, the coder is able to choose the correct code from the Tabular List (Volume 1).

E X A M P L E

Look at the code for accelerated hypertension. Note that the code for accelerated hypertension (401.0) is listed only under the column for a malignant condition.

Verify the code for accelerated hypertension in the Tabular List (Volume 1). Without using the table, the coder would not have been able to code this diagnosis, because Volume 1 does not specify the term *accelerated*. Unless the coder knew that "accelerated hypertension" is always coded as a malignant condition, it would have been difficult to code.

At the top of the heading, notice the words *malignant, benign,* and *unspecified*. Many people are more familiar with the words *malignant* and *benign* as they pertain to cancer. However, when applied to hypertension, the definitions have a different meaning.

Malignant Hypertension

- Uncommon form of hypertension occurring in approximately 5% of patients with elevated blood pressure
- Generally of an abrupt onset and runs a course measured in months
- Often produces renal failure or cerebral hemorrhage
- Patient generally exhibits blood pressure of 200/140 mm Hg
- Chances for long-term survival depend on early treatment before development of renal insufficiency

Benign Hypertension

- Remains fairly stable over a long course of time without compromising the life span
- Becomes a risk factor if untreated because it may result in coronary heart disease or cerebrovascular disease
- Generally is asymptomatic until complications develop
- Usually treated with antihypertensive drug therapy

Unspecified

The type of hypertension has not been determined by a physician.

Hypertension is often the cause of various forms of heart or vascular disease, but you should not assume that "hypertension with heart disease" is a cause-and-effect relationship. The mention of hypertension with some forms of heart diseases does not necessarily imply a combination condition. The conditions can be combined only if the diagnostic statement showing cause uses the words *due to*. The words *and* or *with* do not imply cause in the diagnostic statement. Also, if hypertensive disease is stated as being present, the combination of codes may also be made. Watch out for the words *due to* and *with*.

With

The mention of hypertension *with* a heart condition should not be interpreted as a combination code resulting in hypertensive heart disease. A combination code is only used if there is a cause- and-effect relationship with the heart condition and the hypertension (see heart condition codes 428.0-428.9, 429.0-429.3, and 429.8-429.9).

Due to

The phrase *due to* is considered synonymous with hypertensive disease.

E X A M P L E

Hypertensive Heart Disease (Heart disease due to Hypertension)
- Because the statements indicate a cause-and-effect relationship for the conditions (heart disease and hypertension), one code covers both statements: 402.90.

Benign Hypertension with Congestive Heart Failure
- Two codes are required to document this statement because there is *no* cause-and-effect relationship. In this statement, you have two separate problems for treatment: 428.0, Congestive heart failure, and 401.1, Benign hypertension.

Benign Hypertension due to Congestive Heart Failure
Because the statement indicates a cause-and-effect relationship for the conditions (heart failure and hypertension), one code covers both statements: 402.11.

 CODING TIP

Do not confuse hypertension with elevated blood pressure. A patient should not be given a diagnosis of hypertension unless it has been confirmed by the physician based on a series of tests and blood pressure readings.

Hypertension versus Elevated Blood Pressure

401-405	Hypertension	Persistent high blood pressure
796.2	Elevated blood pressure	Blood pressure that might have been caused by stress or other problems occurring only during the visit or a procedure

Coding conditions from Chapter 7 of the Tabular List (Volume 1), Diseases of the Circulatory System, can be complex because of the interrelationship of conditions, the specificity of coding guidelines, and the various terms used to describe circulatory conditions.

According to ICD-9-CM, *Official Guidelines for Coding and Reporting*, Hypertension as related to high blood pressure due to an unknown cause is reported using ICD-9-CM code 401, essential hypertension, which is a primary diagnosis. However, when a cause is known, hypertension is referred to as a *secondary condition*. Specific categories are provided to report hypertension in association with other conditions or problems.

E X A M P L E

1. Hypertensive Heart Disease Category 402

   This category is used when a causal relationship is stated (*due to* hypertension) or implied (hypertensive). The use of these terms implies that a cause-and-effect relationship exists. The fifth-digit subclassification for category 402 is used to indicate the presence of heart failure.

   A cause-and-effect relationship between hypertension and heart disease cannot be assumed. You must examine the exact wording of the diagnostic statement to determine if it is a cause-and-effect situation or if it is two coexisting conditions. When the conditions coexist, use two separate diagnostic codes.

   When there is a cause-and-effect condition, the primary diagnosis would be the 402 code with a fifth digit indicating the presence of heart failure and a second code to identify the type of heart failure.

   Example of cause-and-effect coding: Congestive heart failure *due to* hypertension, 402.91 + 428.0

   Example of coexisting conditions (no cause-and-effect relationship): Congestive heart failure *with* benign hypertension, 428.0 + 401.1

2. Hypertension and Kidney (Renal) Disease Category 403

   ICD-9-CM assumes a cause-and-effect relationship when *hypertension* and *renal disease* are listed in the same diagnostic statement. The determining factor for using category 403 is that the renal failure must be a chronic condition. If the renal failure is an acute problem, you would code essential hypertension (401) and acute renal failure (584).

   Example: 403.01, Accelerated hypertension *with* chronic renal failure

3. Hypertension with Renal Disease And Heart Disease Category 404

   Category 404 is used when a heart condition (402) and a chronic kidney condition (403) coexist. The fifth digit specifies whether congestive heart failure, chronic kidney disease, or both are present. Additional codes are required to report the type of heart failure and/or chronic kidney disease.

   Example: Hypertensive congestive heart failure *with* chronic kidney disease, 404.91 + 428.0

4. Secondary Hypertension Category 405

   Secondary hypertension (405) is the result of some other primary disease. When the condition causing the hypertension can be cured or brought under reasonable control, the secondary hypertension may either be stabilized or it may disappear altogether. The underlying cause or condition should be listed as the first or primary code followed by the code for secondary hypertension (405).

   Examples: Hypertension *due to* systemic lupus erythematosus, 710.0 + 405.99; Acromegaly with secondary hypertension, 253.0 + 405.99

NEOPLASM TABLE

In the Tabular List (Volume 1), neoplasms (growths or tumors resulting from abnormal cell activity), are found in Chapter 2. The Index (Volume 2) also has a special listing for neoplasms in the form of a table (Table 1-3). The table is listed under "neoplasm."

TABLE 1-3   Neoplasm Table

Neoplasm	MALIGNANT			Benign	Uncertain Behavior	Unspecified
	Primary	Secondary	Ca in situ			
Neoplasm (continued) bone (periosteum)	170.9	198.5	—	213.9	238.0	239.2

Note: Carcinomas and adenocarcinomas of any type other than intraosseous or odontogenic of the sites listed under "Neoplasm, bone" should be considered as constituting metastatic spread from an unspecified primary site and coded to 198.5 for morbidity coding and to 199.1 for underlying cause of death coding.

Neoplasm	Primary	Secondary	Ca in situ	Benign	Uncertain Behavior	Unspecified
acetabulum	170.6	198.5	—	213.6	238.0	239.2
acromion (process)	170.4	198.5	—	213.4	238.0	239.2
ankle	170.8	198.5	—	213.8	238.0	239.2
arm NEC	170.4	198.5	—	213.4	238.0	239.2
astragalus	170.8	198.5	—	213.8	238.0	239.2
atlas	170.2	198.5	—	213.2	238.0	239.2
axis	170.2	198.5	—	213.2	238.0	239.2
back NEC	170.2	198.5	—	213.2	238.0	239.2
calcaneus	170.8	198.5	—	213.8	238.0	239.2

Source: *International Classification of Diseases, Ninth Revision, Clinical Modification* (ICD-9-CM).

At the beginning of the table, you see information regarding the various types of neoplasms. Neoplasms are broken into four main categories: malignant, benign, uncertain behavior, and unspecified. Under the *malignant* heading there are three categories to describe the types of malignancy: primary, secondary, and ca in situ.

- Malignant: A severe form of neoplasm with the potential for destructive growth and metastasis (shifting to a new site)
- Primary: Original location or presumed site of a malignant neoplasm
- Secondary: Area where a neoplasm metastasizes or spreads to
- Ca in situ: Neoplasms that are contained or confined to the original site or location
- Benign: A nonmalignant neoplasm
- Uncertain behavior: The pathologist has been unable to determine the type of neoplasm from the features that are present.
- Unspecified: The physician has insufficient data to categorize the neoplasm.
- At the beginning of the table, a boxed note appears. Within this note, important directions are identified with an asterisk (*). When the asterisk appears with a specific site in the table, the following rules apply:
  - Squamous cell carcinomas or epidermoid carcinomas should be classified as malignant neoplasms of the skin.
  - Neoplasms identified as papilloma (any type) should be classified as a benign neoplasm of the skin.

When placing these codes on an insurance form, you should always list the primary site and then the secondary site.

Once a neoplasm has been successfully treated, it is inappropriate to use the neoplasm codes for follow-up care. Offices should use codes V10 to V19, which are special V codes associated with neoplasms, for the following situations:

- The primary malignancy has been removed.
- The patient is not receiving chemotherapy or radiotherapy associated with an active neoplasm.
- There is no evidence of any remaining malignancy.

Morphology Codes (M8000/0 to M9970/1)

The morphology of neoplasms appears in Appendix A of the Tabular List. Morphology codes identify the histological type and behavior of a neoplasm. These codes consist of the letter *M* followed by a five-digit number. The first four digits of the code identify the histological type of the neoplasms, and the fifth digit indicates the behavior of the neoplasm. The purpose of M codes is to document statistical information; they are used by researchers, pathologists, and agencies that specialize in cancer care.

E X A M P L E

M8800/3, Sarcoma of femur

The behavior codes indicate the following information:

Code	Description
/0	Benign
/1	Uncertain whether benign, malignant, or borderline malignant
/2	Carcinoma in situ
/3	Malignant, primary site
/6	Malignant, secondary site
/9	Malignant, uncertain whether primary or metastatic site

A complete list of M codes can be found in the Tabular List of ICD-9-CM.

In the physician setting, these codes are not required and should never appear on an insurance claim form. The primary purpose of M codes is to assist in tumor registries, pathology departments, and other agencies specializing in cancer.

 Coding Tip

Morphology codes should ***never*** be used in place of neoplasm codes to report a patient's condition. Morphology codes are never placed on a claim form.

Neoplasm Coding Specifics

There are two basic types of neoplasms: Solid (140-199) and hematopoietic and lymphatic (200-208). In the Alphabetic Index, neoplasms are classified by system, organ, or site. The exceptions to this rule include neoplasms of the lymphatic and hematopoietic systems. These neoplasms should always be coded in categories 200-208, regardless of whether the neoplasm is primary or secondary. Because they are considered widespread and systemic in nature, they do not metastasize and, therefore, would not be coded to category 196.

Other exceptions include malignant melanomas of the skin; lipomas; and common tumors of the bone, uterus, and ovary. Only use category 195, Malignant neoplasms of other and ill-defined sites, when a more specific site cannot be identified.

Code Sequencing

To correctly sequence diagnostic codes, the following three factors should be considered:
- Behavior of the neoplasm
- Site or location of the neoplasm
- Reason for the patient encounter

General Coding Guidelines

- When treatment is directed toward the primary neoplasm, code that neoplasm as the primary or principal diagnosis.
- When treatment is directed only at a secondary site, sequence the metastatic site as the primary or principal diagnosis with the primary site listed as a secondary diagnosis.
- When the malignancy has been excised and the patient is no longer receiving treatment for the condition, use the V code for Personal history of malignant neoplasm to report the diagnosis.
- When a patient with a malignancy receives treatment for an acute condition that may be a result of the malignancy (e.g., anemia or pain), code the acute condition as the primary or principal diagnosis and the malignancy as the secondary diagnosis.
- When treatment is directed at a malignancy (e.g., chemotherapy [V58.1] or radiotherapy [V58.0]), one should code the purpose of the encounter or admission as the primary diagnosis.

Guidelines for Primary Sites

The primary site or origin of the tumor may involve two adjacent sites. To code overlapping boundaries, you should use the fourth-digit subcategory 8. To report therapies following the surgical removal of a neoplasm, code the therapy as the primary diagnosis and the carcinoma as the secondary diagnosis. When the patient is receiving therapy for the removed carcinoma, it is correct to report the neoplasm as though it still exists. For recurring neoplasms that have been surgically removed or eradicated by a therapy procedure, use a primary malignant code unless otherwise directed by the Alphabetic Index. In a diagnostic statement, when cancer is described as "metastatic from" a specific site, a coder should interpret this as the primary neoplasm (i.e., where the neoplasm began).

Guidelines for Secondary Sites

A secondary site is one that the neoplasm has metastasized to from another location. In the diagnostic statement the wording may be listed or stated as "Metastatic to." For neoplasms described as "metastatic to" a specific site, you should interpret the specific site to be a secondary neoplasm for that site.

When the only site that is noted in the diagnostic statement is "metastatic," the following steps must be taken to determine the correct code category:

- Locate the morphologic type of the neoplasm.
- Review subterms for the specific site.
- When a specific site is not included as a subterm, assign a primary code of unspecified site.

Sites Subject to Exception for Secondary Neoplasms

The following sites are classifiable as secondary when not otherwise specified. These are classified to codes 195.0 to 195.8, Malignant neoplasms of other and ill-defined sites.

Bone	Mediastinum
Brain	Meninges
Diaphragm	Peritoneum
Heart	Pleura
Liver	Retroperitoneum
Lymph nodes	Spinal Cord

Also take care to assign the appropriate code for primary or secondary malignant neoplasms of specified or unspecified sites that are included in the diagnostic statement.

E X A M P L E

1. Diagnosis:

Metastatic Carcinoma of the Bone.

Step 1: Look for a subterm of unspecified site; if no entry found, you are referred to "see also" neoplasm by site; the term *malignant* appears after *carcinoma.*

Step 2: Look in the Neoplasm Table for a subterm of unspecified site, then select code 199.1.

Step 3: Review the exception list to determine if bone is included on the list.

Step 4: Because *bone* is on the list, assign it as a secondary code.

2. Diagnosis:

Metastatic Carcinoma of the Lung.

Step 1: Look for a subterm of unspecified site; if no entry found, you are referred to "see also" neoplasm by site; the term *malignant* appears after *carcinoma.*

Step 2: Look in the Neoplasm Table for a subterm of unspecified site, then select code 199.1.

Step 3: Review the exception list to determine if lung is included on the list.

Step 4: Because *lung* is not included in the list, assign a primary site code of 162.9, Malignant neoplasm of bronchus and lung, unspecified.

Quick Reference: Neoplasm Rules and Ranking

- "Metastatic from": Indicates where the neoplasm began, or the primary site (e.g., *Metastatic* carcinoma *from* the lung: 162.9).
- "Metastatic to": Indicates where the neoplasm moved or metastasized to, or a secondary malignant neoplasm (e.g., *Metastatic* carcinoma *to* the brain: 198.3).
- "Metastatic of": Typically refers to a primary site unless the anatomical site is on the exception list and not otherwise specified as primary or secondary (*Metastatic* adenocarcinoma *of* transverse colon: 153.1).
- When treating both a primary and a secondary site, code the primary site first. When there are two primary sites, list both as a primary neoplasm; ranking will depend on the severity of the conditions.
- When treating a secondary site only and the primary site is known, use the secondary site as the first diagnosis code with the primary neoplasm as the secondary code.
- In the case of a malignancy with a complication, first code the reason the patient is seeking care. For example, the patient developed anemia associated with a malignancy and the only treatment is for the anemia; code the anemia as the primary diagnosis followed by the appropriate code for the neoplasm. When a patient is being treated for a neoplasm (e.g., chemotherapy) and develops a complication (e.g., uncontrolled nausea or vomiting), the primary code would be V58.0, Encounter for chemotherapy, followed by the code for the complication.
- Patient receiving chemotherapy or radiation therapy: First use the V code for the therapy followed by the code that identifies the reason for the treatment.
- Admitted for chemotherapy for carcinoma of the ovary: V58.11 + 183.0.
- Assign a personal history code when the primary neoplasm has been eradicated and is no longer under treatment (e.g., Metastatic adenocarcinoma of sacrum, prostatic in origin, patient had previous prostatectomy: 198.5 + V10.46).

ICD-9-CM CODING EXERCISE 3   Coding Applications of ICD-9-CM

Directions: Using Volumes 1 and 2, correctly code the following conditions. List the Index page number for reference.

CODE/PAGE

1. Renal and heart disease due to hypertension   _____

2. Chest pain originating in chest wall   _____

3. Abnormal electrocardiogram   _____

4. Secondary malignant neoplasm of the ovary   _____

5. Lipoma of the kidney   _____

6. Carcinoma in situ, breast   _____

7. Neoplasm of unspecified nature, liver   _____

8. Skin cancer, squamous cell carcinoma of the primary site, eyelid   _____

SUSPECTED CONDITIONS

There may be times in coding when the physician is unable to provide a specific diagnosis that enables you to code the reason the patient sought medical care. The physician might make a statement such as "rule out," "probable cause," or "suspect" as part of the thought process. These words can cause coding problems.

The ICD-9-CM manual does not contain codes to "rule out" a diagnosis or to report "probable cause" situations. Once a code has been assigned to report the patient's condition or problem, the insurance carrier is, in effect, being told that is the reason the patient sought medical care.

When a coder is faced with this type of coding problem, it is best to code for a sign or a symptom. A more specific, clear, descriptive diagnosis can be made when the physician receives more information concerning the patient's problem.

E X A M P L E

A patient comes to the office complaining of headaches. The physician orders tests to "rule out" a possible brain tumor. However, when the claim is submitted to the insurance carrier, code 191.1, Malignant neoplasm of the frontal lobe, is listed as the diagnosis. For this insurance carrier, the patient now has a history of a brain tumor. Because this code is on his or her record, the patient might have trouble obtaining new insurance or be forced to pay a higher premium for coverage. The situation could have been avoided if the office had coded for a sign or symptom (e.g., code 784.0, Pain in the head NOS).

CHRONIC CONDITIONS

Only code a chronic condition when the patient is seeking medical care for that specific condition or problem. It is not necessary to list on the insurance claim form every condition for which the physician has ever treated the patient. A good general rule is to apply only diagnosis codes for specific problems as they affect patient care or for which the patient seeks medical attention.

EXAMPLE
A patient with a history of arthritis saw his family doctor for a sore throat. Do not report the arthritis for this visit unless the physician actually treated the chronic condition of arthritis while treating the problem of the sore throat.

Coding Tip

Coding is often a case of research, trial and error, and plain hard work.

TEST YOUR KNOWLEDGE   Locating a Diagnosis Code

The five rules for locating a diagnosis code are:

1. _____

2. _____

3. _____

4. _____

5. _____

CODING FOR LATE EFFECTS

A late effect is usually an inactive, residual effect or condition produced after the acute portion of an injury or illness has passed. Key phrases such as "due to an old injury" or "due to previous illness" indicate that the problem or condition may be a late effect. If these indicators are not present in the diagnostic statement, the injury or condition may be considered to be a late effect provided sufficient time has elapsed between the original problem condition and the late effect.

To correctly code a late effect, one should first list the code that describes the current problem or condition, then list the code for the original illness or injury that is no longer present in its acute phase.

EXAMPLE
Diagnosis: Malunion of fracture, left arm
Codes: 733.81   Malunion of fracture
905.2   Late effect of fracture of upper extremity (for injuries classifiable to 810-819)

The residual or continuing problem is the malunion of the arm. It would have been incorrect to code the problem as a current or active injury (e.g., code 818.0, Ill-defined fracture of the arm).

Because the example was a fracture, refer to the notes concerning fractures in Volumes 1 and 2. The note in Volume 2 explains that fractures are considered either "closed" or "opened." The note in Volume 1 clarifies the coding process by stating, "A fracture not indicated as closed or open should be classified as closed." Had this example been a current injury, the coder would have known, based on the notes at the beginning of the section for fracture care, that the correct code would have been the one that indicated a closed fracture of the arm.

To locate "late effect" codes, begin by looking in Volume 2 under the main phrase "late effect" to determine if an applicable code is listed for the coding situation. Remember to always verify the code in Volume 1 before using the code.

V CODES

V codes (V01-V82.3) are supplemental classification codes for factors that influence patient care. These codes may be used when the patient sees the doctor without a complaint or problem (e.g., sports examination or employment physical) or to describe circumstances or conditions that could influence patient care (e.g., allergy to penicillin).

V codes are broken down into the following categories in the Tabular List:

V01-V06	Persons with potential health hazards related to communicable disease (e.g., V02, Carrier or suspected carrier of infectious disease)
V07-V09	Persons with need for isolation, other potential health hazards, and prophylactic measures (e.g., V07.1, Desensitization to allergens)
V10-V19	Persons with potential health hazards related to personal and family history (e.g., V14.7, Personal history of allergy to serum or vaccine)
V20-V29	Persons encountering health services in circumstances related to reproduction and development (e.g., V24.2, Routine postpartum follow-up)
V30-V39	Healthy live-born infants according to type of birth (e.g., V30.0, Single live born, in a hospital)
V40-V49	Persons with a condition influencing health status (e.g., V46.1, Patient dependent on respirator)
V50-V59	Persons encountering health services for specific procedures and aftercare (e.g., V58.3, Attention to surgical dressing and sutures)
V60-V69	Persons encountering health services in other circumstances (e.g., V67.4, Follow-up treatment of a fracture)
V70-V83	Persons without a reported diagnosis encountered during examination and investigation of individuals and populations (e.g., V77.5, Special screening for gout)

Another way to understand the use of V codes is to examine the three main types of conditions or categories of the codes.

1. Problems: Something that could affect the patient's overall health status.

Example: V14.0, History of allergy to penicillin

This situation could affect the overall treatment of the patient's problem.

2. Services: When a patient returns for a problem or treatment for something other than illness or injury.

Example: V70.3, Routine vaccination or V03, Routine exam before a student can participate in sports activities at school.

3. Factual Findings: V Codes can be used to describe facts for statistical purposes.

Example: V34, Pregnancy w/multiple births

To locate V codes, you need to use a *keyword list*. In recent years, the publishers of ICD-9-CM have been omitting this vital piece of information. Because ICD-9-CM does not contain a keyword list, you may find it beneficial to develop your own. The following list is provided as an example and as the foundation of a keyword list to assist coders in finding V codes in the alphabetical index.

Admission for	Counseling	History of	Replacement
Aftercare	Dialysis	Maintenance	Screening
Attention to	Donor	Maladjustment	Status
Care (of)	Examination	Newborn	Supervision
Carrier	Fitting of	Observation	Test
Contact	Follow-up	Problem	Transplant
Contraception	Health	Prophylactic	Vaccination

ICD-9-CM CODING EXERCISE 4   Using Keyword List

Directions: The following exercise is designed to help you locate V codes. List the keyword and page number for reference. *Note:* More than one code may apply.

Example: Adjustment of cardiac pacemaker
Keyword: Admission; Page: 30, Volume 2; Code: V53.

DESCRIPTION	KEYWORD	PAGE	CODE
1. Single live birth in hospital			
2. Desensitization to allergies			
3. Examination of donor bone marrow			
4. Fourteen-day-old infant admitted for health supervision due to abandonment			
5. Family planning advice			
6. Panic disorder due to parent-child conflict			
7. Transplantation of heart valve			
8. Observation following automobile accident			

E CODES

What is an "E" Code?

E codes are *optional* codes to show the following:
- Events or circumstances
- Cause of injury or poisoning
- Other adverse effects

CODING TIP

An E code should never be used as a primary or stand-alone code.

The function of an E code is as follows:
- To provide details of an incident or injury
- To help identify the following:
  - Automobile accident liability
  - Worker compensation situations
  - Third-party insurance liability

EXAMPLE

A patient with a diagnosis of a Colles' fracture caused by a fall from a scaffold at a construction site. This situation would be coded as follows:
1. 813.41   Colles' fracture
2. E881.1   Fall from scaffold
3. E849.3   Industrial premises

Based on the previous example, the E Code would clarify which insurance carrier would be responsible for paying the claim by showing how and where the accident occurred. This claim would then be easily identified as a workers' compensation claim.

 CODING TIP

The key to locating E codes may be found in Volume 2 under "Index to External Cause."

The following is a list of the categories of E codes.

Categories of E Codes

E800-E848	Transport accidents (e.g., E843.8, Ground crew fall from aircraft)
E849	Category used to describe place of occurrence with categories E850-E869 (e.g., E849.1, Farm)
E850-E858	Accidental poisoning by drugs, medical substances, and biologicals (e.g., E856, Accidental poisoning by antibiotics)
E860-E869	Accidental poisoning by other solid and liquid substances, gases, and vapors (e.g., E861.5, Accidental poisoning from lead paint)
E870-E876	Misadventures to patients during surgical and medical care (e.g., E871.4, Foreign object left in body during endoscopic exam)
E878-E879	Surgical and medical procedures as the cause of abnormal reaction of patient or later complication, without mention of misadventure at time of procedure (e.g., E878.5, Amputation of limbs)
E880-E888	Accidental falls (e.g., E884.2, Fall from a bed)
E890-E899	Accident caused by fire and flame (e.g., E898.0, Accident caused by burning bed clothes)
E900-E909	Accident due to natural and environmental factors (e.g., E905.6, Sting of jellyfish)
E910-E915	Accident caused by submersion, suffocation, and foreign bodies (e.g., E913.1, Suffocation by plastic bag)
E916-E928	Other accidents (e.g., E917.1, Crushed by crowd)
E929	Late effects of accidental injury (e.g., E929.2, Late effects of accidental poisoning)
E930-E949	Drugs, medicinal substances, and biological substances causing adverse effects in therapeutic use (e.g., E930.0, Adverse effect of penicillin)

E950-E959	Suicide and self-inflicted injury (e.g., E950.1, Suicide by use of barbiturates)
E960-E969	Homicide and injury inflicted by other persons (e.g., E965.7, Assault by letter bomb)
E970-E978	Legal intervention (e.g., E978, Legal execution)
E979	Terrorism (e.g., Terrorism involving firearms)
E980-E989	Injury undetermined accidentally or purposefully inflicted (e.g., E980.1, Poisoning by barbiturates)
E990-E999	Injury resulting from operations of war (e.g., E997.1, Injury due to biological warfare)

ICD-9-CM CODING EXERCISE 5   E Codes

Directions: Locate and list the correct code(s) that describe the following situations.

DESCRIPTION	CODE	PAGE
1. Open wound (laceration) of face, unspecified site, due to circular power saw accident at a farm		
Secondary code (E code)	_____	_____
Location (E code)	_____	_____
2. Post-traumatic convulsion. Patient was in a boating accident 6 months ago that resulted in a skull fracture.		
Contributing code	_____	_____
Late effect (E code)	_____	_____
3. Gunshot wound, complicated, right leg		
Victim of gang shooting	_____	_____
Secondary code (E code)	_____	_____
4. Residual of tuberculosis	_____	_____
5. Late effect of rickets	_____	_____
6. Traumatic arthritis due to left wrist fracture	_____	_____

POISONING AND ADVERSE EFFECTS OF DRUGS

E codes can be used to distinguish between poisoning and the adverse effects of drugs. Most insurance companies do not require a coder to use E codes; however, using these codes can help eliminate lengthy correspondence between the physician and third-party payers.

Drug poisoning usually occurs in one of three ways. The following is a list with a brief description to clarify how poisoning may occur.

The three categories of drug poisoning
- Accidental   Drug or medication was given in error
- Purposeful   Suicide or homicide attempt
- Undetermined   Insufficient data to determine whether the poisoning was accidental or intentional

In addition, drug poisoning can be an adverse effect. An adverse effect occurs when a prescribed drug or medication was properly administered or taken in accordance with the prescribed dosage recommendation but resulted in a reaction (e.g., rash, headache).

TABLE OF DRUGS AND CHEMICALS

The Table of Drugs and Chemicals (Table 1-4) is found in the Index (Volume 2). The table provides the quickest reference to find poisoning and the adverse effects of drugs. As always, verify and code the diagnosis from the Tabular List (Volume 1).

Substance (First Column)

The table provides an alphabetical listing of drugs and substances. Each item listed is followed by codes for particular use and definition.

Poisoning (Second Column)

This column provides a list of codes to identify if the poisoning was by drugs, both medicinal and biological substances (960 to 979).

TABLE 1-4   Table of Drugs and Chemicals

Substance		EXTERNAL CAUSE (E CODE)				
	Poisoning	Accident	Therapeutic Use	Suicide Attempt	Assault	Undetermined
Adalin (acetyl)	967.3	E852.2	E937.3	E950.2	E962.0	E980.2
Adenosine (phosphate)	977.8	E858.8	E947.8	E950.4	E962.0	E980.4
Adhesives	989.89	E866.8	—	E950.9	E962.1	E980.9
ADH	962.5	E858.0	E932.5	E950.4	E962.0	E980.4
Adicillin	960.0	E856	E930.0	E950.4	E962.0	E980.4
Adiphenine	975.1	E855.6	E945.1	E950.4	E962.0	E980.4
Adjunct, pharmaceutical	977.4	E858.8	E947.4	E950.4	E962.0	E980.4
Adrenal (extract, cortex, or medulla) (glucocorticoids) (hormones) (mineralocorticoids)	962.0	E858.0	E932.0	E950.4	E962.0	E980.4
ENT agent	976.6	E858.7	E946.6	E950.4	E962.0	E980.4
Ophthalmic preparation	976.5	E858.7	E946.5	E950.4	E962.0	E980.4
Topical NEC	976.0	E858.7	E946.0	E950.4	E962.0	E980.4
Adrenaline	971.2	E855.5	E941.2	E950.4	E962.0	E980.4
Adrenergic blocking agents	971.3	E855.6	E941.3	E950.4	E962.0	E980.4
Adrenergics	971.2	E855.5	E941.2	E950.4	E962.0	E980.4

External Cause (E Codes)

This category is composed of five columns to show the different circumstances in which a poisoning may occur. These descriptions provide a numerical breakdown for each type of poisoning. These codes classify or specify the cause of a poisoning with the exception of the therapeutic use column.

- Accident
- Therapeutic use
- Suicide attempt
- Assault
- Undetermined

Therapeutic Use

Although the E codes for therapeutic use are listed with poisoning, these codes are not intended to be used to report a poisoning. Codes from this column should be used to report adverse reactions when the correct substances are administered properly. This column is listed with the poisoning codes so that the table did not have to be repeated for just the one column, which saves space in the code book.

 CODING TIP

Late Effects of Poisoning	
Code 909.0	Used to report late effects of drug poisoning
Codes E929.2, E959, E969, and E989	Used to identify external causes of late effects of drug poisoning

---

ICD-9-CM CODING EXERCISE 6   Coding Drug Poisoning

Directions: Using the table in Volume 2, code the scenarios in the following exercise. List the correct classifications and applicable codes.

Example: Lead poisoning from eating paint
Classification: Poisoning; Codes: 984.0 and E861.5

Note: The number of spaces provided is not an indication of the number of codes required.

DESCRIPTION	CLASSIFICATION	CODE(S)
1. Suicide attempt by overdose (amphetamines)	_____	_____
2. Carbon monoxide poisoning due to faulty exhaust system in car	_____	_____
3. Adverse effect from dye in intra-arterial injection	_____	_____

CMS GUIDELINES FOR ICD-9-CM CODING

The Centers for Medicare and Medicaid Services (CMS) developed specific guidelines for physicians to use when reporting diagnoses to a Medicare carrier. This book is designed to provide the coder with a brief descriptive summary for reference purposes only. A complete description of the guidelines is located in the introduction to the ICD-9-CM manual or can be obtained from the CMS web site, *http://www.cms.hhs.gov/*.

Guideline 1

ICD-9-CM code ranges 001.0 through V83 must be used to report the reason for patient care or treatment. When a specific diagnosis is unavailable, the physician may report signs, symptoms, or complaints. To report conditions or circumstances other than disease or injury, the physician may use V codes (V01.0 through V83) to report the reason for the visit.

EXAMPLE
A patient was seen for follow-up of diabetes, adult onset, controlled. Reason for the visit: 250.00

Guideline 2

The primary diagnosis should be the diagnosis, condition, problem, or reason for the encounter. Coders may list any additional codes that describe current, coexisting conditions requiring patient care or treatment. No more than a total of four diagnosis codes may be listed on a CMS-1500 claim form.

If it is necessary to report more than four diagnoses to present a clear picture of the patient's condition, an additional sheet can be attached to the claim form and the word "attachment" stated in block 10-D on the CMS 1500 claim form. For electronic submission, use the note section to list additional diagnoses instead of sending in a separate attachment.

EXAMPLE
A patient was seen for a follow-up examination after surgery. Reason for the visit: V67.0

Guideline 3

ICD-9-CM codes should be reported to the highest level of specificity for a given code.
- Use a three-digit code number when the code does not require a fourth-digit or fifth-digit subclassification.
- Assign four-digit codes only if there is no fifth-digit subclassification for that category.
- Assign the fifth digit of the subclassification code for those subcategories where it exists.

> **EXAMPLE**
>
> **Coding Examples:**
> Third-digit specificity: Acute tonsillitis
> Correct code: 463
> Fourth-digit specificity: Brief depressive reaction
> Correct code: 309.0
> Fifth digit specificity: Macular keratitis
> Correct code: 370.22

Guideline 4

Do not code diagnoses that are documented as "rule out," "probable cause," "suspected," "possible," or "questionable." Code the condition to the highest degree of certainty as supported by the medical record. When a specific condition or problem has not been identified, code symptoms, signs, test results, or other reasons for the visit.

> **EXAMPLE**
>
> Reason for the test: chest pain (786.50) to rule out angina (413.9)
> Correct code: 786.50, Chest pain

Guideline 5

Report a chronic disease or condition only when the patient receives treatment or care for that particular problem or condition.

> **EXAMPLE**
>
> A patient with a history of chronic low back pain (724.2) is seen for forearm laceration (881.00).
> Correct code: 881.00

Guideline 6

Code only the conditions, problems, or diagnoses that currently affect patient care. Do not code conditions that were previously treated and no longer exist.

> **EXAMPLE**
>
> A patient is seen in follow-up for diabetes (adult onset, controlled) and congestive heart failure; the same patient was treated 6 months ago for an incarcerated inguinal hernia.
> Correct code sequencing: 1. 250.00, Diabetes
>   2. 428.0, Congestive heart failure

Guideline 7

Use the postoperative diagnosis when known.

E X A M P L E
Preoperative Dx: Breast mass (611.72)
Postoperative Dx: Fibrocystic breast disease (610.3)
Correct code: 610.3

Guideline 8

When a patient receives ancillary services (e.g., laboratory or radiographic testing), first code the reason for the test—or, if known, the results of the test—followed by the appropriate V code for the type of service provided.

E X A M P L E
Reason for the test: chest pain (786.50) to rule out angina (413.9)
Correct code sequencing: 1. 786.50, Chest pain
2. V72.5, Radiologic examination

Guideline 9

When a patient is receiving only ancillary or therapeutic services, list as the primary diagnosis the appropriate V code, followed by the code for the diagnosis or problem for which the service is being provided.

E X A M P L E
A patient is seen for a third course of chemotherapy infusions.
Correct code sequencing: 1. V58.1, Chemotherapy
2. 188.0, Bladder cancer

ICD-9-CM CODING EXERCISE 7   General Coding Problems

Directions: In the appropriate volumes, look up the following descriptions. List all pertinent codes that accurately describe the condition. More than one code may apply.

DESCRIPTION   CODE(S)

1. Cancer in situ of the ovary   _____   _____

2. Bronchitis   _____   _____

3. Acute pericarditis due to chronic renal failure (uremia)   _____   _____

4. Follow-up examination after surgery   _____   _____

5. Whiplash syndrome   _____   _____

6. Black eye due to fist fight   _____   _____

7. Metastatic carcinoma to the small intestine from the large intestine   _____   _____
    (surgery performed on the large intestine 1 year earlier without
    recurrence)

8. Abnormal thyroid scan   _____   _____

9. Chronic arthritis due to late effect of ankle fracture   _____   _____

10. Jet lag syndrome   _____   _____

ICD-9-CM REVIEW

1. What does the acronym *ICD-9-CM* mean?

    _____

2. Volume 1 is the _____ or _____ listing of codes.

3. Volume 2 is the _____ or _____ listing for codes.

4. Volume 3 is primarily used in _____ and should not be used to code procedures in a private practice.

5. List the three main purposes for using ICD-9-CM.

    A. _____

    B. _____

    C. _____

6. List the appendices found in Volume 1.

    A. _____

    B. _____

    C. _____

    D. _____

    E. _____

7. List the three tables found in the Index.

    A. _____

    B. _____

    C. _____

8. _____ digit subclassification provides information regarding the cause or description of a diagnosis.

9. _____ codes are supplemental classifications for factors that influence patient care.

10. _____ codes should never be used as primary or stand-alone codes.

11. The key to locating E codes may be found in Volume 2, under

_____

12. In the drug table, which series of E codes should not be listed to report poisoning?

_____

_____

LOCATING ICD-9-CM CODES   Practice Exercise

Directions: The following is an exercise to put into practice using ICD-9-CM codes. Locate the code in Volume 2 and verify it in Volume 1.

DESCRIPTION	CODE
1. Headache	_____
2. Internal hemorrhoids	_____
3. Abnormal cervical Pap smear	_____
4. Old healed myocardial infarction	_____
5. Acute pharyngitis	_____
6. Malignant hypertension with congestive heart failure	_____
7. Second-degree burn, back of hand	_____
8. Cancer in situ of the ovary	_____
9. Small intestinal diverticulosis due to unspecified peritonitis	_____
10. Abnormal thyroid scan	_____
11. Acute suppurative otitis media with spontaneous rupture of ear drum	_____
12. Urinary frequency, rule out bladder tumor	_____
13. Prolonged labor (first stage) with third-degree perineal tear, delivery of healthy twins	_____
14. Chronic obstructive pulmonary disease with acute respiratory failure	_____
15. Progressive systemic sclerosis of multiple sites with lung involvement	_____

2

Diagnostic Coding: International Classification of Diseases, 10th Revision, Clinical Modification (ICD-10-CM)

CHAPTER OUTLINE

KEY TERMS

Term	Definition
Manifestation code	A display or characteristic signs or symptoms of an illness. Also known as an asterisk (*) code in some editions of ICD-10.
CDC	Centers for Disease Control.
Classification	Standard grouping of diseases by a set of principles.
CM	Clinical modification.
CMS	Centers for Medicare and Medicaid Services.
Default code	A code located in the Index that refers to a condition most commonly associated with the main term. An unspecified code where a higher level of specificity is not presented.
ICD-10-CM	*International Classification of Disease, Tenth Edition, Clinical Modification.*
ICD-10-PCS	*International Classification of Disease, Tenth Edition, Procedural Coding System.*
NEC	Not elsewhere classified: A category of codes to be used only when the coder lacks the information required to code the term to a more specific category.

Place holder	Usually a fifth digit character that is an "x" that must be used for correct code selection.
Sequela	Morbid condition following as a consequence of a disease.
Specificity	Applying the highest level of code based on the documentation of patient care.
Underlying cause	Typically a patient's main condition. In some editions of ICD-10 these codes are also referred to as a dagger (†) code.
WHO	World Health Organization.

OBJECTIVES

After completing this chapter, readers should be able to:

- Have a rudimentary understanding of the new coding system ICD-10-CM.
- Apply the basic steps studied in Chapter 1 for application with the new coding system.
- Be able to identify and code correct diagnosis based on documented **specificity.**
- Recognize and use the tables in the ICD-10-CM Index.
- Understand the differences between ICD-9 and ICD-10 coding systems.
- Correctly enter ICD-10-CM codes on a claim form.

This chapter is designed to introduce the reader to the new **ICD-10-CM** coding system that is scheduled for implementation on October 01, 2013 as the only diagnosis coding system used by the United States.

The Health Insurance Portability and Accountability Act of 1996 (HIPAA) was passed to set standards for electronic health care transactions. The ICD-10-CM is part of the HIPAA regulations for electric claims processing and transmitting.

Although diagnosis coding (ICD) is not easy, it is essential to good reporting of services provided to enhance reimbursements received. As stated in the previous chapter on ICD-9-CM, it is easier to locate codes when you have a good working knowledge of medical terminology, basic anatomy and physiology, and a fundamental understanding of the ICD-9-CM and ICD-10-CM coding conventions and applications.

HISTORY

Traditionally, the World Health Organization **(WHO)** revises ICD code books once every 10 years. The newest version (ICD-10) was originally released in 1992. The United States did not adopt the new code set because offices were in a learning process for correct usage of ICD-9-CM coding. Additionally, our computer systems were not equipped to accept the new coding format because we had just created the format for fourth- and fifth-digit coding required by ICD-9-CM. Additionally, there were concerns regarding changes for specific use in the United States for the Clinical Modifications required to meet our needs and standards.

According to government officials, the new coding system (ICD-10-CM) will go into effect as of October 01, 2013. At that time, only the 10th edition will be the accepted system to report a diagnosis. The government is currently working to complete the translation and revision of ICD-10-CM and to upgrade computer software to accommodate the new format.

THE MEANING OF CLASSIFICATION

There are many diseases, and one needs to establish a common language for reporting and data analysis. Standard grouping of diseases by a set of principles is called classification, and it allows:
- Easy storage, retrieval and analysis of data
- Comparison and transmission of data between hospitals, provinces and countries
- Comparison in the same location across different time period

FOR COMPARISON AND COMMUNICATION

Agreeing on the definitions of groups at a regional, national, and international level enables comparison of results and merging of information from different sources.

Each individual case is assigned to exactly one category (group). The categories do not overlap (i.e., they are mutually exclusive), and there is a category for every case.

The International Classification of Diseases is designed to serve as a way to capture mortality and morbidity data for reporting for public health, epidemiology, and treatment, and allows comparison of frequencies—for example causes of death from the community level up to the whole world.

ICD is the international standard for this purpose, with all WHO member states having committed to report causes of death and illness to WHO since 1967 (nomenclature regulations). The ICD (International Statistical **C**lassification of **D**iseases and Related Health Problems) is a classification that is used in 194 countries. It has been developed internationally since 1891. ICD coding has had 10 major revisions with the most recent changes being ICD-10.

The United States has set an implementation date of October 1, 2013, for the new diagnosis code system, ICD-10-CM, to go into effect. coding professionals should start familiarizing themselves with the classification system to prepare for its future use.

WHAT IS ICD-10-CM?

ICD-10-CM is a clinical modification of the World Health Organization's ICD-10, which consists of a diagnostic system. ICD-10-CM includes the level of detail needed for morbidity classification and diagnostic specificity. It also provides code titles and language that complement accepted clinical practice. As with ICD-9-CM, ICD-10-CM is maintained by the National Center for Health Statistics.

The system consists of more than 68,000 codes, compared to approximately 13,000 ICD-9-CM codes. ICD-10-CM codes have the potential to reveal more about quality of care, so that data can be used in a more meaningful way to better understand complications, better design clinically robust algorithms, and better track the outcomes of care. ICD-10-CM incorporates greater specificity and clinical detail to provide information for clinical decision making and outcomes research.

COMPARING ICD-9-CM AND ICD-10-CM

ICD-10-CM differs from ICD-9-CM in its organization and structure, code composition, and level of detail.

ICD-9-CM	ICD-10-CM
▪ Consists of three to five characters	▪ Consists of three to seven characters
▪ First digit is numerical or alphabetical (E or V)	▪ First digit is alphabetical
▪ Second, third, fourth, and fifth digits are numerical	▪ All letters used except U
	▪ Second and third digits are numerical
▪ Always at least three digits	▪ Fourth, fifth, sixth, and seventh digits can be alphabetical or numerical
▪ Decimal placed after the first three characters	▪ Decimal placed after the first three characters when a fourth digit is present

Code structure of ICD-10-CM versus ICD-9-CM

ICD-10-CM codes may consist of up to seven digits, with the seventh-digit extensions representing visit encounters or sequelae for injuries and external causes.

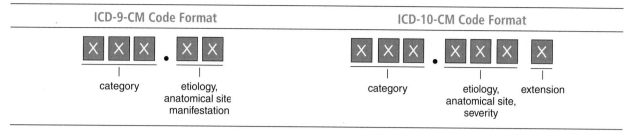

ICD-10-CM Structure

ICD-10-CM has an index and tabular list similar to those of ICD-9-CM. However, the ICD-10-CM index is much longer. As with ICD-9-CM, ICD-10-CM uses an indented format for both the index and tabular list. Categories, subcategories, and codes are contained in the tabular list.

Coding professionals will need to:

Monitor the National Center for Health Statistics web site *(http://www.cdc.gov/nchs)* for any new versions of the guidelines, index, and tabular list before implementation.

As with ICD-9-CM, proper coding relies on use of the guidelines, which house all information about the coding conventions for ICD-10-CM, general use guidelines, and chapter-specific guidelines for the tabular list. Coding guidelines are also in the index.

The two parts of the ICD-10-CM index are the index to diseases and injury and index to external causes of injury. The table of drugs and chemicals and the neoplasm table are housed in the index to diseases and injury.

The former V codes are now Z codes contained in Chapter 21, "Factors Influencing Health Status and Contact with Health Services."

Differences Between ICD-10-CM and ICD-9-CM

ICD-10-CM differs from ICD-9-CM in its organization and structure, code composition, and level of detail. The table above provides a comparison of the two classification systems.

ICD-10-CM codes may consist of up to seven digits, with the seventh digit extensions representing visit encounter or sequela for injuries and external causes. The difference in code structure is shown in the figure above.

Organizational Changes

While ICD-10-CM has the same type of hierarchical structure as ICD-9-CM, some differences are seen in the organization, including:

- ICD-10-CM consists of 21 chapters.
- Some chapters include the addition of a sixth character.
- ICD-10-CM includes full code titles for all codes (no references back to common fourth and fifth digits).
- V and E codes are no longer supplemental classifications.
- Sense organs have been separated from nervous system disorders.
- Injuries are grouped by anatomical site rather than injury category.
- Postoperative complications have been moved to the procedure-specific body system chapter.

New Features

ICD-10-CM has numerous new features allowing for a greater level of specificity and clinical detail. These include:

- Combination codes for conditions and common symptoms or manifestations
- Combination codes for poisonings and external causes
- Added laterality
- Added extensions for episode of care
- Expanded codes (injury, diabetes, alcohol and substance abuse, postoperative complications)
- Inclusion of trimester in obstetrics codes and elimination of fifth digits for episode of care
- Expanded detail relevant to ambulatory and managed care encounters
- Changes in time frames specified in certain codes
- External cause codes no longer a supplementary classification

ICD-10-CM also includes added standard definitions for two types of excludes notes.

Excludes 1

A type 1 Excludes note is a pure excludes. It means "NOT CODED HERE!" An Excludes1 note indicates that the code excluded should never be used at the same time as the code above the Excludes1 note. An Excludes1 is used when two conditions cannot occur together, such as a congenital form versus an acquired form of the same condition. For example, B06 Rubella [German measles] has an Excludes1 of congenital rubella (P35.0).

Excludes 2

A type 2 Excludes note represents "NOT INCLUDED HERE." An Excludes2 note indicates that the condition excluded is not part of the condition it is excluded from but a patient may have both conditions at the same time. When an Excludes2 note appears under a code it is acceptable to use both the code and the excluded code together. For example, J04.0, Acute laryngitis has an Excludes2 of chronic laryngitis (J37.0).

There are three volumes that comprise ICD-10:

- Volume 1—The Tabular List
- Volume 2—The Alphabetical Index
- Volume 3—PCS

Let's take a look at each one in detail.

Volume 1, the Tabular List, is an alphanumeric listing of diseases, disease groups, and health-related problems. It contains inclusion and exclusion notes and some coding rules.

E X A M P L E

Malignant Neoplasm of Gum

C03	**Malignant neoplasm of gum**	

    Includes: alveolar (ridge) mucosa
                        gingiva

    Excludes: malignant odontogenic neoplasms (C41.0–C41.1)

C03.0   **Upper gum**

C03.1   **Lower gum**

C03.9   **Gum, unspecified**

C04   **Malignant neoplasm of floor of mouth**

C04.0   **Anterior floor of mouth**
               Anterior to the premolar-canine junction

INTERNATIONAL CLASSIFICATION OF DISEASES

3.1.2   **Use of the tabular list of inclusions and four-character subcategories**

Inclusion terms

Within the three- and four-character rubrics[1], there are usually listed a number of other diagnostic terms. These are known as "inclusion terms" and are given, in addition to the title, as examples of the diagnostic statements to be classified to that rubric. They may refer to different conditions or be synonyms. They are not a subclassification of the rubric.

Inclusion terms are listed primarily as a guide to the content of the rubrics. Many of the items listed relate to important or common terms belonging to the rubric.

In Volume 2, the Alphabetical Index, is an alphabetical list of the diseases and conditions that have codes in the Tabular List.

ALPHABETICAL INDEX TO DISEASES AND NATURY OF INJURY

A

Aarskog's syndrome Q87.1
Abandonment T74.0
Abasia (-astasia) (hysterical) F44.4
Abdomen, abdominal – *see also condition*
– acute R10.0
– convulsive equivalent G40.8
– muscle deficiency syndrome Q79.4
Abdominalgia R10.4
Abduction contracture, hip or other
  joint – *see* Contraction, joint

Abnormal, abnormality—*continued*
– autosomes NEC—*continued*
– – fragile site Q95.5
– basal metabolic rate R94.8
– biosynthesis, testicular androgen E29.1
– blood level (of)
– – cobalt R79.0
– – copper R79.0
– – iron R79.0
– – lithium R78.8

There are more entries in the Index than there are in the Tabular List because some diseases have more than one name and some diseases are grouped under one code. Not all of the names that appear for a code will be found in the Tabular listing. Always trust the index to guide you to the most appropriate code in the Tabular List.

Volume 2, Alphabetical Index also contains:

- Guidance on selecting the appropriate codes for many conditions not displayed in the Tabular List
- A Table of Neoplasms
- An Index of external causes of injury
- A Table of drugs and chemicals

E X A M P L E

Kristi has ruptured her spleen during a skiing accident.
Which volume will you refer to *first* to find the code that represents her problem?

Volume 1—Tabular List

S36 Injury of intra-abdominal organs
    Code also any associated open wound (S31.–)
       the appropriate seventh character is to be added to each code from category S36
A initial encounter
D subsequent encounter
S sequela*

Volume 2—Alphabetical List

Rupture, ruptured-*continued*
  perineum-*continued*
    complicating delivery-*continued*
      first degree O70.0
  sigmoid (nontraumatic) K63.1
    fetus or newborn P78.0
    obstetric trauma O71.5
    traumatic #36.5
  spinal cord (*see also* Injury, spinal cord, by region) T09.3
    fetus or newborn (birth injury) P11.5
  spleen (traumatic) #36.0
    birth injury P15.1
    congenital (birth injury) P15.1
    due to *Plasmodium vivax* malaria B51.0[†] D77

*Sequela: Morbid condition following as a consequence of a disease.

Summary

Volumes 1 and 2 have to be used together to correctly find codes for each case (e.g., cause of death or diagnosis).

The basic process is to first check the Index for a code representing your disease. Then confirm your choice in the Tabular List. Trying to find the correct code in Volume 1 without first checking the Index may result in an incorrect code being assigned.

CODING SYSTEM OBJECTIVES

The new classification system provides significant improvements though greater detailed information and the ability to expand in order to capture additional advancements in clinical medicine. The ICD-10 coding system is divided into two parts.

- ICD-10-CM   The diagnosis classification system developed by the Centers for Disease Control and Prevention for use in all U.S. health care treatment settings. Diagnosis coding under this system uses three to seven alphabetical and numerical digits and full code titles. The format or layout of the codes is much the same as ICD-9-CM.

- ICD-10-PCS   The procedure classification system developed by the Centers for Medicare & Medicaid Services (CMS) for use in the United States for inpatient hospital settings and hospital billing only. This coding system uses seven alphabetical or numerical digits unlike the three or four numerical digits used in the ICD-9-CM system.

WHY THE NEED FOR CHANGE?

The current system, ICD-9-CM:

- Does not provide the necessary detail to report medical conditions or the procedures and services performed in hospitalized patients
- Current coding system is 30 years old
- Contains outdated and obsolete terminology
- Uses outdated codes that produce inaccurate, limited data
- Is inconsistent with current medical practice
- Does not accurately describe the diagnoses and inpatient procedures for care provided in the 21st century

The following examples are provided to illustrate the completeness and preciseness of ICD-10-CM code selections versus ICD-9-CM coding selections.

E X A M P L E

Example: Mechanical complication of other vascular device, implant, graft

ICD-9-CM (only one code) | | **ICD-10-CM (156 codes)** |
|---|---|---|---|
| 996.1 | Mechanical complication | T82.310* | Breakdown aortic |
| | | T82.311* | Breakdown carotid arterial |
| | | T82.328* | Displacement of other vascular grafts |

*A few examples of the ICD-10-CM codes are provided for illustration.

Pressure ulcer codes of the lower back

ICD-9-CM (nine location codes)
Show broad location—not depth or stage

ICD-10-CM (125 codes)
More specific location with depth & stage

707.03	Pressure ulcer lower back	L89.131*	Pressure ulcer of right lower back, stage I
		L89.132*	Right lower back, stage II
		L89.144*	Left lower back, stage IV

Example: Hospital Procedure Coding: angioplasty

ICD-9-CM (only one code) | | **ICD-10-CM (854 codes)** |
|---|---|---|---|
| 39.50 | Angioplasty | 047K04Z* | Dilation rt. femoral artery drug-eluting intraluminal device, open |
| | | 047K0ZZ* | Dilation rt. femoral artery open |
| | | 047K3DZ* | Dilation rt. femoral artery w/intraluminal device, percutaneous approach |

*A few examples of the ICD-10-PSC codes provided for illustration only.

ICD-9-CM VS ICD-10-CM CHAPTER COMPARISONS

	ICD-9-CM	ICD-10-CM	
Chapter I	001-139	A00-B99	Certain Infectious and Parasitic Diseases
Chapter II	140-239	C00-D49	Neoplasms
Chapter III	240-279 (Endocrine)	D50-D89	Diseases of the Blood and Blood-Forming Organs and Certain Disorders Involving the Immune Mechanism
Chapter IV	280-289 (Blood)	E00-E89	Endocrine, Nutritional, and Metabolic Diseases
Chapter V	290-319	F01-F99	Mental and Behavioral Disorders
Chapter VI	320-389	G00-G99	Diseases of the Nervous System
Chapter VII	390-459 (Circulatory)	H00-H59	Diseases of the Eye and Adnexa
Chapter VIII	460-519 (Respiratory)	H60-H95	Diseases of the Ear and Mastoid Process
Chapter IX	520-579 (Digestive)	I000-I99	Diseases of the Circulatory System
Chapter X	580-629 Genitourinary	J00-J99	Diseases of the Respiratory System
Chapter XI	630-677 (Pregnancy)	K00-K94	Diseases of the Digestive system
Chapter XII	680-709 (Skin)	L00-L99	Diseases of the Skin and Subcutaneous Tissue
Chapter XIII	710-739 (Musculoskeletal)	M00-M99	Diseases of the Musculoskeletal System and Connective Tissue
Chapter XIV	740-759 (Congenital)	N00-N99	Diseases of the Genitourinary System
Chapter XV	760-779 (Perinatal)	O00-O99	Pregnancy, Childbirth, and the Puerperium Period
Chapter XVI	780-799 (Signs)	P00-P96	Certain Conditions Originating in the Perinatal Period
Chapter XVII	800-999 (Injury)	Q00-Q99	Congenital Malformations
Chapter XVIII	V01-V89 V-Codes (Health Status)	R00-R99	Symptoms, Signs, and Abnormal Clinical and Laboratory Findings Not Elsewhere Classified
Chapter XIX	E000-E999 E-Codes (External Causes)	S00-T88	Injury, Poisoning, and Certain Other Consequences of External Causes
Chapter XX		V00-Y99	External Causes of Morbidity (Originally E Codes)
Chapter XXI		Z00-Z99	Factors Influencing Health Status and Contact with Health Services (Originally V Codes)

ICD-9-CM VERSUS ICD-10-CM FORMATS

ICD-9-CM	ICD-10-CM
▪ Tabular	▪ Tabular
▪ Alphabetical index	▪ Alphabetical index
▪ Hospital procedures	▪ Hospital procedures (PCS)
▪ 19 chapters	▪ 21 chapters
▪ Numerical coding system	▪ Alphanumeric coding system
▪ Fourth- and fifth-digit specificity	▪ Sixth- and seventh-digit specificity
▪ Category for unspecified codes	▪ Limited use of unspecified codes
▪ Supplementary classifications for V and E Codes	▪ New chapters for eye and ear
	▪ New chapter for V code
	▪ New chapter for E codes

CHANGES and SIMILARITIES

In addition to the expansion capabilities of the new coding system, the supplementary classifications of the V and E codes have been converted into distinct chapters. (See Chapters XX and XXI.)

ICD-10 has kept the appendices (A-E).

The new coding system still consists of three volumes.
- Volume 1—Tabular List of Diseases and Injuries
- Volume 2—Alphabetical Index
- Volume 3—Procedures

All coders, without regard to the location of the services or type of services provided, must use the ICD-10-CM to report services on or after October 1, 2013.

The switch to ICD-10-CM will not impact CPT or HCPCS coding; therefore, coders who are currently using CPT or HCPCS codes to report physician services will continue doing so even after ICD-10 is implemented.

Volume 2 still contains the following information:
- Index to Disease
- Neoplasm Table
- Table of Drugs and Chemicals
- Index to External Causes (formerly referred to as E codes)

The Tabular List contains categories, subcategories and codes. Characters for categories may be either a letter or a number. All categories are 3 characters. A three-character category that has no further sub-classification is equivalent to a code. Not all codes will have four to seven more digits.

CATEGORY: Three-Digit Character

The first three characters classify a disease or an injury of similar circumstance within a particular category.

Example:
Code E11: Diabetes mellitus without mention of complication type 2 or unspecified type

Subcategory:

A subcategory is either four or five characters.

Each subdivision after a category is a subcategory.

Code Selection

A code is only a valid code when all subdivisions have been applied as appropriate.

Example: Type 2 diabetes mellitus with severe nonproliferative diabetic retinopathy

Category: E11

Subcategory: E11.3

Completed code: E11.34

NOTE: This code is not complete because it requires another subcategory character to further identify complications of the retinopathy such as E11.34. In ICD-9-CM this was referred to as a subclassification because the extra characters were used to supply even more clinical detail about the patient's condition.

JUST A WORD ABOUT VOLUME 3 (ICD-10-PCS)

Volume 3 is a tabular alphabetical and numerical listing used by hospitals to report inpatient care. This means that if you work for a physician practice and your physician goes to the hospital to perform procedures or other patient-related services, you only code from Volumes 1 and 2. The bottom line is that you would never code from Volume 3, PCS.

 Special Note

It is inappropriate to use codes from the ICD-10-PCS on physician claim forms. The only group that should use the PCS version is hospital personnel who are coding hospital claims.

HOSPITAL PROCEDURAL CODE COMPARISONS	
ICD-9-CM	**ICD-10-PCS**
Includes diagnostic information in the procedure description	Exclusion of diagnostic information from the procedure description
Five-digit code number	Alphanumerical structure with each character having up to 34 different values. The following defines the seven characters to identify a procedure or service. - First: specifies the section - Second: root operation or type - Third: defines the service - Fourth: body part - Fifth: approach - Sixth: device - Seventh: qualifier
	Requires specification of the precise body part and operation

E X A M P L E						
CODE: 094GBDZ Dilation eustachian tube, right with intraluminal device, perorifice intraluminal						
DEFINING THE CHARACTERS						
0	9	4	G	B	D	Z
Section	Body System	Root or Type	Body Part	Approach	Device	Qualifier
Surgical	Ears	Dilation	Right Eustachian Tube	Per Orifice Intraluminal	Intraluminal Device	None

ICD-10-CM CONVENTIONS

The great news is that ICD-10 will be following the same rules, guidelines, and conventions you have learned while working with ICD-9-CM. However, to keep us on our toes and to hold our interest, ICD-10-CM does have a few surprises that were not found in ICD-9.

To allow for future expandability, ICD-10 has incorporated the use of **"placeholders"** within the codes. The placeholder is usually a fifth digit character and is an "X." When a placeholder exists, the X must be used in order for the code to be considered a valid diagnosis code.

An example of placeholder coding is seen in the poisoning, adverse effects, and underdosing codes, categories T36-T50.

E X A M P L E
T40.5   Poisoning by adverse effect of and underdosing of cocaine

As was determined in the first chapter, ICD-9-CM, when coding for substances such as poison the intent or reason for the poisoning must be listed when known. Therefore code T40.5 is an invalid code because it requires more characters or digits to complete the code to the highest level of specificity.

Additionally, some codes require a seventh character and that the seventh character be applicable to all codes within that code set. That character must be always be the seventh character and visible in the seventh character field on the claim form. To solve the problem, when a code does not have six characters, a placeholder X must be used to fill in any empty characters.

Based on this new information, how would you code the following?

E X A M P L E
Poisoning by adverse effect of and underdosing of cocaine for intentional self-harm, first encounter.
ANSWER: T40.5x2A

 R E M I N D E R

Where a place code exists, an X must be used in order for the code to be a valid code.
Always code to the highest level of specificity for a valid code.

Exclude Notes

ICD-9-CM uses only one type of exclusion note to let the coder know which types of illnesses are not located within that category. ICD-10-CM has two types of exclusions.

Exclusion 1:   This is a pure exclusion note. It means "not coded here." Any code in the exclusion note should never be coded at the same time as the code listed.

Exclusion 2:   Indicates that the excluded condition is not part of the condition represented by the code; however, the patient may have both conditions at the same time.

EXAMPLE: CODE J39.9

Code has an Exclusion 1.
-You can never use code J68.0 when you use code J39.9. The two codes cannot be reported at the same encounter.

Code also has an Exclusion 2.
-Cystic fibrosis (E84) is not included with this code and can be separately reported at the same encounter if both are documented.

Default Codes

Default codes are located in the ICD-10-CM index. **Default codes** refer to a condition that is most commonly associated with the main term or is the unspecified code when more specific information is not provided to code to a higher level of specificity.

E X A M P L E
Bronchitis, J40.
This is the highest level of specificity to report bronchitis when more detailed information is not available.

LOCATING CODES

Developing good research habits is the key to correct coding. There are five basic steps to locating the correct diagnosis code. When these steps are followed, the coder will be successful in locating even the most elusive codes.

- Correctly identify the main term or condition to be coded.
- Use the Index to locate the condition or problem.
- Refer to all notes, and review the information given while following all instructions or cross references.
- Locate and confirm the correct code in the Tabular List and review all notes and information to select the correct code.
- Place codes in correct sequence when using multiple diagnoses. The main or primary diagnosis should always be coded as the condition or reason that caused a patient to seek medical care.

E X A M P L E
Patient with a history of peptic ulcers (K27.0) was seen in the office for acute pharyngitis (J02.9). Because the ulcer is part of patient history and does not affect the patient's care, you would need only to report the reason for the visit, which is Pharyngitis (J02.9).

ICD-10-CM CODING EXERCISE 1   Using the Conventions

1.   What is the complete code to report Pain, acute of the right hip joint?

_____

_____

2.   What, if any, differences exist between an Exclusion 1 and Exclusion 2?

_____

_____

3.   Explain the term Default code.

_____

_____

4.   What has become of the supplementary classifications (V and E codes) in ICD-10-CM?

_____

_____

5.   To allow for future expandability, ICD-10 has incorporated the use of placeholders within the codes. Explain placeholder.

_____

_____

6.   Code the following diagnoses to the highest levels of specificity.

_____

_____

    a.   Macrotia ear

    b.   Banti's disease with cirrhosis

    c.   Wright's syndrome

    d.   Trench mouth

    e.   Bilateral renal hypoplasia

ICD-10-CM CHAPTER CODING SPECIFICS

CHAPTER 1: CERTAIN INFECTIOUS AND PARASITIC DISEASES

(A00-B99)

You will need to check the inclusion and exclusion notes at chapter, block, category, and subcategory levels carefully.

A range of codes from this chapter are used with codes from other chapters, where this instruction is given.

Codes B95-B97 should never be used for primary coding. In other words, they should not be used for underlying cause of death or main condition.

Chapter II: Neoplasms (C00-D49)

INTERNATIONAL CLASSIFICATION OF DISEASES

	Malignant		In situ	Benign	Uncertain or unknown behavior
	Primary	Secondary			
Neoplasm, neoplastic—*continued*					
– – cervix (uteri)	C53.9	C79.8	D06.9	D26.0	D39.0
– – canal	C53.0	C79.8	D06.0	D26.0	D39.0
– – squamocolumnar junction	C53.8	C79.8	D06.7	D26.0	D39.0
– – stump	C53.8	C79.8	D06.7	D26.0	D39.0

Chapter II, Neoplasms, is used to code all types of neoplasm, tumor, and cancer. Neoplasms are a form of new abnormal growth in organs and tissues. The cells do not develop as an organized part of the site where they form and may spread to other parts of the body in a process called metastasis.

Neoplasms are classified according to the site affected and the way they behave, which can be malignant, benign, in situ, or uncertain or unknown.

Excluded from this chapter are benign polyps—, most of which are coded to the chapter of the body system in which they are found.

The code sets in Chapter II are organized according to behavior, with the section for malignant neoplasms, C00-C97, being the largest. These codes are further divided into subcode sets based on the site of the neoplasm. Only code a malignant neoplasm from this code set if the documentation clearly states that it is a primary site. If the documentation does not state whether a malignant neoplasm is primary or not, the neoplasm must be assumed to be primary.

Codes for in situ and benign neoplasms follow malignant neoplasms, followed by codes for neoplasms of uncertain or unknown behavior.

Where a neoplasm is described as affecting overlapping or contiguous sites that would normally be coded individually within the same three-character category, a .8 fourth character should be used instead (see note 5 at the beginning of the chapter).

For example, a diagnosis of primary malignant neoplasm of the oropharynx (lateral and posterior walls) should be coded to C10.8 if the originating site is not identified, rather than using C10.2 and C10.3 together.

C10	**Malignant neoplasm of oropharynx**
	Excludes: tonsil (C09.–)
C10.0	**Vallecula**
C10.1	**Anterior surface of epiglottis**
	Epiglottis, free border [margin]
	Glossoepiglottic fold (s)
	Excludes: epiglottis (suprahyoid portion) NOS (C32.1)
C10.2	**Lateral wall of oropharynx**
C10.3	**Posterior wall of oropharynx**
C10.4	**Branchial cleft**
	Branchial cyst [site of neoplasm]
C10.8	**Overlapping lesion of oropharynx**
	(See note 5 at the beginning of this chapter.)
	Junctional region of oropharynx
C10.9	**Oropharynx, unspecified**

The Index sometimes provides help with locating the correct site code even if the site is not specified in the diagnosis. For example, a diagnosis of glioma must be coded to C71.9, Malignant neoplasm of brain unspecified, unless there is more detail available about the part of the brain affected.

In some cases the site of the cancer is completely unknown and the Index entry under the morphological type does not provide a default code. This may also occur where the patient has metastases but the treating physician does not know where the cancer started. In such cases, use the code C80, Malignant neoplasm without specification of site, which you will find in the table of neoplasms under Neoplasm, metastatic, primary site unknown.

When you need to code a patient who has two primary cancers at the same time, you can either:

- Code each cancer individually, or
- Use the code C97, Malignant neoplasms of independent (primary) multiple sites.

C25.0 Malignant neoplasm of head of pancreas

C16.1 Malignant neoplasm of fundus of stomach

C97 Malignant neoplasms of independent (primary) multiple sites

Your choice will depend on how the data will be used and the requirements of the users for specificity regarding cancer sites.

Lymphomas, leukemias, and hematopoietic neoplasms are located using the Index directly, without reference to the table of neoplasms. To code these diagnoses, use the Index to find the morphological type.

For example, acute lymphocytic leukemia is found in the Index under the lead term Leukemia with code C91.0, which can be confirmed in the Tabular List.

Chapter III: Diseases of the Blood and Blood-Forming Organs (D50-D89)

Chapter III is a short chapter that is used to code diseases of the blood and blood-forming organs and certain disorders of the immune system. This includes diseases of:

- The erythrocytes (red blood cells)—for example, anemia
- The leukocytes (white blood cells)—for example, granulocytosis
- The blood-clotting mechanism and thrombocytes (platelets)—for example, hemophilia
- Certain aspects of the immune system—for example, sarcoidosis

---

Note: Vegans eat no meat, fish, or dairy products. There are other forms of pernicious anemia, but because this patient's condition arises from diet, his diagnosis is coded to D51.3, Other dietary vitamin B_{12} deficiency anemia.

Chapter IV: Diseases of the Endocrine System (E00-E89)

Chapter IV is used to code diseases of the endocrine system and various nutritional and metabolic diseases. This includes conditions such as:

- Diseases of the glands—the thyroid, parathyroid, pituitary, and adrenal glands
- Diabetes
- Malnutrition, obesity, and other hyperalimentation such as the excess consumption of vitamins
- Metabolic disorders—that is, disorders in the body's ability to process chemicals and nutrients for use by cells

Diabetes mellitus
(E10–E14)

Use additional external cause code (Chapter XX), if desired, to identify drug, if drug-induced.

The following fourth-character subdivisions are for use with categories E10–E14:

.0   **With coma**
   Diabetic:
   • Coma with or without ketoacidosis
   • Hyperosmolar coma
   • Hypoglycemic coma
   Hyperglycemic coma NOS

The type of diabetes is captured at the three-character level. A fourth character is chosen from the list at the start of the block to record the diabetic complications present, if any. Most diabetes codes require a second code from another chapter to specify the diabetic manifestation. Diabetes coding has been changed to reflect manifestations so that the coder no longer has to report two codes when reporting the patient's condition.

EXAMPLE	
Examples	
E10.610	Type 1 diabetes mellitus with diabetic neuropathic arthropathy
E11.341	Type 2 diabetes mellitus with severe nonproliferative diabetic retinopathy with macular edema

Chapter V: Mental and Behavioral Disorders (F00-F99)

Chapter V is used to code mental and behavioral disorders. It includes:

- Disorders with an organic origin, where disease or injury causes the mental or behavioral condition
- Conditions caused by substance abuse
- Psychotic and delusion conditions such as schizophrenia
- Mood disorders such as depression and mania
- Behavioral and personality disorders, including those caused by stress or traumatic events
- Developmental disorders, such as hyperactivity and mental retardation

Unique to Chapter V are the detailed glossary descriptions.

These define the contents of the categories and are designed to explain to physicians and certifiers how mental and behavioral disorders are classified and to help medical personnel how to document using the correct ICD-10 terminology. They are not intended for use by coders to interpret the signs and symptoms of a documented disorder.

F00∗ **Dementia in Alzheimer's disease (G30.–†)**
Alzheimer's disease is a primary degenerative cerebral disease of unknown etiology with characteristic neuropathological and neurochemical features. The disorder is usually insidious in onset and develops slowly but steadily over a period of several years.

F00.0∗ **Dementia in Alzheimer's disease with early onset (G30.0†)**
Dementia in Alzheimer's disease with onset before the age of 65, with a relatively rapid deteriorating course and with marked multiple disorders of the higher cortical functions.

Diabetes mellitus
(E10–E14)

Use additional external cause code (Chapter XX), if desired, to identify drug, if drug-induced.

- Code sets F10-F19 contains codes for disorders caused by the use of substances that affect the mind, such as alcohol or heroin. The three-character codes identify the type of substance. The fourth characters listed at the start of the block are common to all the three-character codes and identify the clinical state of the patient. For example, a patient suffering from delirium tremens as a result of alcohol withdrawal would be coded to F10.231.

Note that the use of non–dependence-producing substances, such as painkillers, is excluded from this block, being coded to F55 instead.

Chapter VI: Diseases of the Nervous System (G00-G99)

Chapter VI, containing the codes G00-G99, is used to code diseases of the nervous system, which consists of the brain and spinal cord (the central nervous system) and the cranial and spinal nerves (the peripheral nervous system).

The chapter contains a large number of manifestation or asterisk (*) categories, because many underlying conditions can cause nervous system disorders. Examples include conditions caused by infectious diseases (Chapter I), circulatory disorders (Chapter IX), and external causes such as injury or drugs (Chapter XX).

Chapter VII: Diseases of the Eye and Adnexa (H00-H59)

Chapter VII is a short chapter containing the codes H00-H59.

Used to code diseases of the eye and the adnexa, which consists of the structures that surround the eye, such as the lacrimal (tear) glands and ducts, the extraocular muscles (the muscles around the eye), and the eyelids.

Contains several asterisk categories because a number of diseases coded to other chapters have manifestations that occur in the eye.

Example: Eye conditions associated with infectious diseases (Chapter I) and diabetes (Chapter IV)

Code sets H00-H06 is used for disorders of the eyelid, lacrimal system, and orbit.

Conditions include hordeolum (or stye), which is a nodular granuloma of the eyelid, and chalazion, which is an inflamed oil gland in the eyelid.

Disorders of the eyelid as a result of another disease are coded to H03 with an additional code from Chapter I to identify the type of infection.

The section includes the lacrimal system affecting the eye's ability to produce and drain tears, as well as disorders of the orbit.

H15-H22 contains codes for disorders of the sclera, cornea, iris, and ciliary body.
Example: Keratoconjunctivitis due to herpes virus infection is coded to B00.5† for the herpes virus infection and H19.1* for the keratoconjunctivitis.

H30-H36 is for disorders of the choroid and retina.

H40-H42, is specifically for coding glaucoma.

> Example: Choroidal degeneration would be coded to H31.1. Glaucoma resulting from being hit by a baseball bat would be coded to H40.3, Glaucoma secondary to eye trauma, with an additional code, W21.11 from Chapter XX, for the external cause (being struck by an item of sports equipment).

Codes H43-H44 are for coding disorders of the vitreous body (the vitreous chamber) and of the globe of the eye.

> Included are problems with the transparent jelly-like substance (the vitreous humor) that fills the interior of the eyeball and with the eyeball itself.

> > Example: A patient who has a retained foreign body in his eye from an old injury would be coded to H44.7, Retained (old) intraocular foreign body, nonmagnetic.

H46-H47 contains codes for disorders of the optic nerves and visual pathways.

> Different problems, such as total loss of vision in one or both eyes or a loss of a particular visual field, are the result of disease or damage at different parts of the visual pathway.

> > Example: A compression of the optic nerve would be coded to H47.0, Disorders of optic nerve, not elsewhere classified.

Code sets H49-H52 are used to code problems with the eye's muscles, movements, and ability to focus. Conditions coded here include strabismus, myopia, diplopia, and astigmatism.

> Example: Intermittent monocular esotropia would be coded to H50.3, Intermittent heterotropia.

Code sets H53-H54 are used to code visual disturbances and blindness.

> This code set contains a supporting table that describes how low vision and blindness are measured to determine which code is appropriate. However, this table contains information that is now quite dated. As when coding any other disease, it is preferable for coders to rely on specific diagnostic documentation from clinicians, not on documented measurements.

Chapter VII contains codes H55-H57, which are used for other disorders of the eye and adnexa, including:

- Conditions of the eye that cannot be assigned to a more specific category
- Certain eye disorders that are the result of surgery or other procedures

> Example: Keratopathy following cataract surgery is coded to H59.01, Keratopathy (bullous aphakic) following cataract surgery.

ICD-10-CM CODING EXERCISE 2 Chapters 1-7

Directions: Review each statement and code to the highest level of specificity.

1. Diabetes insipidus
2. Senile dementia in Alzheimer's disease
3. Elderly male with chronic congestive enlargement of spleen
4. Major depression, single, mild
5. Tobacco dependence, cigarettes with withdrawal
6. Fourteen-year-old boy with hypergammaglobulinemia
7. Food poisoning with vomiting
8. Infant boy with hereditary sickle cell anemia
9. Common migraine with blurred vision

Note: Two codes are required to identify all presenting conditions. This is an example of multiple coding because there is not a single code that contains both conditions.

10. Adult male with hypothyroidism resulting from thyroiditis
11. Adult female with carcinoma of the colon and anemia caused by bleeding from the tumor
12. Cryptococcal meningitis

Note: In some editions of ICD-10 dual reporting codes are identified by a dagger (†) for the underlying cause (primary condition) and the manifestation is identified by an asterisk (*).

Chapter VIII: Diseases of the Ear and Mastoid Process (H60-H95)

There are only four code sets in this chapter.

Code sets are arranged anatomically so that diseases of the outer ear come first, the middle ear and mastoid second, then the inner ear, and finally other disorders of the ear.

H60-H62: Diseases of the external ear

Included are conditions such as primary otitis externa and otitis externa resulting from conditions coded elsewhere in the ICD-10.

H65-H75: Diseases of the middle ear and mastoid

Code H67* is used to code middle ear infections resulting from diseases classified to other chapters of the ICD-10.

H80-H83: Disorders of the inner ear

Ménière's disease is coded here, as are various other vertiginous syndromes related to the inner ear.

Dizziness or vertigo not otherwise specified is not coded in this code set.

H90-H94: Other disorders of the ear

Use to code different types of hearing loss and deafness

Different codes are used to identify deafness that is unilateral or bilateral, or different types of hearing loss in each ear.

Chapter IX: Diseases of the Circulatory System (I00-I99)

The circulatory system consists of the vessels that carry blood around the body (veins, arteries, and capillaries), the muscles that control the blood flow, such as the heart, and the lymphatic system that drains lymph from tissues and transfers it to the blood. The chapter also contains several asterisk categories for conditions of the circulatory system that result from disorders coded to other chapters. Examples include conditions associated with infectious diseases, such as toxoplasmosis (Chapter I), and endocrine disorders, such as thyroiditis (Chapter IV).

The first code set, I00-I02, is used to code acute rheumatic fever. It is further split into codes for rheumatic fever with or without heart involvement, followed by rheumatic chorea. (Chorea is a condition where there are rapid, involuntary movements.)

I05-I09 is used to report chronic rheumatic heart diseases. These codes are organized according to the heart valve affected.

The next code sets contains codes for conditions where the patient has high blood pressure, or hypertension. Note that hypertension in pregnancy is among the forms of hypertensive disease excluded from this chapter.

Examples of conditions coded to I10-I15 are:
- High blood pressure, coded to I10 Essential (primary) hypertension
- Hypertensive heart and renal disease with renal failure, coded to I13.1
- Hypertension secondary to endocrine disorders, coded to I15.2

Code sets I20-I25 are used to code ischemic heart disease—that is, conditions where the blood supply to the heart muscle is reduced. There are codes here for angina, myocardial infarction, and atherosclerosis of the coronary arteries.

There is an important note at the beginning of this block that explains what the term *duration* means when used for morbidity and mortality coding. Also notice the "use additional" note for the presence of hypertension.

Code sets I30-I52 are for all other types of ischemic heart disease. You will find the nonrheumatic heart diseases in this block, together with infective conditions, heartbeat irregularities, and various forms of heart failure.

The last code set includes circulatory conditions that arise following surgery or a procedure. The category for hypotension (low blood pressure) is included here, and there is one category in this block containing asterisk codes.

Chapter X: Diseases of the Respiratory System (J00-J99)

This section is organized into codes for upper respiratory conditions, lower respiratory conditions, and other diseases of the respiratory system. Codes are organized anatomically, with conditions of higher anatomical sites first.

For example, J00-J06, Acute Upper Respiratory Infections, start with infections in the nose and end with infections in the larynx. The chapter starts with a note that tells you that conditions occurring in more than one site should be classified to the lower anatomical site.

The chapter includes conditions caused by certain infections and some external agents, such as in occupational exposure, so you need to check the inclusion and exclusion notes at chapter, block, category, and subcategory levels carefully.

With some codes in Chapter X, a further code may be used to identify an infection with which the respiratory disease is associated, or the infectious agent that caused the condition.

For example, with code J15, Bacterial pneumonia, not elsewhere classified, there are several fourth-digit characters to identify the bacteria responsible for the infection, and J17* is an asterisk category for pneumonia resulting from a disease that is coded to another chapter, such as Chapter I, Certain Infectious and Parasitic Diseases.

Chapter XI: Diseases of the Digestive System (K00-K94)

This chapter is often referred to as the alimentary or gastrointestinal tract.

The chapter is structured with the diseases of the upper digestive system first (starting with diseases of the oral cavity, glands, and jaw), then the lower digestive system, and then other digestive system conditions.

There are eight exclusions at the chapter level. These mainly relate to diseases that are captured in the special diseases chapter.

Diseases in the special diseases chapter take precedence over the body system chapters.

If you are coding a hernia, you will need to refer to the note at the beginning of block K40-K46, explaining how hernias with both gangrene and obstruction should be classified as hernia with gangrene.

Chapter XII: Diseases of the Skin and Subcutaneous Tissue (L00-L99)

This chapter contains ten exclusions at chapter level and six asterisk categories. It includes conditions caused by certain conditions coded to other chapters.

For example, in the first code sets, L00-L08, an additional code from Chapter I can be used to record the agent responsible for the infection. To code staphylococcal infection of the skin of the leg, two codes would be required:

- L08.9 Local infection of skin and subcutaneous tissue, unspecified
- B95.8 Unspecified staphylococcus as the cause of diseases classified to other chapters.

Papulosquamous disorders, L40-L45, are disorders characterized by papules (pimples) that are usually red with a variable amount of scaling on the surface. Therefore code L40.1 would be used to report generalized pustular psoriasis.

Code sets L60-L75 are used to report diseases of skin appendages such as nails, hair, hair follicles, sebaceous glands, and sweat glands.

To code for nonscarring alopecia (hair loss) and premature greying of hair, two codes would be required:

- L65.9 Nonscarring hair loss, unspecified
- L67.1 Variations in hair color

Chapter XIII: Diseases of the Musculoskeletal System and Connective Tissue (M00-M99)

Use these code sets to report diseases of the musculoskeletal system and connective tissue (e.g., ligaments and tendons) that are not the result of injury. To report conditions that are the result of injury, see Chapter XIX, Injury, Poisoning, and Certain Other Consequences of External Causes.

This chapter contains several categories for conditions of the musculoskeletal system that are coded to the special diseases chapters, such as endocrine disorders (Chapter IV). The distinctive feature of Chapter XIII is the use of optional fifth characters to provide a site subclassification. You will find the main list at the start of the chapter. Instead of using the chapter level site codes, the three categories M23, M40-M54 (except M50 and M51), and M99 have their own site subclassifications.

Be sure to read all notes and descriptions carefully because some codes in this chapter are site-specific and will not require a site subclassification.

Codes M00-M25 are used to code arthropathies and contain diseases affecting limb joints. Within this code set, codes are further broken down into four subgroups, each one for a specific type of arthropathy. Here you will find infective, inflammatory, degenerative, and other diseases of joints.

Codes M30-M36 contain descriptions for autoimmune and collagen diseases. Specifically excluded from here are autoimmune disorders that affect single organs or single cell types, whereas systemic conditions are included.

E X A M P L E
■ Lupus erythematosus with lung involvement M32.1† J99 (although a single organ is involved, the underlying condition is systemic) ■ Lupus erythematosus > L93.0 (affects the red blood cells only, therefore excluded)

Codes M40-M54 are for diseases affecting the spine. It has three subcode sets, each one for a specific type of dorsopathy. The code sets start with a list of supplementary subclassification codes for the site affected. Some of the codes are for the areas where the different spinal curves meet, such as the cervicothoracic region.

Examples of conditions coded here are ankylosing spondylitis, coded at M45; sciatica, coded at M54.3; and various forms of curvature of the spine, coded within the subcode sets M40-M43.

To report soft tissue disorders see codes M60-M79. These are diseases that affect muscles, tendons, and synovium (the soft tissue that lines the noncartilaginous surfaces in some joints). This code set has a further breakdown into three subsets based on the structure affected. There are a number of categories within this code set that can use the site codes from the beginning of the chapter.

To report acquired deformities of the musculoskeletal system see codes M95-M99. These are postprocedural disorders. For instance, to report a fracture of the femur following the insertion of a hip joint replacement, use code M96.66.

Chapter XIV: Diseases of the Genitourinary System (N00-N99)

There are 11 sections in this chapter, structured according to the different sites and then the diseases that affect the genitourinary system. There are eight exclusions that mainly relate to diseases that are captured in the special diseases chapter.

Codes N00-N08 contain diseases affecting the glomeruli with a list of fourth character subdivisions that provides details of morphological changes.

Codes N10-N16 are used to report renal tubulointerstitial disease involving structures in the kidney outside the glomerulus.

Codes N17-N19 are for the different kinds of renal failure. There are a lot of exclusions in this code set with a "use additional" note reminding you to add an external cause code if the renal failure has been caused by an external agent.

Use codes N40-N53 to report diseases affecting the different organs of the male genital system. Codes N60-N65 contain diseases affecting both male and female breasts.

Codes N70-N77 cover inflammatory diseases of the female pelvic organs. Many of these codes have a "use additional" note to code the organism that is causing the inflammation or infection. Codes N80-N98 describe noninflammatory disorders of the female genital tract that are related to structural problems and include endometriosis.

ICD-10-CM CODING EXERCISE 3   Chapters 8-14

1. Patient is completely blind in one eye and has impaired vision in the other
2. Rheumatic mitral valve insufficiency
3. Allergic dermatitis due to exposure to the sun
4. Common migraine with blurred vision

Note: Two codes are required to identify all presenting conditions. This is an example of multiple coding, because there is not a single code that contains both conditions.

5. Bleeding peptic ulcer with hemorrhage
6. Myocardial infarction with hypertension, initial episode of care
7. Patient with postencephalitic parkinsonism
8. Actinic keratosis
9. Scintillating scotoma (a visual disturbance preceding migraine)
10. Urinary tract infection with vaginitis NOS

Note: Two codes are required to identify all presenting conditions. This is an example of multiple coding because there is not a single code that contains both conditions.

11. Food poisoning NOS with vomiting

Note: Two codes are required to identify all presenting conditions. This is an example of multiple coding as there is not a single code that contains both conditions.

12. Cardiomyopathy due to excessive alcohol

Chapter XV: Pregnancy, Childbirth, and the Puerperium (O00-O99)

There are eight code sets in the chapter, broadly arranged according to when the condition is recorded as occurring—during pregnancy, delivery, or the puerperium. There are no manifestation (asterisk) categories in this section.

O00-O08 is the code set for pregnancies with abortive outcomes. It includes codes for abnormal products of conception as well as pregnancies that are aborted before 20 weeks of gestation. Additionally there is a special note at the fourth character subdivisions for series O03-O06. These subdivisions provide detail on whether the abortion was incomplete or complete, and whether or not there were any associated complications.

Series O30-O48 is a large category containing codes for many of the conditions that may require care being given to the mother. It includes codes for conditions such as multiple fetuses, malpresentation of the fetus, disproportion and other structural abnormalities in the maternal pelvis or organs, and fetal abnormalities. These are all conditions that affect the fetus and could lead to delivery problems. When the condition is recorded as leading to difficulties during labor and delivery, use code set O60-O77. To report complications in the puerperium or the postpartum period, see code series O85-O92.

Chapter XVI: Certain Conditions Originating in the Perinatal Period (P00-P96)

This chapter contains 10 code sets, structured according to the various conditions that occur in the perinatal period, with some codes containing conditions specific to certain body systems.

The first code sets, P00-P04, are for fetuses and newborns affected by maternal factors and by complications of pregnancy, labor, and delivery. Many of the conditions in this series are actually the mother's conditions. They are here in this chapter to show that the problem the mother incurred during the pregnancy, labor, or delivery had an effect on the infant in some way. When you code cases where the infant has been affected by the condition affecting the mother you will need two codes, one for the effect on the infant and the other code—from series P00-P04—to show the cause.

Chapter XVII: Congenital Malformations, Deformations, and Chromosomal Abnormalities (Q00-Q99)

A congenital condition is one that is discovered at the time of birth or shortly afterward. Congenital conditions are not necessarily inherited (genetic) ones, although genetic conditions are included in the chapter.

This section is not to be used to report inborn errors of metabolism, which are coded to Chapter IV: Endocrine, Nutritional, and Metabolic Diseases. Also excluded are acquired malformations and abnormalities, such as acquired deformities or acquired deafness.

To report various malformations of the eye, ear, face, and neck, see codes Q10-Q18.

Code sets Q80-Q89 relate to various syndromes and conditions affecting a number of different systems including the skin, breast, and multiple systems.

The conditions in Q90-Q99 all result from chromosomal abnormalities, and they often include abnormalities that affect a number of body systems in the one syndrome. (Chromosomes are pieces of human DNA, which controls development.)

This series includes codes for various trisomies, monosomies, and other abnormalities of the chromosome structure.

Chapter XVIII: Symptoms, Signs, and Abnormal Clinical and Laboratory Findings (R00-R99)

Codes from this section are used when no definitive diagnosis has been made for a particular case. It is very important to read the notes at the beginning of this chapter because they provide explanations as to what is coded in this chapter and give examples of the type of situations in which you would assign a code from this chapter.

The chapter contains 13 code sets. The first seven sets contain codes for symptoms and signs for specific body systems. The eighth set is for general symptoms and signs that are not specific to a body system. The next four sets are for abnormal findings found on the diagnostic testing of a patient where no diagnosis has been made.

The final code set is R95-R99, Ill-defined and unknown causes of mortality. Included in this series are some codes for the death of a patient. It is very rare for one of these codes to be assigned for morbidity coding. They should only be assigned when there is no information at all as to the cause of the patient's death.

Chapter XIX: Injury, Poisoning, and Certain Other Sequences of External Causes (S00 -T88)

Most code sets in this chapter require a seventh character extension. With the exception of fractures, most of these codes require information as to whether this is an initial encounter (A), subsequent encounter (D), or sequela (S).

(A) Initial encounter. Use this extension while the patient is receiving active treatment for the injury.

  Example: Surgery, emergency care, evaluation and treatment by a new physician

(D) Subsequent encounter. Use this extension after the patient has received active treatment but is now receiving routine care during the healing or recovery phase.

  Example: Cast change or removal of internal or external devices, medication adjustments, other aftercare or follow-up visits

(S) Use for complications or conditions that occur as a direct result of the injury.

  Example: Formation of scarring after a burn

The remaining guidelines that pertain to this chapter are the same as those that were discussed in the chapter on ICD-9-CM coding.

Chapter XX: External Cause of Morbidity (V01- Y99)

Codes from this chapter are used to explain:

- Events or circumstances
- Cause of injury or poisoning
- Other adverse effects

These codes are considered "companion codes" to Chapter XIX because they provide more detail for injury prevention and planning purposes. In the ICD-9-CM version these codes were considered supplementary codes or optional use codes. They were referred to as E codes. However, in ICD-10, these codes are now to be used to provide extra information and are no longer considered to be optional.

More than one external cause code may be used per claim to further describe the events surrounding the injury or poisoning.

Just as there are late effect codes for injuries, you will find that in this section there are also late effects to report circumstances.

Chapter XXI: Factors Influencing Health Status and Contact with Health Services (Z00-Z99)

Chapter XXI is a special chapter that contains codes used to describe health care services provided to patients who may or may not be ill. A note at the beginning of the chapter explains the purpose of the codes and how they should be used. The first part of the chapter is structured according to the type of health service being provided to the patient. The rest is structured according to the health status of the patient.

Code set Z00-Z13 is for patients encountering health services for examination and investigation.

Code set Z20-Z29 is for persons with potential health hazards related to communicable diseases. These are used for patients who are admitted to hospital who have come into contact with a certain disease, are a carrier of a disease, need immunization against a disease, or may require prophylactic treatment against a disease.

Code set Z30-Z39 is to report services for patients encountering health services in circumstances related to reproduction (e.g., Z37, Outcome of Delivery and Z38, Liveborn infants according to place of birth).

Code set Z55-Z65 is for patients with potential health hazards related to socioeconomic and psychological circumstances. The categories in this block consist of circumstances rather than actual diseases that can cause the person to have health problems.

Code set Z70-Z76 is for patients encountering health services in other circumstances. There are a number of codes in this set for patients undergoing counseling. Additionally, there are codes for lifestyle issues and circumstances that are beyond a patient's control.

The final code set, Z77-Z99, is for coding persons with potential health hazards related to family and personal history and certain conditions influencing health status.

ICD-10-CM CODING EXERCISE 4   Chapters 15-22

1. Diverticulitis, congenital
2. Colles' fracture, initial care
3. Yellow jaundice
4. Ruptured tubal pregnancy with an embolism
5. Pregnancy complicated by cervical incompetence
6. Follow-up examination after surgery
7. Obstructed labor due to a breech presentation
8. Infant born with cystic lung disease
9. Agenesis of the eye

Note: Agenesis is a condition in which part of the body fails to develop in the embryo.

ICD-10-CM CODING EXERCISE 5   End of Chapter Review

1. Type 2 diabetes, caused by obesity, with foot ulcer
2. Subacute thyroiditis
3. Congenital iodine deficiency syndrome, neurological type, and associated mild mental retardation
4. Alcoholic with alcoholic liver sclerosis with esophageal varices without bleeding
5. A patient with epilepsy treated with carbamazepine that resulted in aplastic anemia
6. Patient with spasmodic torticollis, a condition causing involuntary twisting of the neck
7. Cryptophthalmos syndrome
8. Duchenne muscular dystrophy
9. Puncture wound with foreign body of unspecified part of thorax
10. Ganglion on a tendon in the wrist, unspecified
11. Acute rheumatic pericarditis
12. Patient with thyrotoxic myopathy
13. Cerebrospinal fluid leak from spinal puncture
14. Allergic urticaria
15. Type 1 diabetes mellitus with diabetic cataract
16. Petit mal epilesy
17. Carpal tunnel syndrome
18. Idiopathic gouty arthritis of the right knee
19. Idiopathic osteoporosis with a pathological facture of the tibia, initial encounter
20. Pneumonia due to whooping cough
21. Single spontaneous vaginal delivery, live-born male infant, vertex position

3

Service and Procedural Coding: Current Procedural Terminology (CPT)

Radiology

Pathology

    Medicare and Pathology/
    Laboratory

Injections

    Immunizations (90281 to 90749)

    Therapeutic or Diagnostic
    Injections (96365 to 96379)

Allergy Injections (95115 to
    95180)

Tests and Diagnostic Studies

Cardiology (92950 to 93799)

Otorhinolaryngology (92502
    to 92598)

Pulmonary Tests (94010 to
    94799)

Psychiatry (90801 to 90899)

Ophthalmology (92002 to 92499)

    Special Service Codes (99000
    to 99091)

KEY TERMS

Term	Definition
Adjunct Codes	Codes used to record additional services.
AMA	American Medical Association.
Audit	A process to determine if the information sent to the insurance company is supported by the documentation in the medical record.
Biopsy	Removal of a small amount of tissue to determine the extent of a disease or to determine a diagnosis.
Bundling Services	Combining lesser services with a major service so that one charge will include the variety of services.
CCI	Correct Coding Initiative: Bundling edits created by CMS to combine various component items with a major service or procedure.
CMS	Centers for Medicare and Medicaid Services: The federal agency responsible for maintaining and monitoring the Medicare program, beneficiary services, and Medicaid and state operations (formerly Health Care Financing Administration [HCFA] until 2001).
Comorbidity	An ongoing condition that exists with another condition for which the patient is receiving treatment.
Component Billing	Billing for each item or service provided to a patient in accordance with insurance carriers' policies.
CPT	Current Procedural Terminology. Nomenclature published by the AMA as a means to describe services rendered to a patient through the use of numerical codes.
CPT Code	Procedural description with a five-digit identifying code number.
Diagnostic Services	Services performed to determine or establish a patient's diagnosis.
E&M Codes	Evaluation and Management codes used to report patient visits, consults, hospital care, and so on.
Endoscopic Procedure	A procedure performed through an existing orifice with an endoscope to visualize an abnormality or to determine the extent of a disease.
Global Period	Specific time frames assigned to a code by an insurance company before additional payment will be made following a surgical procedure (e.g., 10 days, 90 days).
Global Procedures	Major surgical procedures that typically have a follow-up period of 30, 60, 90, or 120 days before you may begin to bill the patient for services related to the original procedure.
HCPCS	Healthcare Common Procedure Coding System: A coding system designed by CMS to report patient services that uses codes from CPT and other sources of alphanumeric codes.
HIPAA	Health Insurance Portability and Accountability Act: An act passed in 1996 to set standards for electronic health care transactions and to protect the privacy and security of patients' health information.
Major Procedure	A packaged procedure that includes the operation, local infiltration, digital blocks, and follow-up care for a specific number of days.
Medicare Part A	A national health insurance program for persons over the age of 65 years and qualified disabled or blind persons regardless of income, administered by CMS to cover the cost of hospitalizations and nursing facility charges.
Medicare Part B	An elective coverage program offered by CMS for aged and disabled patients to provide benefits for physician and other medical services as part of the Medicare program. This program has a monthly premium that must be paid by the beneficiary to keep the policy in good standing.

Minor Procedures	Services identified by AMA as a starred procedure. For Medicare, these include services with either 0 or 10 days of follow-up care.
Modality	Any physical agent applied to produce therapeutic changes to biological tissues (e.g., thermal, acoustic, mechanical).
POS Codes	Place service (e.g., office, hospital) codes: A complete list of these codes is found in the introduction section of the professional version of the CPT manual.
Ranking Codes	Listing services in their order of importance by dates of service and values. Codes are usually ranked by value from highest to lowest charges.
RVU	Relative value unit: A method to calculate fees for services. A unit is translated into a dollar value using a conversion factor or dollar multiplier. The assigned value is generally based on three factors: physician work component, overhead practice expense, and malpractice insurance.
Superbill	A form designed by a medical practice listing the most frequently used diagnosis and procedure codes.
Therapeutic Services	Services performed for treatment of a specific condition.
Unbundling Services	Listing services or procedures as separate billable components. Although this practice may generate more revenue, it is often an incorrect reporting technique that could result in an insurance company auditing a practice or asking for refunds of paid monies.
UPIN	Unique Personal Identification Number.

OBJECTIVES

To use a tool, one must understand its language, format, and purpose. This chapter has been developed as a guide to help the coder achieve a better understanding of the various methods available in locating correct codes for maximum appropriate reimbursement. After completing this chapter, readers should be able to:

- Explain the structure, format, and conventions used in CPT (Current Procedural Terminology).
- Identify CPT codes and explain their application within a medical office.
- Locate and use the appendices of CPT.
- Assign correct Evaluation and Management (E&M) codes.
- Apply modifiers with an understanding of their importance in coding.
- Identify services and procedures included in a surgical package.
- Define the difference between a consult and a referral.
- Identify and use the HCPCS (Healthcare Common Procedure Coding System) for Medicare claims.
- Translate written documentation into a numerical language.
- Identify and code services for entry on an insurance claim form.

INTRODUCTION

This chapter provides an introduction to procedural coding. The more you know about coding, the better your chances for succeeding in your chosen field. In today's world, more emphasis is placed on coding than ever before in the history of the medical profession. Practices are seeking trained coders to keep pace with the ever-changing rules and mandates. Therefore, the more informed the coder becomes, the more valuable his or her services will be.

CPT—THE HIPAA STANDARD CODE SET

The **Health Insurance Portability and Accountability Act (HIPAA)** national standard code set for procedures is the **Current Procedural Terminology,** more commonly referred to as **CPT**. This code set was established in 1966 by the **American Medical Association (AMA)** to serve as a uniform language describing services and procedures performed by physicians and other health care professionals. CPT serves as a guide that helps the coder accurately report medical, surgical, or diagnostic services rendered to a patient. It is composed of five-digit numerical codes with descriptive explanations. CPT serves as a dependable, nationally mandated communication tool used by physicians, insurance companies, and patients.

PURPOSE

The purpose of this book is to teach you convention and guideline applications as they pertain to AMA guidelines for coding applications. The purpose of CPT coding is to provide a means to report services to the patient. **CPT codes** often serve as a time use chart to track patient encounters or services. The patient's medical record is the source for procedure codes that comply with regulations.

The care provided to a patient is documented in his or her medical record in terms of the services rendered. This documentation is a legal record of both the diagnoses and the procedures for a patient. The medical office documents every meeting with a patient by documenting the patient's name, the encounter date and reason, the physician's examination results, tests that were ordered, the diagnosis, the plan of care or notes on treatments that were performed, and the instructions given to the patient.

It is important for the coder to remember that using a CPT code does not guarantee that the provider will receive payment from the insurance company. It is often said, "If it is not documented, it did not happen," meaning that Medicare and commercial carriers examine the medical necessity of services before payment. Therefore, if the physician performed a service, it must be documented in the medical record. If a carrier doubts that there is adequate medical necessity, it may conduct an **audit** of the documentation. In such a review, the carrier examines the medical record to ensure that the diagnosis and procedure codes are correctly linked and that services were provided at the correct level. If the service is not documented, the carrier will deny payment for the service even if a correct CPT code is used.

TRAINING AND ADVANCEMENT

When you begin your career in the medical community, you will find that reimbursement and coding applications might be influenced by such factors as the following:
- AMA guidelines for coding applications
- **Centers for Medicare and Medicaid Services (CMS)** mandates for procedural coding
- Individual insurance company rules and regulations

Certifications

Many coders, after gaining basic experience on the job, seek certification as a coder. Certification is granted after the coder passes a national test of coding knowledge, and it increases the coder's value to the practice. Two organizations offer coding certification.

The American Academy of Professional Coders grants the following certifications:
- Certified Professional Coder (CPC)
- Certified Professional Coder-Hospital (CPC-H)

For more information contact the American Academy of Professional Coders, 309 West 700 South, Salt Lake City, UT 84101; 800-626-2633, http://www.aapc.com.

The American Health Information Management Association offers the three following coding certifications:
- Certified Coding Associate (CCA), intended as a starting point for a career as a coder
- Certified Coding Specialist (CCS)
- Certified Coding Specialist-Physician-based (CCS-P)

For more information contact the American Health Information Management Association (AHIMA), 919 North Michigan Avenue, Suite 1400, Chicago, IL 60611-1683; 312-787-2672, *http://www.ahima.org.*

UNDERSTANDING CPT

CPT was established in 1966 by the AMA to serve as a uniform language describing the services and procedures performed by physicians and other health care professionals. CPT serves as a guide to accurate reporting of medical, surgical, or diagnostic services rendered to a patient. It consists of five-digit numerical codes with descriptive explanations. CPT serves as a dependable, nationally accepted communication tool used by physicians, insurance companies, and patients. CPT is the HIPAA standard code set for reporting procedures.

CPT is updated and published every November to meet the constantly changing demands of the medical industry. As new codes are added, the older, obsolete codes are revised or deleted from the manual. Several factors must be considered before determining if a code should or should not be included in the updated edition of the CPT manual. Two key factors are as follows:

- The procedure or service must be commonly performed by physicians nationwide.
- The procedure or service must be consistent with current medical practice.

Note that the inclusion or exclusion of a code or description from CPT does not necessarily affect reimbursement for the procedure. Reimbursement policies are determined by individual third-party payers based on contract agreements and special clauses.

Code descriptions may be changed or added to CPT when a physician writes to the AMA asking that a new code be entered into the manual or an older code be expanded based on new methods and terminology. The inclusion or deletion of a code is a lengthy process involving the cooperation of the AMA, physicians, and medical societies.

The CPT manual contains six categories that are listed in numerical order, with the exception of the Evaluation and Management (E&M) codes. Because all practices use these E&M codes, the AMA has placed them in the front of the book for easy access.

CPT CODING SECTIONS

Introduction Category	Code Sections
Category I Codes	
Evaluation and Management	99201 to 99499
Anesthesia	00100 to 01999
	99100 to 99140
Surgery	10021 to 69990
Radiology	70010 to 79999
Pathology and Laboratory	80048-89356
Medicine	90281 to 99199
	99500 to 99602
Category II	0001F TO 7025F
Category III	0019T TO 0259T

WHAT IS A CPT CODE?

A CPT code is a five-digit numerical code used to describe the professional services of a physician or other caregiver. Professional services may include medical, surgical, radiology, pathology or laboratory, anesthesiology, or evaluation and management services.

CPT codes are used by the following:

- Those who work with the business side of medicine
- Those who report professional services and procedures provided to the patient
- Those who work with outpatient facility services for Medicare or Medicaid claims

Information contained in the introduction explains the intent of the coding system while providing insight into the formats and terminologies used. Additional definitions are provided for CPT update requests, guidelines, modifier applications, and unlisted services or procedures.

CPT CODE COMPONENTS

Correct Use

The CPT coding system is a means of communicating to third-party payers exactly what the physician did to or for a patient. Correct use of the codes will help the practice receive, in a timely manner, the full reimbursement allowed for work performed by the physician.

Numerical Code

A numerical code is a unique five-digit numerical code that is assigned to each procedure, service, or supply provided by a physician and included in the CPT book.

E X A M P L E
Numerical Codes 25120, 95831

Descriptor

A descriptor accompanies the code in the book and describes the procedure, service, or supply.

E X A M P L E	
Codes	**Descriptors**
25120	Excision or curettage of bone cyst or benign tumor of radius or ulna (excluding head or neck of radius and olecranon process)
95831	Muscle testing, manual (separate procedure), extremity (excluding hand) or trunk report

CATEGORY I CODES

E&M (99201 to 99499)

E&M codes are listed first in the manual, as a matter of convenience, because they are the codes most commonly used by all medical practices. These codes are based on levels of service or treatment and the location in which the service was provided. A few examples of applications for E&M codes are office visits, hospital visits, and consultations.

Anesthesia (00100 to 01999)

The anesthesia codes were developed to report the administration of anesthesia. These codes include local, general, and regional anesthesia; the administration of fluids and blood as related to anesthesia; and other supportive services, such as preoperative and postoperative visits.

Surgery (10021 to 69990)

Surgery is the largest section in CPT. Codes are listed in numerical order by anatomical site. Codes in this section are used to report services for incision, excision, repair, reconstruction, and revision.

Radiology (70010 to 79999)

The radiology section includes codes for diagnostic and therapeutic radiology, nuclear medicine, computed tomography (CT scan), magnetic resonance imaging (MRI), and ultrasonography.

Pathology and Laboratory (80048 to 89399)

Pathology and laboratory codes are used to report services provided by physicians, pathologists, or technologists under the responsible supervision of a physician. These codes are used for diagnostic studies, tests, consultations, toxicology, hematology, immunology, and anatomical or surgical pathology.

Medicine (90281 to 99607)

The medical services codes are used to report services for injections, psychiatry, ophthalmology, otorhinolaryngology, pulmonary, allergy, neurology, and special services.

 CODING TIP

> The listing of a service in a particular section does not limit its use to a specialty. Any code in the manual may be used by any physician if that code accurately describes the services or procedures the physician rendered to the patient.

CATEGORY II CODES

Codes in this section are supplemental tracking codes that can be used for measuring performance. The purpose of these codes is to reduce the need for record abstraction and chart review, thereby minimizing the administrative burden on health care providers and professionals. These codes facilitate data collection about the quality of care by coding certain measures that have been agreed upon as contributions to good patient care.

The use of these codes is optional. The codes are not required for correct coding, and they may not be used as a substitute for Category I codes. Note that because these codes describe components that are typically included in an E&M service or test results that are part of a laboratory procedure, there is no reimbursement value associated with them.

EXAMPLE
1000F   Tobacco use assessed

CATEGORY III CODES

Because of advances in technology and procedure development, the AMA has created another code series, the Category III codes. These codes are listed in the back of the CPT manual before Appendix A. These codes are temporary codes used for emerging technology, services, and procedures. Category III codes were established to more accurately capture information lacking in established codes and to eliminate overuse of the unlisted codes.

E X A M P L E
0030T   Antiprothrombin antibody

Unlike Category I codes, which are revised only once a year, Category II and III codes are updated semiannually in January and July. Updates can be obtained via the AMA/CPT web site (*www.ama-assn.org/go/cpt*).

In the following exercise, you will become familiar with the various sections of CPT. With time and experience, the coder is able to identify a particular code section by the first two digits of the procedure code.

CPT CODING EXERCISE 1   Coding Classification

Directions: Based on the information for classification of various code types just described, list the sections where you would find the following codes.

Example: Code: 99242; Section: Medical section; Code range: 90281 to 99600

CODE	SECTION	CODE RANGE
1. 35501	_____	_____
2. 84234	_____	_____
3. 64575	_____	_____
4. 90802	_____	_____
5. 77305	_____	_____
6. 01400	_____	_____
7. 97750	_____	_____
8. 27370	_____	_____
9. 15002	_____	_____
10. 99215	_____	_____

CPT CODING AND MEDICARE

Medicare did not adopt CPT coding until 1986. In 1986, CMS (formerly HCFA) developed a multilevel coding system to describe services and procedures. CMS named this coding system the Healthcare Common Procedure Coding System, more commonly referred to as **HCPCS** (sometimes pronounced "hick pix").

Level I

This section is based on CPT codes established by the AMA. The AMA CPT manual lists more than 8000 codes that describe procedures and services provided by physicians.

Level II

This section, referred to as National Use Codes, contains codes created by Medicare as a supplement to the CPT manual. This publication lists more than 2000 codes for reporting supplies, services, or procedures that are not contained in the CPT manual developed by the AMA.

Level II codes differ from CPT in that they are alphanumeric codes. These codes begin with letters of the alphabet (A to V) followed by four numbers (e.g., A0001). Level II codes are generally accepted for reporting services nationwide because they were designed with set descriptions and guidelines for use.

Because level II HCPCS is a national coding set for Medicare carriers, copies may be purchased from the same companies that sell ICD-9-CM and CPT coding manuals. Unlike the CPT manuals, HCPCS level II codes are updated throughout the year. The updated or revised codes are published in the Medicare newsletters for your state and are available on the Internet.

CPT FORMAT

It is important to understand how to use CPT correctly. The introduction to CPT provides instructions for using the manual. The introduction explains the format, the definitions of levels of service, and the symbols used; it also provides general instructions about using the manual. Each section also includes explanations pertinent to a particular chapter or subchapter that should be read before coding from that section.

Section Arrangement

Within each of the six sections of CPT, there is a repetitive, consistent structure.

Section	Identifies the service and code range (e.g., Surgery)
Subsection	Identifies the type of service (e.g., Integumentary)
Heading	Identifies anatomical setting (e.g., Skin, subcutaneous and accessory structures)
Subheading	Identifies the service (e.g., Incision and drainage)

Indented Format

CPT codes and definitions have been developed as stand-alone descriptions. However, to save space, CPT uses semicolons and indented text to abbreviate some procedure definitions.

A procedure description containing a semicolon **(;)** is divided into two parts:

1. The wording before (to the left of) the semicolon is considered the common language of the code.
2. The wording following (to the right of) the semicolon is a unique description pertinent only to that specific code.

Codes that immediately follow the code with the semicolon share the common language portion of the definition. The code shares the common portion of the definition. The codes immediately following are indented so you can easily see that they count as the wording to the right of the semicolon.

E X A M P L E	
10021	Fine-needle aspiration; without imaging guidance
10022	With imaging guidance

 CODING TIP

The correct, full definition for code 10022 is "Fine-needle aspiration; with imaging guidance."

Coders unfamiliar with this format could double-bill the service by listing the base code and the indented code. Had the documentation stated "Fine-needle aspiration; with imaging guidance," you would have listed CPT code 10022 on the claim form.

Guidelines

Guidelines are notes that appear at the beginning of each section to define terms or items for correct interpretation and reporting. To code correctly, the coder should read and be familiar with all guidelines.

E X A M P L E
Guidelines at the beginning of the E&M section define terms used to report E&M codes and documentation requirements.

Notes

Notes appear at the beginning of a series of codes to provide explanations for use or to clarify the intent of the code.

E X A M P L E
Under "Applications of Casts and Strapping," the note alerts the coder that these codes are for replacement services only.

Guidelines for Using Notes

- Notes that appear immediately after a heading or subheading apply to all entries in that heading or subheading.
- Notes that appear in parentheses apply in general to the entry immediately above it or immediately below it.
- Notes that appear at the end of a series of codes may apply either to all of the preceding series or to only the code immediately above it.
- A note in a block of type may apply to all entries beneath it as in the beginning of a heading or subheading, or it may apply to all of the preceding section.

Parenthetical Instructions

To draw the coder's attention to important information, CPT provides additional coding information in the form of statements in parentheses. Within a parenthetical statement, the coder might be directed to another code or to information that an additional code might be used to report the service.

E X A M P L E
(For hammertoe operation or interphalangeal fusion, see 28285.)

Symbols

CPT uses symbols to alert the coder to changes or special aspects of a code. The circle, triangle, and inverted triangles are used to highlight text only for a specific publication. In the next edition of CPT, these symbols will be used to highlight different coding information that has been updated or newly created.

CPT SYMBOLS

Symbol	Function
●	A circle or dot identifies a new code.
▲	A triangle identifies a revised code.
►◄	Highlights new and revised text other than the procedure descriptors for ease in comparing the older data with the new or updated information.
+	Indicates an add-on code (e.g., +15787 . . . Abrasion; each additional four lesions or less).
⊘	Used to identify codes exempt from modifier -51 (e.g., ⊘20660, Application of cranial tongs, caliper, or stereotactic frame, including removal [separate procedure]).
;	A semicolon is used to save space (e.g., 20670, Removal of implant; superficial [e.g., buried wire, pin, or rod] [separate procedure]).
◎	Bull's-eye: This bull's-eye symbol was added to indicate those procedures in which the provision of moderate sedation services is considered to be inherent and, therefore, not separately reported by the same physician performing the primary service.
⚡	Lightning bolt: This convention was added to highlight products that are awaiting U.S. Food and Drug Administration (FDA) approval (e.g., 90661, Influenza virus vaccine, derived from cell cultures).
#	Number sign is used to identify codes listed out of numerical sequence. See Appendix N.

Add-On Procedures (+)

Add-on codes are for procedures that are always performed during the same operative session as another surgery and are never performed separately. These codes are inherently secondary codes. The CPT manual highlights these codes by listing a plus (+) sign before the code and adding the phrase "each additional" or "list separately in addition to primary procedure."

		E X A M P L E

CPT code	Add-on	Definition
11200	11201	Removal of skin tags, multiple fibrocutaneous tags, any area; up to and including 15 lesions each additional 10 lesions (list separately in addition to code for primary procedure)
19125	19126	Excision of breast lesion identified by preoperative placement of radiological marker; single lesion, each additional lesion separately identified by a radiological marker (list separately in addition to code for primary procedure)

Unlisted Procedure Codes

Within each section and subsection, codes are provided to use when a description or code does not completely or accurately describe the service or procedure provided by the physician. These codes are unlisted procedures codes. They are easy to identify because they are listed as the last code in each section and usually end with the digits "99" or "9." A complete list of unlisted procedure codes for each of the major six categories is provided in the notes or guidelines at the beginning of each category.

Coders must exercise particular care when using these codes, because reimbursement may be lower than anticipated. To provide a third-party payer with sufficient information to determine reimbursement, operative notes or any other supporting documentation should accompany these codes.

E X A M P L E
Many offices have a policy of charging patients for missed appointments. A regular office visit code cannot be used to record a missed appointment because these codes are for face to face encounters. In this circumstance, the coder would use the following code:
Code 99499   Unlisted E&M Service

APPENDIXES

The AMA has developed 13 appendices to assist the coder in the coding process. These appendixes are found in the back of the CPT manual after the medical section and Category III codes.

CPT APPENDIXES

Appendix	Description
A	Complete listing of CPT modifiers with detailed descriptions.
B	Summary of additions, deletions, and revisions for the current year.
C	Clinical examples of E&M codes.
D	Summary of CPT add-on codes, which are identified by a + symbol.
E	Summary of CPT codes exempt from Modifier -51 reporting rules. These codes are identified by a Ø symbol.
F	Summary of CPT codes exempt from Modifier 63, Procedures performed on infants weighing less than 4 kg.
G	Summary of CPT codes that include Moderate (Conscious) Sedation. These codes are identified by the bull's-eye symbol (◎).
H	Alphabetical Index of Performance Measures by Clinical Condition or Topic.

I	Genetic Testing Code Modifiers.
J	Electrodiagnostic Medicine Listing of Sensory, Motor, and Mixed Nerves.
K	Products pending FDA approval. These codes are identified by a lightning bolt symbol (⚡).
L	Vascular Families. The addition of this appendix is to assist coders in the selection of first, second, third, and beyond third-order branch arteries using the aorta as the entry point.
M	Cross-walk to deleted CPT codes. This appendix is provided as a summary of deleted codes for 2006 that have been cross-walked to the 2007 CPT codes.
N	Summary of resequenced CPT codes.

INDEX

The AMA has listed procedures in alphabetical order at the back of the CPT manual. To find a code quickly, you should refer to this index.

 CODING TIP

Do not code from the index. Only use the index as a reference to help you find the correct code in the Tabular List.

The index offers the following four primary classes of main entries or ways to look up a code:
1. Name of procedure or service (e.g., Endoscopy)
2. Organ part or anatomical site (e.g., Colon)
3. Patient's condition (e.g., Abscess)
4. Symptom, common abbreviation, or eponym (the name of person who developed the procedure or service)
   - Symptom (e.g., Laceration repair, tongue)
   - Common abbreviation (e.g., EEG)
   - Eponym (e.g., McBride procedure)

For each entry, a specific code or a range of codes may be provided to start the search for the exact code. To locate a code in the index, the coder should do the following:
1. Identify the service or procedure performed.
2. Identify the organ involved.
3. Identify the condition or keyword.

The following page contains a short coding exercise to illustrate the various aspects involved in using the index. Refer to the index to locate the correct code.

CPT CODING EXERCISE 2   Index Guide

Directions: Find the code in the index. Underline the keyword used to find the code.

Example: Description: Consultation, x-ray; Code (s): 76140

DESCRIPTION   CODE(S)

1.   Procedure or service: arthrodesis, knee   _____

2.   Body part or organ: heart transplant   _____

3.   Condition: appendix surgery   _____

4.   Symptom: laceration repair of the tongue   _____

5.   Eponym: McCannel suture   _____

6.   Common abbreviation: electrocardiogram, 12 lead with interpretation and report   _____

THE CODING PROCESS

General Guidelines

- Review information and identify services and procedures to code.
- Review and understand the content of the terms contained in the medical record.
- Select and locate key terms in the index.
- Locate the code in the body of the book.
- Read the notes for using the codes, and select the most appropriate code.
- Apply any relevant modifiers.

Coding Tip

Be sure to have the following appropriate resource materials handy when coding:
- Medical dictionary
- Anatomy and physiology books
- Medical reference tools

If you are having problems understanding a specific procedure, such as anatomical site, technique, or extent of the procedure, seek assistance from clinical personnel.

MODIFIERS

The AMA developed modifiers to be used with codes to explain various aspects of coding. Modifiers help clarify codes and may maximize reimbursement. A complete list of CPT modifiers is found in Appendix A of the CPT manual.

In the HCPCS code list, Medicare has also developed level II modifiers to be used in addition to the CPT modifiers. The national modifier codes are AA thru ZZ. Two or more modifiers may be used with one code to give the most accurate description possible for that service. The modifier that has the greatest impact on reimbursement should be listed immediately after the CPT code.

Functions of a Modifier

The primary functions of modifiers are as follows:
- To record a service or procedure that has been modified but not changed in its identification or definition
- To explain special circumstances or conditions of patient care
- To indicate repeat or multiple procedures
- To show cause for higher or lower costs while protecting charge history data

CPT modifiers are reported with a two-digit numerical code added to the five-digit CPT code (e.g., 99201-57).

HCPCS level II modifiers are two-character alphabetical and/or alphanumeric codes added to the five-digit CPT code (e.g., 78814-TC).

Modifiers

All of the modifiers are listed with examples of correct coding applications.

Unusual Procedural Services

-22 When the service provided is greater than the time or service usually required for the procedure.

Example: A surgical procedure that usually takes 1 hour took 3 hours. A report or summary should accompany the claim to explain the reason for the increase in charges.

Correct Coding: 58180-22 (Supracervical abdominal hysterectomy)

Unusual Anesthesia

-23 Occasionally, a procedure that usually requires either no anesthesia or local anesthesia must be done under general anesthesia because of unusual circumstances. This circumstance is reported by adding modifier -23 to the procedure code of the basic service.

Example: During a sigmoidoscopic procedure, the patient required general anesthesia.

Correct Coding: 45330 Sigmoidoscopy, flexible

45330-23 General anesthesia applied

Unrelated Evaluation and Management Service by the Same Physician during a Postoperative Period

-24 Use this modifier when the physician needs to indicate that an E&M service was performed during a postoperative period for a reason (or reasons) unrelated to the original procedure.

Example: A patient had gallbladder surgery but came to the office because of a cold 3 weeks following the procedure (same physician). By using this modifier, the coder alerts the carrier that the office visit was not related to the surgical procedure. The physician will then be paid for the visit pertaining to the cold.

Correct Coding: 99213-24 (Established patient office visit)

Significant, Separately Identifiable E&M Service by the Same Physician on the Day of a Procedure

-25 This modifier indicates that on the day a procedure or other service was performed, the patient's condition required a significant, separately identifiable E&M service above and beyond the usual preoperative and postoperative care associated with the procedure that was performed.

Example: A patient was seen for a sore throat and the removal of a wart. Both services (the office visit and the procedure) should be coded, because the reason for the office visit (sore throat) was unrelated to the reason for the surgery.

Correct Coding: 17110 Wart removal

99213-25 Office visit

Professional Component

-26 Certain procedures are a combination of a physician component and a technical component. To report only the physician component, add this modifier to the CPT code number.

Example: The patient has had a chest x-ray, and the physician is only interpreting the film.

Correct Coding: 71010 Radiology examination, chest, single

71010-26 Interpretation only

Mandated Services

-32 This modifier applies to services related to mandated treatments or testing (e.g., third-party payer, governmental, legislative, or regulatory requirement).

Example: Mandated service

Correct Coding: 99243-32 Outpatient consultation, mandated

Anesthesia by Surgeon

-47 Use this modifier to code for the services of regional or general anesthesia when this service is provided by the surgeon. Do not use it to code local anesthesia.

Example: The surgeon who drained the patient's cyst also administered a regional anesthetic.

Correct Coding: 40801-47 Drainage of abscess, cyst, hematoma, vestibule of mouth; with application of anesthesia by the surgeon

Bilateral Procedure

-50 When the same procedure is performed on both sides of the body, use this modifier to indicate that service. The modifier is appended to the second procedure.

Example: The patient had two hernias, one in the right groin and one in the left groin that were repaired at the same operative session.

Correct Coding: 49520 Repair recurrent inguinal hernia, right side

49520-50 Repair recurrent inguinal hernia, left side

Multiple Procedures

-51 When multiple procedures other than E&M services are performed on the same day or during the same operative session by the same provider. The services are reported as follows:

Example: The surgeon removed the patient's uterus and also cut an opening into the bladder to drain it.

Correct Coding: Primary procedure: 58150 Supracervical abdominal hysterectomy

Secondary procedure: 51040-51 Cystostomy with drainage

Reduced Services

-52 Under certain circumstances, a service or procedure is partially completed. This modifier alerts the carrier that a reason exists for a lower than usual charge. The reduced services modifier will protect the charge data for the practice.

Example: 93923, Noninvasive physiological studies of upper or lower extremity arteries, multiple levels or with provocative functional maneuvers, complete bilateral study (e.g., segmental blood). The study was performed on a patient with a history of amputation of the extremity.

Correct Coding: 93923-52 Noninvasive physiological studies of upper or lower extremity arteries

Discontinued Procedure

-53 The physician may elect to terminate a procedure due to extenuating circumstances or because it threatens the well-being of the patient. Note: This modifier is not used to report the elective cancellation of a procedure before the patient's anesthesia induction and/or surgical preparation in the operating suite.

Example: The physician began a colonoscopy but had to discontinue the procedure because the patient had not been properly prepped.

Correct Coding: 45378-53 Colonoscopy, discontinued

Surgical Care Only

-54   This modifier indicates that one physician performed a surgical procedure and another physician provided preoperative and/or postoperative management.

Example: The physician performed only the laminectomy.

Correct Coding: 63250-54   Laminectomy, surgical procedure only

Postoperative Management Only

-55   This modifier indicates that a physician other than the surgeon provided the postoperative care.

Example: A physician other than the surgeon provided the postoperative management of the laminectomy.

Correct Coding: 63250-55   Laminectomy, postoperative management

Preoperative Management Only

-56   This modifier indicates that a physician other than the surgeon provided the preoperative evaluation of the patient.

Example: A physician, other than the surgeon, performed the preoperative evaluation before the patient was admitted for a laminectomy.

Correct Coding: 63250-56   Laminectomy, preoperative management

Decision for Surgery

-57   Use this modifier for an E&M service that results in the initial decision to perform surgery. It applies only to major procedures (i.e., those with a 90-day global period) when surgery is performed within 24 hours of the decision for the surgery.

Example: During the encounter with the surgeon, the decision was made to perform surgery the next day.

Correct Coding: 99203-57   Initial office visit with decision for surgery made at the time of the visit

Staged or Related Procedure or Service by the Same Physician during the Postoperative Period

-58   This modifier is used when the physician needs to indicate that a procedure or service performed during the postoperative period was planned prospectively at the time of the original procedure (staged), was more extensive than the original procedure, or was performed for therapy following a diagnostic surgical procedure.

Example: The patient had a breast biopsy. The results indicated a need for a partial mastectomy. The service was scheduled within the 10-day global period of the biopsy.

Correct Coding: 19160-58   Mastectomy, partial

Distinct Procedural Service

-59   This modifier indicates that a procedure or service was distinct or independent from other services performed on the same day. It is used to identify procedures or services that are not normally reported together but are appropriate under the circumstances. This may represent a different patient encounter, different site or organ system, separate lesion, or separate injury not ordinarily encountered or performed on the same day by the same physician.

Example: Removal of a lesion from the arm and another from the back.

Correct Coding: 11601   Excision, malignant lesion (first lesion)

11601-59   Excision, malignant lesion (second lesion)

Two Surgeons

-62   Under certain circumstances, two surgeons (usually with different skills) may be required to manage a surgical procedure.

Example: A laminectomy was performed by a neurosurgeon and an orthopedic surgeon. Each bills the same CPT code with modifier -62.

Correct Coding: 63250-62   Laminectomy, two surgeons

Procedure Performed on an Infant Weighing Less Than 4 kg

-63   In some cases, the small size of a neonate or infant significantly increases the complexity and physician work components required for a procedure. This modifier is used only for procedures on patients in this circumstance.

Example: The patient is a 3-kg infant who requires an enterectomy, resection of small intestine.

Correct Coding: 44120-63   Enterectomy, resection of small intestine; single resection and anastomosis

Surgical Team

-66   Use this modifier when highly complex procedures (i.e., those requiring the concomitant services of several physicians, often of different specialties, plus other highly skilled, specially trained personnel and various types of complex equipment) are carried out under the "surgical team" concept.

Example: A heart transplantation required the skills of a highly trained cardiovascular team.

Correct Coding: 33945-66   Heart transplant, with or without recipient cardiectomy

Repeat Procedure by Same Physician

-76   Use this modifier when a physician needs to indicate that a procedure or service was repeated subsequent to the original service on the same day.

Example: The patient had an ECG (93000) in the morning with a repeat ECG in the afternoon.

Correct Coding: 93000-76   ECG, repeat procedure

Repeat Procedure by Another Physician

-77   This modifier indicates that a procedure had been performed by another physician on the same day and was repeated by a different physician.

Example: The patient had an ECG (93000) at the primary care physician's office and was sent to a cardiologist who repeated the ECG on the same day.

Correct Coding: 93000-77   ECG, repeat procedure

Return to the Operating Room for a Related Procedure

-78   This modifier indicates that another procedure, related to the first procedure, was performed during the initial procedure's postoperative period and required a return to the operating room.

Example: The patient had abdominal surgery. Three days after surgery an infection occurs in the wound site, requiring the patient to return to the operating room for debridement of the wound site.

Correct Coding: 11000-78   Debridement of necrotic tissue, related procedure

Unrelated Procedure or Service in a Postoperative Period

-79   When a patient is seen by the same physician for an unrelated problem or condition during the postoperative period, use this modifier.

Example: A patient has a Maze procedure for the treatment of atrial fibrillation (33253) and goes home. The wound site is healing well. Two weeks later, the patient is seen by the same physician for pericardiotomy for removal of a foreign body (33020). Because the second procedure is within the global period for the original surgery, attach modifier -79 to the second procedure.

Correct Coding: 33020-79   Pericardiotomy

Surgical Assistant

-80   This modifier identifies the services of another physician who acts as a second pair of hands for a surgical procedure.

Example: A patient undergoes intestinal fistula closure (44640), requiring the assistance of another physician to complete. The primary surgeon would report the service as 44640. To report the services of the assistant, add modifier -80 to the same code.

Correct Coding: 44640-80   Closure of intestinal fistula (Surgical assisting coding only)

Minimum Assistant Surgeon

-81   Use this modifier for a procedure that does not normally require a surgical assistant but because of extenuating circumstances requires the services of another physician for a short time.

Note: Many commercial insurance companies allow this modifier to be used when assistance is provided by personnel other than an MD or DO. For Medicare carriers, you must use modifier -AS to report services provided by an assistant who is not an MD or DO.

Example: A patient treated for gingivitis requiring a gingivectomy (41820, excision gingiva, each quadrant) required the assistance of another physician for a short period of time. Note: This modifier may also be used to report surgical assistance of a nurse practitioner or physician assistant based on insurance company policies.

Correct Coding: 41820-81   Gingivectomy, excision gingiva, each quadrant

Assistant Surgeon

-82   Use this modifier when a qualified resident surgeon is not available. This modifier is typically reserved for teaching hospitals and teaching physician services.

Example: A teaching physician required assistance to close an intestinal fistula. At the time of the procedure, a resident was not available to provide assistance. Another teaching physician had to assist with the procedure.

Correct Coding: 44640-82   Closure of intestinal fistula

Reference (Outside) Laboratory

-90   This modifier is used when laboratory procedures are performed by a party other than the treating or reporting physician. Use this modifier with only the 80000 code series.

Example: A patient with Conn's disease is scheduled for aldosterone studies in the morning and in the afternoon to compare the results of electrolyte excretion by the kidneys.

Correct Coding: 82088-90   Aldosterone

Repeat Clinical Diagnostic Laboratory Test

-91   Use this modifier to indicate a repeat of the same laboratory test on the same day to obtain subsequent (multiple) test results.

Note: This modifier may not be used when tests are performed to confirm initial results; when specimen testing problems or equipment failure occur; or for any other reason when a normal, one-time, reportable is all that is required. This modifier may not be used when other code(s) describe a series of test results (e.g., glucose tolerance testing, evocative/suppression testing).

Correct Coding: 82088   Aldosterone

                          82088-91   Aldosterone

Alternate Laboratory Platform Testing

-92   Use this modifier when laboratory testing is performed using a kit or transportable instrument.

Correct Coding: 86701   HIV testing

                          86701-92   HIV testing

E&M CODES

Medical services are based on several components to establish the correct level of service for each visit. The E&M codes represent a way to clarify services provided by physicians and other caregivers.

Many practices make the mistake of using only one or two codes to report levels of service for patient care. By not having a complete understanding of coding based on the various levels of care, the practice may not be obtaining the full benefit of these codes.

It is important, when using levels of service codes, to document the actual service(s) provided to the patient. Many practices err in using higher code levels without the necessary supporting documentation. The caregiver's notes are the only source or record that describes the actual services provided to a patient. When such documentation is incomplete, the level of service that can be billed is often lower than the actual level of service provided.

 CODING TIP

Coding's Golden Rule
If it is not documented, it did not happen.
If it is not documented, you cannot code it.

Levels of service codes (E&M) are broken down into subsections based on the following:
- Actual location or type of service (e.g., office, hospital, nursing home)
- Content or level of service (e.g., minimal, consult, new patient)
- Nature of the presenting problem (e.g., disease, condition, illness)
- Time typically required for the completion of the service (e.g., 10 minutes, 30 minutes)

 CODING TIP

Regardless of the location where the service is provided, the definition of the service level and the required components to use that level of service remain the same based on the specific criteria listed with each code description.

Knowing the sections in which a code may be found is a key factor in quickly locating the correct code for a specific type of service. However, a code may not be restricted to a particular location. The following information is designed to help the coder understand correct applications for each of the E&M services.

Where May Services be Performed?

In some cases, codes are restricted for use based on the place of service (POS) or where the actual care was provided. The following guidelines show where and how services may be performed and how they are to be coded. As always, code selection is based on these two factors: POS and level of service supported by the documentation.

Outpatient Services (99201 to 99215)
- The physician's office (primarily used for initial examinations or follow-up visits)
- Outpatient departments of hospitals or clinics

Observation Services (99217 to 99236)
- Hospital service for the purpose of observing a patient
- Used to report the "first encounter when designated as observation status"

Inpatient Care (99221 to 99239)
- Hospital admission or confinement
- Level consists of admission, daily hospital care, and discharge visits

Consultations (99241 to 99255)
- Outpatient and hospital settings
- Used when a physician is asked to give advice or an opinion on a patient's care

Emergency Department Services (99281 to 99288)

- An emergency room is defined as an organized, hospital-based facility for the provision of unscheduled, episodic services available 24 hours a day.
- No distinction is made between new and established patients.

Nursing Facilities (99304 to 99318)

Skilled Nursing Facilities

- Requires an outlined plan of treatment
- Patients usually have a diagnosis of a curable but acute illness requiring observation and care by trained medical personnel.
- Patients are expected to have complete recovery, partial recovery, or rehabilitation.

Nursing Home

- The patient usually has an illness or disease that is not curable.
- The problem or condition requires regular care and case management on an infrequent or custodial basis.
- Requires minimal physician services for treatment

Home Visit Services (99341 to 99350)

- Services are provided in a private residence.
- Includes, but is not limited to, the patient's home based on medical necessity

LEVEL OF SERVICE

When you use the E&M codes, it is important to choose the correct level of service based on the description given in the CPT manual. The definitions for levels of care have six components, three key components and three contributory factors.

The three key components are as follows:
1. The extent of the history
2. The extent of the examination
3. The complexity of the decision-making

The other three factors are contributory factors. They are as follows:
1. Counseling and coordination of care
2. Nature of the presenting problem (i.e., the diagnosis)
3. Time

Next we will see what the key components are and how they work in defining the level of service for E&M coding.

DOCUMENTING HISTORY

Within the guidelines, there are four types of history: problem-focused, expanded problem-focused, detailed, and comprehensive. Each type of history includes some or all of the following elements: a chief complaint (CC); history of present illness (HPI); review of systems (ROS); and past, family, and/or social history (PFSH). The extent of each type of history that is obtained and documented depends on the clinical judgment of the physician and the nature of the presenting problem.

Table 3-1 shows the levels of the elements (HPI, ROS, and PFSH) for each type of history. A given type of history must include a CC plus the other three elements as listed in the table.

TABLE 3-1   History Table Criteria

Types of History	History of Present Illness (HPI)	Review of Systems (ROS)	Past, Family, and/or Social History (PFSH)
Problem-focused	Brief (1-3 elements)	N/A	N/A
Expanded problem-focused	Brief (1-3 elements)	Problem pertinent (1 system)	N/A
Detailed	Extended (4 or more)	Extended (2-9 systems)	Pertinent (1 factor)
Comprehensive	Extended (4 or more)	Complete (10 systems)	Complete (based on code)

N/A, Not applicable.
Source: U.S. Department of Health and Human Services, Centers for Medicare and Medicaid Services.

Chief Complaint (CC)

The CC is the reason the patient is seeing the physician or service provider.

 CODING TIP

A chief complaint must be indicated for all levels of service.

To qualify for a given type of history, **all three elements in the table must be met.**

History of Present Illness (HPI)

The HPI is a chronological description of the development of the patient's present illness from the first sign or symptom or from the previous encounter to the present. It includes the following elements: location, quality, severity, duration, timing, context, modifying factors, and associated signs and symptoms.

Brief and extended HPIs are distinguished by the amount of detail needed to accurately characterize the clinical problem(s). A brief HPI consists of one to three elements from the list. An extended HPI consists of four or more elements from the list.

Defining the Elements of the HPI

Location
Determine if the pain is diffused or localized, unilateral or bilateral, fixed or migratory.

Quality
Because some diseases or conditions produce specific patterns of complaints, encourage the patient to describe the symptoms. Use words such as sharp, dull, throbbing, or stabbing; constant or intermittent; acute or chronic; and stable, improving, or worsening.

Severity
Define the severity of the discomfort, sensation, or pain. The physician may suggest a numbering scale for the patient to describe the pain based on a scale of 1 to 10. Minimal or no pain could be 1, and severe or the worst pain would be 10. Severity may be measured by nonverbal signs of discomfort such as lying still or pacing the floor. To measure the quality of pain, use comparisons to previous experiences such as pin sticks or labor.

Duration and Timing

Establish the onset of symptoms or problems. Establish if it is nocturnal, diurnal, or continuous. Look for repetitive patterns of symptoms.

Context

Obtain a description of what the patient is doing or the patient's locality when the signs begin. Is the patient resting or active? When is the problem aggravated or relieved?

Modifying Factors

What has the patient done in an attempt to obtain relief? What makes the condition better or worse? If the patient used over-the-counter drugs, what happened?

Associated Signs or Symptoms

Look for any associated signs or symptoms the patient has experienced such as sweating or nausea.

Review of Systems (ROS)

ROS is an inventory of body systems that the physician obtains through a series of questions to identify signs or symptoms that the patient may be experiencing or has experienced. For the purposes of an ROS, the following systems are recognized for review: constitutional symptoms (e.g., fever, weight loss), eyes, ears, nose, mouth, throat, cardiovascular, respiratory, gastrointestinal, genitourinary, musculoskeletal, integumentary (skin and breasts), neurological, psychiatric, endocrine, hematological/lymphatic, and/or allergic/immunological.

A *problem-pertinent* ROS inquires about the system directly related to the problem(s) identified in the HPI. An *extended* ROS inquires about the system directly related to the problem(s) identified in the HPI *and* a limited number of additional systems. A *complete* ROS inquires about the system(s) directly related to the problem(s) identified in the HPI plus all additional body systems.

Characteristics of a System Review

Constitutional

Constitutional review covers any unusual symptoms or problems the patient has or is experiencing. Examples include night sweats, extreme fatigue, and problems when exercising.

Eyes

Identify the date of the last examination. For patients older than 50 years, determine the last glaucoma check. Obtain information on corrective lenses, infections, or injuries.

Ears, Nose, Throat, and Mouth

Ask about the last hearing test; experiences with nose bleeds or drainage; history of sore throat; ringing of the ears; last dental examination; and a description of the teeth.

Cardiovascular

Determine if the patient has had chest pain, palpitations, murmurs, or hypertension.

Respiratory

Ask about the history of asthma, respiratory problems, chronic coughing, and history of pneumonia or bronchitis.

Gastrointestinal

Inquire about problems with indigestion, burning sensations, or reflux; problems with nausea or vomiting; changes in bowel activity or stool color/consistency; history of hemorrhoids; and laxative use.

Genitourinary

Determine if patient has had any changes in urinary frequency patterns, painful urination, incontinence, bed-wetting problems, or an increase or decrease in urinary output.

Musculoskeletal

Obtain a history of fractures, cramping, joint swelling or stiffness, and chronic pain. Inquire about problems walking or rising.

Integumentary

Note any scarring, moles, or lesions. Ask for the date and result of the last mammogram or breast examination; problems with nipple pain, itching, or discharge; and any history of breastfeeding.

Neurologic

Inquire about problems with fainting, seizures, memory loss, or disorientation; any speech dysfunctions; and problems with concentration.

Endocrine

Ask about thyroid disease; diabetes; any unexplained changes in weight or height; increased thirst or urinary output; and problems with goiter.

Hematologic or Lymphatic

Ask about problems with anemia, fatigue, easy bruising, blood transfusions, and so on.

Allergic or Immunologic

Cover allergy histories, frequent sneezing, itching, and so on.

Psychiatric

Obtain a history of psychiatric treatment or conditions.

Past, Family, and/or Social History (PFSH)

The PFSH consists of a review of three areas: past history, family history, and social history. The *past history* consists of the patient's experiences with illness, operations, injuries, and treatments. The family history is a review of medical events in the patient's family, including diseases that may be hereditary or that place the patient at risk. The *social history* is an age-appropriate review of past and current activities. For the categories of subsequent hospital care, follow-up inpatient consultations, and subsequent nursing facility care, CPT requires only an interval history. It is not necessary to record information about the PFSH.

A *pertinent PFSH* is a review of the history area(s) directly related to the problem(s) identified in the HPI. A *complete PFSH* is a review of two or all three of the PFSH history areas, depending on the category of the E&M service. A review of all three history areas is required for services that by their nature include a comprehensive assessment or reassessment of the patient. A review of two of the three history areas is sufficient for other services.

Review History Criteria by Type

Problem-Focused History

- CC (why the patient is being seen)
- Brief HPI or problem (How long has the patient had the condition? A day? A week? A year?)

<table>
<tr><td align="center">E X A M P L E</td></tr>
<tr><td>A 10-year-old boy complaining of a sore throat and headache that he has been experiencing for the past 24 hours sees his physician.</td></tr>
</table>

Expanded Problem-Focused History

- CC (the reason a patient is seeing the physician)
- Brief HPI (How long has the problem been present?)
- Problem pertinent to system review (Has the patient had this problem or condition before?)

<table>
<tr><td align="center">E X A M P L E</td></tr>
<tr><td>A 6-year-old girl with a history of chronic ear infections comes to the office because her ear has been draining for 1 to 2 days.</td></tr>
</table>

Detailed History

- CC (current diagnosis and any contributing diagnoses or problems)
- Extended HPI (How long has the patient had the problem or condition?)
- Extended system review (information contributing to the history of illness that could affect treatment or care)
- Pertinent PFSH
- Past history (e.g., patient medications)
- Family history (e.g., parents alive or deceased; congenital medical problem within the family)
- Social history (e.g., smoker; how many packs per day and for how long?)

<table>
<tr><td align="center">E X A M P L E</td></tr>
<tr><td>A 16-year-old male with a 3-day history of acute eye infection (conjunctivitis) sees the physician. The physician takes an extensive history to determine allergies or exposure to harmful substances, previous problems with the eyes, and whether the patient has used any medications to treat the problem.</td></tr>
</table>

Comprehensive History

- CC (current or contributing diagnosis)
- Extended history of present illness (length of time the condition or complaint has been present)
- Complete system review
- Past treatments
- Medications used to treat problem
- Any associated problems

- Complete PFSH
- Any related or contributing health problems (e.g., diabetes, heart disease)
- Social history (e.g., smoker, married or single, drinker)
- Family history (e.g., parents living or deceased and their cause of death, number of siblings and their general health status, and the history of family disease or mental conditions)
- Contributory conditions (e.g., past surgeries, illness, hospitalizations, or allergies; last menstrual period; and problems related to current illness)

E X A M P L E

A 60-year-old man with an onset of chest pain that radiates down to the left arm and painful breathing.

DOCUMENTING EXAMINATION CRITERIA

The extent of the examination and documentation of the service depends on the clinical judgment of the physician and is limited by the nature of the presenting problem (the diagnosis). For example, a patient who is seen for a sore throat would not require a complete physical examination (e.g., a rectal or pelvic examination) because the diagnosis does not justify that extent of service. Examinations range from limited examinations of single body areas to general multisystem examinations to complete single-organ system examination.

At this time, in selecting the examination portion of a service, you have two criteria tables from which to choose. Because the 1994 table (Table 3-2) is simplistic in its design, it is easier to use for coding. However, because it is vague, this could lead you to overcode a service. The revised tables from 1997 (Table 3-3) are based on bullet points or elements that better define each phase of the physical examination.

TABLE 3-2   1994 Examination Criteria

Problem-focused	A limited examination of the affected body area or organ
Expanded problem-focused	A limited examination of the affected body area or organ system and other symptomatic or related organ system(s)
Detailed	An extended examination of the affected body area(s) and other symptomatic or related system(s)
Comprehensive	A general multisystem examination or complete examination of a single-organ system

Source: U.S. Department of Health and Human Services, Centers for Medicare and Medicaid Services.

TABLE 3-3   1997 Multisystem Examination Criteria

Problem-focused	Performance and documentation of *one to five elements* identified by a bullet (■) in one or more organ system(s) or body area(s)
Expanded problem-focused	Performance and documentation of *at least six elements* identified by a bullet (■) in one or more organ system(s) or body area(s)
Detailed	At least *six organ systems or body areas* with at least *two elements* identified by a bullet (■) for each system or area

Comprehensive	Performance and documentation of at least *nine organ systems or body areas* with the following:
	  ■ All elements of the examination identified by the bullet
	  ■ *At least two elements* identified by a bullet (■) for each area or system for a total of 18 elements

Source: U.S. Department of Health and Human Services, Centers for Medicare and Medicaid Services.

In an ideal environment the physician should document services based on the 1997 tables; however, use the 1994 tables for code selection.

At this point, you may be wondering why there are two different tables for one coding area. The answer is that the AMA and CMS have not been able to decide the best way to capture examination information. Therefore, coders have a choice of using either the 1994 table or the 1997 table to select examination levels. In other words, you can choose between the tables and use the one that allows you to select the highest possible level of service based on the documentation.

☑ R E M I N D E R

In choosing examination levels, you may choose from the 1994 table or the 1997 table.

Table 3-4 is an example of the information required to be performed for a multi system examination.

TABLE 3-4   1997 Multisystem Examination Table

System or Area	Examination Elements
Constitutional	■ Measurement of any three of the following seven vital signs: (1) sitting or standing blood pressure, (2) supine blood pressure, (3) pulse rate and regularity, (4) respiration, (5) temperature, (6) height, (7) weight (might be measured and recorded by ancillary staff) ■ General appearance of the patient (e.g., development, nutrition, body habitus, deformities, attention to grooming)
Eyes	■ Inspection of conjunctivae and lids ■ Examination of pupils and irises (e.g., reaction to light and accommodation; size and symmetry) ■ Ophthalmoscopic examination of optic discs (e.g., size, C/D ratio, appearance) and posterior segments (e.g., vessel changes, exudates, hemorrhages)
Ears, nose, mouth, and throat	■ External inspection of ears and nose (e.g., overall appearance, scars, lesions, masses) ■ Otoscopic examination of external auditory canals and tympanic membranes ■ Assessment of hearing (e.g., whispered voice, finger rub, tuning fork) ■ Inspection of nasal mucosa, septum, and turbinates ■ Inspection of lips, teeth, and gums ■ Examination of oropharynx: oral mucosa, salivary glands, hard and soft palates, tongue, tonsils, and posterior pharynx
Neck	■ Examination of neck (e.g., masses, overall appearance, symmetry, tracheal position, crepitus) ■ Examination of thyroid (e.g., enlargement, tenderness, mass)
Respiratory	■ Assessment of respiratory effort (e.g., intercostal retractions, use of accessory muscles, diaphragmatic movement) ■ Percussion of chest (e.g., dullness, flatness, hyperresonance) ■ Palpation of chest (e.g., tactile fremitus) ■ Auscultation of lungs (e.g., breath sounds, adventitious sounds, rubs)
Cardiovascular	■ Palpation of heart (e.g., location, size, thrills) ■ Auscultation of heart with notation of abnormal sounds and murmurs; examination of the following: 　■ Carotid arteries (e.g., pulse amplitude, bruits) 　■ Abdominal aorta (e.g., size, bruits) 　■ Femoral arteries (e.g., pulse amplitude, bruits) 　■ Pedal pulses (e.g., pulse amplitude) 　■ Extremities for edema or varicosities

TABLE 3-4   1997 Multisystem Examination Table—cont'd

System or Area	Examination Elements
Chest (breasts)	■ Inspection of breasts (e.g., symmetry, nipple discharge) ■ Palpation of breasts and axillae (e.g., masses or lumps, tenderness)
Gastrointestinal (abdomen)	■ Examination of abdomen with notation of presence of masses or tenderness ■ Examination of liver and spleen ■ Examination for presence or absence of hernia ■ Examination of anus, perineum, and rectum, including sphincter tone, presence of hemorrhoids, rectal masses ■ Obtain stool sample or occult blood test when indicated
Genitourinary	Male: ■ Examination of the scrotal contents (e.g., hydrocele, spermatocele, tenderness of cord, testicular mass) ■ Examination of the penis ■ Digital rectal examination of prostate gland (e.g., size, symmetry, nodularity, tenderness) Female: Pelvic examination (with or without specimen collection for smears and cultures), including the following: ■ Examination of external genitalia (e.g., general appearance, hair distribution, lesions) and vagina (e.g., general appearance, estrogen effect, discharge, lesions, pelvic support, cystocele, rectocele) ■ Examination of urethra (e.g., masses, tenderness, scarring) ■ Examination of bladder (e.g., fullness, masses, tenderness) ■ Cervix (e.g., general appearance, lesions, discharge) ■ Uterus (e.g., size, contour, position, mobility, tenderness, consistency, descent, or support) ■ Adnexa or parametria (e.g., masses, tenderness, organomegaly, nodularity)
Lymphatic	Palpation of lymph nodes in two or more of the following areas: ■ Neck ■ Axillae ■ Groin ■ Other
Musculoskeletal	■ Examination of gait and station ■ Inspection and/or palpation of digits and nails (e.g., clubbing, cyanosis, inflammatory conditions, petechiae, ischemia, infections, nodes) Examination of joints, bones, and muscles of one or more of the following six areas: (1) head and neck; (2) spine, ribs, and pelvis; (3) right upper extremity; (4) left upper extremity; (5) right lower extremity; and (6) left lower extremity. The examination of a given area includes the following: ■ Inspection and/or palpation with notation of presence of any misalignment, asymmetry, crepitation, defects, tenderness, masses, or effusions ■ Assessment of range of motion with notation of any pain, crepitation, or contracture ■ Assessment of stability with notation of any dislocation (luxation), subluxation, or laxity ■ Assessment of muscle strength and tone (e.g., flaccid, cogwheel, spastic) with notation of any atrophy or abnormal movements
Skin	■ Inspection of skin and subcutaneous tissue (e.g., rashes, lesions, ulcers) ■ Palpation of skin and subcutaneous tissue (e.g., induration, subcutaneous nodules, tightening)

Continued

TABLE 3-4   1997 Multisystem Examination Table—cont'd

System or Area	Examination Elements
Neurologic	▪ Testing of cranial nerves with notation of any deficits ▪ Examination of deep tendon reflexes with notation of pathological reflexes (e.g., Babinski) ▪ Examination of sensation (e.g., by touch, pin, vibration, proprioception)
Psychiatric	▪ Description of patient's judgment and insight Brief assessment of mental status, including the following: ▪ Orientation to time, place, and person ▪ Recent and remote memory ▪ Mood and affect (e.g., depression, anxiety, agitation)

C/D, Cup/disc.
Source: U.S. Department of Health and Human Services, Centers for Medicare and Medicaid Services.

TABLE 3-5   1997 Single-System Criteria Table

Problem-focused	Performance and documentation of *one to five elements* identified by a bullet (▪) whether in a shaded or unshaded box
Expanded problem-focused	Performance and documentation of *at least six elements* identified by a bullet (▪) whether in a shaded or unshaded box
Detailed	Performance and documentation of *at least 12 elements* identified by a bullet (▪) whether in a shaded or unshaded box
Eye and psychiatric	Performance and documentation of *at least nine elements* identified by a bullet (▪) whether in a shaded or unshaded box
Comprehensive	All elements identified by a bullet (▪) whether in a shaded or unshaded box ▪ Shaded box: Every element ▪ Unshaded: At least one element is expected

Source: U.S. Department of Health and Human Services, Centers for Medicare and Medicaid Services.

When reporting a single-system examination level, specific criteria (Table 3-5) must be documented for that system. Instead of listing the documentation requirements per specialty, CMS and AMA decided to break out the requirements by organ system. To qualify for a level of service for a single-organ system examination, the following requirements of content and documentation must be met.

In addition to the multisystem examination, there are 10 specialty examination tables (see Tables 3-6 to 3-15). Any physician may use any of the tables regardless of specialty if the examination meets the documentation requirements for a given table.

Tables 3-6 through 3-15 describe the criteria requirements for the specialty organ systems. Remember that when determining the extent of the examination, you may choose from the 1994 table, the 1997 multisystem table, or any of the single-system tables. As with any coding scenario, the extent or level to be coded is based on the extent of the documentation.

TABLE 3-6   Cardiovascular Examination

Constitutional	■ Measurement of any three of the following seven vital signs: (1) sitting or standing blood pressure, (2) supine blood pressure, (3) pulse rate and regularity, (4) respiration, (5) temperature, (6) height, (7) weight (might be measured and recorded by ancillary staff) ■ General appearance of the patient (e.g., development, nutrition, body habitus, deformities, attention to grooming)
Respiratory	■ Assessment of respiratory effort (e.g., intercostal retractions, use of accessory muscles, diaphragmatic movement) ■ Auscultation of lungs (e.g., breath sounds, adventitious sounds, rubs)

Cardiovascular	■ Palpation of heart (e.g., location, size and forcefulness of the point of maximal impact, thrills, lifts, palpable S3 or S4)
	■ Auscultation of heart, including sounds, abnormal sounds, and murmurs
	■ Measurement of blood pressure in two or more extremities when indicated (e.g., aortic dissection, coarctation)
	Examination of the following:
	    ■ Carotid arteries (e.g., waveform, pulse amplitude, bruits, apical-carotid delay)
	    ■ Abdominal aorta (e.g., size, bruits)
	    ■ Femoral arteries (e.g., pulse amplitude, bruits)
	    ■ Pedal pulses (e.g., pulse amplitude)
	    ■ Extremities for peripheral edema or varicosities

Gastrointestinal (abdomen)	■ Examination of abdomen with notation of presence of masses or tenderness ■ Examination of liver and spleen ■ Obtain stool sample for occult blood test from patients who are being considered for thrombolytic or anticoagulant therapy

Neurological/psychiatric	Brief assessment of mental status, including the following:
	    ■ Orientation to time, place, and person
	    ■ Mood and affect (e.g., depression, anxiety, agitation)

Eyes	■ Inspection of conjunctivae and lids (e.g., xanthelasma)
Ears, nose, mouth, and throat	■ Inspection of teeth, gums, and palate ■ Inspection of oral mucosa with notation of presence of pallor or cyanosis
Neck	■ Examination of jugular veins (e.g., distention; a, v, or cannon a waves) ■ Examination of thyroid (e.g., enlargement, tenderness, mass)
Musculoskeletal	■ Examination of the back with notation of kyphosis or scoliosis ■ Examination of gait with notation of ability to undergo exercise testing and/or participation in exercise programs ■ Assessment of muscle strength and tone (e.g., flaccid, cogwheel, spastic) with notation of any atrophy and abnormal movements
Extremities	■ Inspection and palpation of digits and nails (e.g., clubbing, cyanosis, inflammation, petechiae, ischemia, infections, Osler's nodes)
Skin	■ Inspection and/or palpation of skin and subcutaneous tissue (e.g., stasis dermatitis, ulcers, scars, xanthomas)

Source: U.S. Department of Health and Human Services, Centers for Medicare and Medicaid Services.

TABLE 3-7   Ears, Nose, and Throat Examination

System or Area	Examination Elements
Constitutional	■ Measurement of any three of the following seven vital signs: (1) sitting or standing blood pressure, (2) supine blood pressure, (3) pulse rate and regularity, (4) respiration, (5) temperature, (6) height, (7) weight (might be measured and recorded by ancillary staff) ■ General appearance of the patient (e.g., development, nutrition, body habitus, deformities, attention to grooming) ■ Assessment of ability to communicate (e.g., use of sign language or other communication aids), quality of voice
Head and face	■ Inspection of head and face (e.g., overall appearance, scars, lesions, masses) ■ Palpation and/or percussion of face with notation of presence or absence of sinus tenderness ■ Examination of salivary glands ■ Assessment of facial strength
Ears, nose, mouth, and throat	■ Otoscopic examination of external auditory canals and tympanic membranes, including pneumo-otoscopy with notation of mobility of membranes ■ Assessment of hearing with tuning forks and clinical speech reception thresholds (e.g., whispered voice, finger rub) ■ External inspection of ears and nose (e.g., overall appearance, scars, lesions, masses) ■ Inspection of nasal mucosa, septum, and turbinates ■ Inspection of lips, teeth, and gums ■ Examination of oropharynx: oral mucosa, hard and soft palates, tongue, tonsils, and posterior pharynx (e.g., asymmetry, lesions, hydration of mucosal surfaces) ■ Inspection of pharyngeal walls and pyriform sinuses (e.g., pooling of saliva, asymmetry, lesions) ■ Examination by mirror of larynx, including the condition of the epiglottis, false vocal cords, true vocal cords, and mobility of larynx (use of mirror not required in children) ■ Examination by mirror of nasopharynx, including appearance of the mucosa, adenoids, posterior choanae, and eustachian tubes (use of mirror not required in children)
Neck	■ Examination of neck (e.g., masses, overall appearance, symmetry, tracheal position, crepitus) ■ Examination of thyroid (e.g., enlargement, tenderness, mass)
Eyes	■ Test ocular motility, including primary gaze alignment
Respiratory	■ Inspection of chest, including symmetry, expansion, and/or assessment of respiratory effort (e.g., intercostal retractions, use of accessory muscles, diaphragmatic movement) ■ Auscultation of lungs (e.g., breath sounds, adventitious sounds, rubs)
Cardiovascular	■ Auscultation of heart with notation of abnormal sounds and murmurs ■ Examination of peripheral vascular system by observation (e.g., swelling, varicosities) and palpation (e.g., pulses, temperature, edema, tenderness)
Lymphatic	■ Palpation of lymph nodes in neck, axillae, groin, and/or other locations

Neurological/psychiatric	■ Test cranial nerves with notation of any deficits
	■ Brief assessment of mental status, including the following:
	  ■ Orientation to time, place, and person
	  ■ Mood and affect (e.g., depression, anxiety, agitation)

Source: U.S. Department of Health and Human Services, Centers for Medicare and Medicaid Services.

TABLE 3-8   Eye Examination

System or Area	Examination Elements
Eyes	■ Test visual acuity (does not include determination of refractive error) ■ Gross visual field testing by confrontation ■ Test ocular motility, including primary gaze alignment ■ Inspection of bulbar and palpebral conjunctivae ■ Examination of ocular adnexae, including lids (e.g., ptosis or lagophthalmos), lacrimal glands, lacrimal drainage, orbits, and preauricular lymph nodes ■ Examination of pupils and irises, including shape, direct and consensual reaction (afferent pupil), size (e.g., anisocoria), and morphology ■ Slit-lamp examination of the corneas, including epithelium, stroma, endothelium, and tear film ■ Slit-lamp examination of the anterior chambers, including depth, cells, and flare ■ Slit-lamp examination of the lenses, including clarity, anterior and posterior capsule, cortex, and nucleus ■ Measurement of intraocular pressures (except in children and patients with trauma or infectious disease) Ophthalmoscopic examination through dilated pupils (unless contraindicated) of the following: 　■ Optic discs, including size, C/D ratio, appearance (e.g., atrophy, cupping, tumor elevation), and nerve fiber layer 　■ Posterior segments, including retina and vessels (e.g., exudates and hemorrhages)
Neurological/psychiatric	Brief assessment of mental status, including the following: ■ Orientation to time, place, and person ■ Mood and affect (e.g., depression, anxiety, agitation)

C/D, Cup/disc.
Source: U.S. Department of Health and Human Services, Centers for Medicare and Medicaid Services.

TABLE 3-9   Genitourinary Examination

System or Area	Examination Elements
Constitutional	■ Measurement of any three of the following seven vital signs: (1) sitting or standing blood pressure, (2) supine blood pressure, (3) pulse rate and regularity, (4) respiration, (5) temperature, (6) height, (7) weight (might be measured and recorded by ancillary staff) ■ General appearance of the patient (e.g., development, nutrition, body habitus, deformities, attention to grooming)
Gastrointestinal (abdomen)	■ Examination of abdomen with notation of presence of masses or tenderness ■ Examination for presence or absence of hernia ■ Examination of liver and spleen ■ Obtain stool sample for occult blood test when indicated
Genitourinary	Male: ■ Inspection of anus and perineum Examination (with or without specimen collection for smears and cultures) of genitalia, including the following: 　■ Scrotum (e.g., lesions, cysts, rashes) 　■ Epididymides (e.g., size, symmetry, masses) 　■ Testes (e.g., size, symmetry, masses) 　■ Urethral meatus (e.g., size, location, lesions, discharge) 　■ Penis (e.g., lesions, presence or absence of foreskin, foreskin retractability, plaque, masses, scarring, deformities) Digital rectal examination, including the following: 　■ Prostate gland (e.g., size, symmetry, nodularity, tenderness) 　■ Seminal vesicles (e.g., symmetry, tenderness, masses, enlargement) 　■ Sphincter tone, presence of hemorrhoids, rectal masses

Continued

TABLE 3-9   Genitourinary Examination—cont'd

System or Area	Examination Elements
	Female: Includes at least seven of the following 11 elements identified by bullets: ■ Inspection and palpation of breasts (e.g., masses or lumps, tenderness, symmetry, nipple discharge) ■ Digital rectal examination, including sphincter tone, presence of hemorrhoids, rectal masses Pelvic examination (with or without specimen collection for smears and cultures), including the following: ■ External genitalia (e.g., general appearance, hair distribution, lesions) ■ Urethral meatus (e.g., size, location, lesions, prolapse) ■ Urethra (e.g., masses, tenderness, scarring) ■ Bladder (e.g., fullness, masses, tenderness) ■ Vagina (e.g., general appearance, estrogen effect, discharge, lesions, pelvic support, cystocele, rectocele) ■ Cervix (e.g., general appearance, lesions, discharge) ■ Uterus (e.g., size, contour, position, mobility, tenderness, consistency, descent, support) ■ Adnexa/parametria (e.g., masses, tenderness, organomegaly, nodularity) ■ Anus and perineum
Neck	■ Examination of neck (e.g., masses, overall appearance, symmetry, tracheal position, crepitus) ■ Examination of thyroid (e.g., enlargement, tenderness, mass)
Respiratory	■ Assessment of respiratory effort (e.g., intercostal retractions, use of accessory muscles, diaphragmatic movement) ■ Auscultation of lungs (e.g., breath sounds, adventitious sounds, rubs)
Cardiovascular	■ Auscultation of heart with notation of abnormal sounds and murmurs ■ Examination of peripheral vascular system by observation (e.g., swelling, varicosities) and palpation (e.g., pulses, temperature, edema, tenderness)
Chest (breasts)	(See Genitourinary [Female])
Lymphatic	■ Palpation of lymph nodes in neck, axillae, groin, and/or other locations
Skin	■ Inspection and/or palpation of skin and subcutaneous tissue (e.g., rashes, lesions, ulcers)
Neurological/psychiatric	Brief assessment of mental status, including the following: ■ Orientation to time, place, and person ■ Mood and affect (e.g., depression, anxiety, agitation)

Source: U.S. Department of Health and Human Services, Centers for Medicare and Medicaid Services.

TABLE 3-10   Hematological/Lymphatic/Immunological Examination

System or Area	Examination Elements
Constitutional	■ Measurement of any three of the following seven vital signs: (1) sitting or standing blood pressure, (2) supine blood pressure, (3) pulse rate and regularity, (4) respiration, (5) temperature, (6) height, (7) weight (might be measured and recorded by ancillary staff) ■ General appearance of the patient (e.g., development, nutrition, body habitus, deformities, attention to grooming)
Ears, nose, mouth, and throat	■ Otoscopic examination of external auditory canals and tympanic membranes ■ Inspection of nasal mucosa, septum, and turbinates ■ Inspection of teeth and gums ■ Examination of oropharynx (e.g., oral mucosa, hard and soft palates, tongue, tonsils, posterior pharynx)

TABLE 3-10 Hematological/Lymphatic/Immunological Examination—cont'd

System or Area	Examination Elements
Respiratory	■ Assessment of respiratory effort (e.g., intercostal retractions, use of accessory muscles, diaphragmatic movement) ■ Auscultation of lungs (e.g., breath sounds, adventitious sounds, rubs)
Cardiovascular	■ Auscultation of heart with notation of abnormal sounds and murmurs ■ Examination of peripheral vascular system by observation (e.g., swelling, varicosities) and palpation (e.g., pulses, temperature, edema, tenderness)
Gastrointestinal (abdomen)	■ Examination of abdomen with notation of presence of masses or tenderness ■ Examination of liver and spleen
Head and Face	■ Palpation and/or percussion of the face with notation of presence or absence of sinus tenderness
Eyes	■ Inspection of conjunctivae and lids
Neck	■ Examination of neck (e.g., masses, overall appearance, symmetry, tracheal position, crepitus) ■ Examination of thyroid (e.g., enlargement, tenderness, mass)
Lymphatic	■ Palpation of lymph nodes in neck, axillae, groin, and/or other locations
Extremities	■ Inspection and palpation of digits and nails (e.g., clubbing, cyanosis, inflammation, petechiae, ischemia, infections, nodes)
Skin	■ Inspection and/or palpation of skin and subcutaneous tissue (e.g., rashes, lesions, ulcers, ecchymoses, bruises)
Neurological/ psychiatric	■ Brief assessment of mental status, including the following: ■ Orientation to time, place, and person ■ Mood and affect (e.g., depression, anxiety, agitation)

Source: U.S. Department of Health and Human Services, Centers for Medicare and Medicaid Services.

TABLE 3-11 Musculoskeletal Examination

System or Area	Examination Elements
Constitutional	■ Measurement of any three of the following seven vital signs: (1) sitting or standing blood pressure, (2) supine blood pressure, (3) pulse rate and regularity, (4) respiration, (5) temperature, (6) height, (7) weight (might be measured and recorded by ancillary staff) ■ General appearance of the patient (e.g., development, nutrition, body habitus, deformities, attention to grooming)
Musculoskeletal	■ Examination of gait and station Examination of joint(s), bone(s), and muscle(s)/tendon(s) of four of the following six areas: (1) head and neck; (2) spine, ribs, and pelvis; (3) right upper extremity; (4) left upper extremity; (5) right lower extremity; and (6) left lower extremity. The examination of a given area includes the following: ■ Inspection, percussion, and/or palpation with notation of any misalignment, asymmetry, crepitation, defects, tenderness, masses, or effusions ■ Assessment of range of motion with notation of any pain (e.g., straight leg raising), crepitation, or contracture ■ Assessment of stability with notation of any dislocation (luxation), subluxation, or laxity ■ Assessment of muscle strength and tone (e.g., flaccid, cogwheel, spastic) with notation of any atrophy or abnormal movements **Note:** For the comprehensive level of examination, all four of the elements identified by a bullet must be performed and documented for each of four anatomical areas. For the three lower levels of examination, each element is counted separately for each body area. For example, assessing range of motion in two extremities constitutes two elements.

Continued

TABLE 3-11   Musculoskeletal Examination—cont'd

System or Area	Examination Elements
Skin	▪ Inspection and/or palpation of skin and subcutaneous tissue (e.g., scars, rashes, lesions, café-au-lait spots, ulcers) in four of the following six areas: (1) head and neck, (2) trunk, (3) right upper extremity, (4) left upper extremity, (5) right lower extremity, and (6) left lower extremity **Note:** For the comprehensive level, the examination of all four anatomical areas must be performed and documented. For the three lower levels of examination, each body area is counted separately. For example, inspection and/or palpation of the skin and subcutaneous tissue of two extremities constitutes two elements.

Neurological/ psychiatric	▪ Test coordination (e.g., finger/nose, heel/knee/shin, rapid alternating movements in the upper and lower extremities, evaluation of fine motor coordination in young children)
	▪ Examination of deep tendon reflexes and/or nerve stretch test with notation of pathological reflexes (e.g., Babinski)
	▪ Examination of sensation (e.g., by touch, pin, vibration, proprioception); brief assessment of mental status, including the following:
	    ▪ Orientation to time, place, and person
	    ▪ Mood and affect (e.g., depression, anxiety, agitation)

Cardiovascular	▪ Examination of peripheral vascular system by observation (e.g., swelling, varicosities) and palpation (e.g., pulses, temperature, edema, tenderness)
Lymphatic	▪ Palpation of lymph nodes in neck, axillae, groin, and/or other locations
Extremities	▪ See Musculoskeletal and Skin

Source: U.S. Department of Health and Human Services, Centers for Medicare and Medicaid Services.

TABLE 3-12   Neurological Examination

System or Area	Examination Elements
Constitutional	▪ Measurement of any three of the following seven vital signs: (1) sitting or standing blood pressure, (2) supine blood pressure, (3) pulse rate and regularity, (4) respiration, (5) temperature, (6) height, (7) weight (might be measured and recorded by ancillary staff) ▪ General appearance of the patient (e.g., development, nutrition, body habitus, deformities, attention to grooming)
Eyes	▪ Ophthalmoscopic examination of optic discs (e.g., size, C/D ratio, appearance) and posterior segments (e.g., vessel changes, exudates, hemorrhages)

Musculoskeletal	▪ Examination of gait and station
	Assessment of motor function, including the following:
	    ▪ Muscle strength in upper and lower extremities
	    ▪ Muscle tone in upper and lower extremities (e.g., flaccid, cogwheel, spastic) with notation of any atrophy or abnormal movements (e.g., fasciculation, tardive dyskinesia)

Neurological	Evaluation of higher integrative functions, including the following:
	    ▪ Recent and remote memory
	    ▪ Attention span and concentration
	    ▪ Language (e.g., naming objects, repeating phrases, spontaneous speech)
	    ▪ Fund of knowledge (e.g., awareness of current events, past history, vocabulary)
	Test the following cranial nerves:
	    ▪ Second cranial nerve (e.g., visual acuity, visual fields, fundi)
	    ▪ Third, fourth, and sixth cranial nerves (e.g., pupils, eye movements)
	    ▪ Fifth cranial nerve (e.g., facial sensation, corneal reflexes)
	    ▪ Seventh cranial nerve (e.g., facial symmetry, strength)
	    ▪ Eighth cranial nerve (e.g., hearing with tuning fork, whispered voice, and/or finger rub)
	    ▪ Ninth cranial nerve (e.g., spontaneous or reflex palate movement)

TABLE 3-12 Neurological Examination—cont'd

System or Area	Examination Elements
	- 11th cranial nerve (e.g., shoulder shrug strength) - 12th cranial nerve (e.g., tongue protrusion) - Examination of sensation (e.g., by touch, pin, vibration, proprioception) - Examination of deep tendon reflexes in upper and lower extremities with notation of pathological reflexes (e.g., Babinski) - Test coordination (e.g., finger/nose, heel/knee/shin, rapid alternating movements in the upper and lower extremities, evaluation of fine motor coordination in young children)
Cardiovascular	- Examination of carotid arteries (e.g., pulse amplitude, bruits) - Auscultation of heart with notation of abnormal sounds and murmurs - Examination of peripheral vascular system by observation (e.g., swelling, varicosities), and palpation (e.g., pulses, temperature, edema, tenderness)
Extremities	See Musculoskeletal

C/D, Cup/disc.
Source: U.S. Department of Health and Human Services, Centers for Medicare and Medicaid Services.

TABLE 3-13 Psychiatric Examination

System or Area	Examination Elements
Constitutional	- Measurement of any three of the following seven vital signs: (1) sitting or standing blood pressure, (2) supine blood pressure, (3) pulse rate and regularity, (4) respiration, (5) temperature, (6) height, (7) weight (might be measured and recorded by ancillary staff) - General appearance of the patient (e.g., development, nutrition, body habitus, deformities, attention to grooming)

Psychiatric	- Description of speech, including rate, volume, and articulation; coherence; and spontaneity with notation of abnormalities (e.g., perseveration, paucity of language)
	- Description of thought processes, including rate of thoughts, content of thoughts (e.g., logical vs. illogical, tangential), abstract reasoning, and computation
	- Description of associations (e.g., loose, tangential, circumstantial, intact)
	- Description of abnormal or psychotic thoughts, including hallucinations, delusions, preoccupation with violence, homicidal or suicidal ideation, and obsessions
	- Description of the patient's judgment (e.g., concerning everyday activities and social situations) and insight (e.g., concerning psychiatric condition)
	Complete mental status examination, including the following:
	Orientation to time, place, and person
	  - Recent and remote memory
	  - Attention span and concentration
	  - Language (e.g., naming objects, repeating phrases)
	  - Fund of knowledge (e.g., awareness of current events, past history, vocabulary)
	  - Mood and affect (e.g., depression, anxiety, agitation, hypomania, liability)

Musculoskeletal	- Assessment of muscle strength and tone (e.g., flaccid, cogwheel, spastic) with notation of any atrophy and abnormal movements - Examination of gait and station

Source: U.S. Department of Health and Human Services, Centers for Medicare and Medicaid Services.

TABLE 3-14   Respiratory Examination

System or Area	Examination Elements
Constitutional	<ul><li>Measurement of any three of the following seven vital signs: (1) sitting or standing blood pressure, (2) supine blood pressure, (3) pulse rate and regularity, (4) respiration, (5) temperature, (6) height, (7) weight (might be measured and recorded by ancillary staff)</li><li>General appearance of the patient (e.g., development, nutrition, body habitus, deformities, attention to grooming)</li></ul>
Ears, nose, mouth, and throat	<ul><li>Inspection of nasal mucosa, septum, and turbinates</li><li>Inspection of teeth and gums</li><li>Examination of oropharynx (e.g., oral mucosa, hard and soft palates, tongue, tonsils, posterior pharynx)</li></ul>
Neck	<ul><li>Examination of neck (e.g., masses, overall appearance, symmetry, tracheal position, crepitus)</li><li>Examination of thyroid (e.g., enlargement, tenderness, mass)</li><li>Examination of jugular veins (e.g., distention; a, v, or cannon a waves)</li></ul>
Respiratory	<ul><li>Inspection of chest with notation of symmetry and expansion</li><li>Assessment of respiratory effort (e.g., intercostal retractions, use of accessory muscles, diaphragmatic movement)</li><li>Percussion of chest (e.g., dullness, flatness, hyperresonance)</li><li>Palpation of chest (e.g., tactile fremitus)</li><li>Auscultation of lungs (e.g., breath sounds, adventitious sounds, rubs)</li></ul>
Cardiovascular	<ul><li>Auscultation of heart, including sounds, abnormal sounds, and murmurs</li><li>Examination of peripheral vascular system by observation (e.g., swelling, varicosities) and palpation (e.g., pulses, temperature, edema, tenderness)</li></ul>
Gastrointestinal (abdomen)	<ul><li>Examination of abdomen with notation of presence of masses or tenderness</li><li>Examination of liver and spleen</li></ul>
Lymphatic	<ul><li>Palpation of lymph nodes in neck, axillae, groin, and/or other locations</li></ul>
Musculoskeletal	<ul><li>Assessment of muscle strength and tone (e.g., flaccid, cogwheel, spastic) with notation of any atrophy and abnormal movements</li><li>Examination of gait and station</li></ul>
Extremities	<ul><li>Inspection and palpation of digits and nails (e.g., clubbing, cyanosis, inflammation, petechiae, ischemia, infections, nodes)</li></ul>
Skin	<ul><li>Inspection and/or palpation of skin and subcutaneous tissue (e.g., rashes, lesions, ulcers)</li></ul>
Neurological/psychiatric	Brief assessment of mental status, including the following:<ul><li>Orientation to time, place, and person</li><li>Mood and affect (e.g., depression, anxiety, agitation)</li></ul>

Source: U.S. Department of Health and Human Services, Centers for Medicare and Medicaid Services.

TABLE 3-15   Skin Examination

System or Area	Examination Elements
Constitutional	▪ Measurement of any three of the following seven vital signs: (1) sitting or standing blood pressure, (2) supine blood pressure, (3) pulse rate and regularity, (4) respiration, (5) temperature, (6) height, (7) weight (might be measured and recorded by ancillary staff) ▪ General appearance of the patient (e.g., development, nutrition, body habitus, deformities, attention to grooming)
Ears, nose, mouth, and throat	▪ Inspection of lips, teeth, and gums ▪ Examination of oropharynx (e.g., oral mucosa, hard and soft palates, tongue, tonsils, posterior pharynx)
Skin	▪ Palpation of scalp and inspection of hair of scalp, eyebrows, face, chest, pubic area (when indicated), and extremities ▪ Inspection and/or palpation of skin and subcutaneous tissue (e.g., rashes, lesions, ulcers, susceptibility to and presence of photo damage) in four of the following five areas: (1) head and neck; (2) chest, breasts, and back; (3) abdomen; (4) genitalia; (5) extremities **Note:** For the comprehensive level, the examination of all four anatomic areas must be performed and documented. For the three lower levels of examination, each body area is counted separately. For example, inspection and/or palpation of the skin and subcutaneous tissue of the head and neck and extremities constitutes two areas. ▪ Inspection of eccrine and apocrine glands of skin and subcutaneous tissue with identification and location of any hyperhidrosis, chromhidrosis, or bromhidrosis
Eyes	▪ Inspection of conjunctivae and lids
Neck	▪ Examination of thyroid (e.g., enlargement, tenderness, mass)
Cardiovascular	▪ Examination of peripheral vascular system by observation (e.g., swelling, varicosities) and palpation (e.g., pulses, temperature, edema, tenderness)
Gastrointestinal (abdomen)	▪ Examination of liver and spleen ▪ Examination of anus for condyloma and other lesions
Lymphatic	▪ Palpation of lymph nodes in neck, axillae, groin, and/or other locations
Extremities	▪ Inspection and palpation of digits and nails (e.g., clubbing, cyanosis, inflammation, petechiae, ischemia, infections, nodes)
Neurological/psychiatric	Brief assessment of mental status, including the following: ▪ Orientation to time, place, and person ▪ Mood and affect (e.g., depression, anxiety, agitation)

Source: U.S. Department of Health and Human Services, Centers for Medicare and Medicaid Services.

Examination

A *problem-focused* examination is limited to the affected body area or organ system in question (e.g., ear, nose).

EXAMPLE

An office visit for a patient who has been treated for athlete's foot. The physician is evaluating the effectiveness of the medication.

An *expanded problem-focused* examination includes the affected body area or organ system and other symptomatic or related organ systems (e.g., heart, lung).

EXAMPLE

A periodic examination of a patient undergoing follow-up for high blood pressure and headaches who takes multiple medications.

A *detailed* examination covers the affected body area(s) and other symptomatic or related organ systems and includes an examination of a patient who is seen with multiple problems or conditions, with a review of the affected body areas.

EXAMPLE

A review of a patient with abnormal weight loss, depression, and lower back pain.

A *comprehensive* examination comprises a complete single-system specialty examination or a complete multisystem examination that includes at least eight body areas or organ systems.

EXAMPLE

A patient being seen for uncontrolled diabetes and high cholesterol count is complaining of fatigue, dizziness, and rectal bleeding. The patient has noticed a decrease in appetite and has trouble sleeping.

DECISION-MAKING

Medical decision-making defines the steps a physician will take to treat the patient based on the specific diagnosis and treatment options, any tests that should be performed, and the amount of risk involved in the care and treatment of the patient. Because there are so many variables that must be considered for patient care, this section typically requires the skills of medical personnel.

Before a coder can determine the extent or level of the decision-making process, the three following questions must be answered. In addition, the coder must always ask if there are any contributing factors that could affect treatment:

- How many diagnoses or possible treatment options pertain to the visit?
- How many tests have been ordered, or what information has been reviewed (e.g., laboratory, x-ray)?
- What is the patient's risk for disease worsening (morbidity) or risk of dying (mortality)?

To qualify for a type of decision-making, two out of the three elements in the decision-making criteria table (Table 3-16) must be met or exceeded.

EXAMPLE

A patient had two diagnoses, review of two laboratory tests, and one x-ray and was at low risk of complication. The decision-making process is low complexity.

Rationale: Diagnosis = Limited   Complexity = Moderate   Risk = Low

Take the two highest (complexity and risk). The lowest of the two highest renders the decision-making process low complexity.

TABLE 3-16   Decision Making Criteria

Types of Decision Making	Number of Diagnoses or Management Options	Amount or Complexity of Data to be Reviewed	Risk of Complications and/or Morbidity or Mortality
Straightforward	Minimal	Minimal/none	Minimal
Low complexity	Limited	Limited	Low
Moderate complexity	Multiple	Moderate	Moderate
High complexity	Extensive	Extensive	High

Source: U.S. Department of Health and Human Services, Centers for Medicare and Medicaid Services.

TEST YOUR KNOWLEDGE   Decision-Making

1.   Number of diagnoses or treatment options is multiple, with an extensive amount of data to be reviewed on a high-risk patient.

     Decision-making: _____

2.   Number of diagnoses or management options is limited; complexity is moderate; risk is high.

     Decision-making: _____

Number of Diagnoses or Management Options

The number of possible diagnoses and the number of management options that must be considered are based on the following physician determinations:
- Number and types of problems addressed during the encounter
- Complexity of establishing a diagnosis
- Management decisions

Generally, decision-making with respect to a diagnosed problem is easier than that for an identified but undiagnosed problem. The number and type of diagnostic tests used could be an indicator of the number of possible diagnoses. Problems that are improving or resolving are less complex than those that are worsening or failing to change as expected. The need to seek advice from others is another indicator of the complexity of diagnostic or management problems.

Amount and/or Complexity of Data to be Reviewed

The amount and complexity of data to be reviewed are based on the types of diagnostic testing ordered or reviewed. A decision to obtain and review old medical records or to obtain history from sources other than the patient increases the amount and complexity of the data to be reviewed.

Discussion of contradictory or unexpected test results with the physician who performed or interpreted the test is an indication of the complexity of the data being reviewed. On occasion, the physician who ordered a test may personally review the image, tracing, or specimen to supplement information from the physician who prepared the test report or interpretation. This is another indication of the complexity of the data being reviewed.

Risk Factors

The risk of significant complications, morbidity, or mortality is based on the risks associated with the presenting problem(s), the diagnostic procedures(s), and the possible management options. Table 3-17 gives examples of items within each of the three categories for determining risk.

Risk is only one part of the decision-making process. However, to choose the type of risk, look at the three columns in Table 3-17. The highest of any of the three equals the risk factor.

TABLE 3-17   Table of Risk

Level of Risk	Presenting Problem	Diagnostic Procedure(s) Ordered	Management Options
Minimal	One self-limiting or minor problem (e.g., cold, insect bite)	■ Laboratory test with venipuncture ■ Chest x-ray ■ ECG/EEG ■ Urinalysis ■ KOH preparation ■ Ultrasound	■ Rest ■ Gargles ■ Elastic bandage ■ Superficial dressing
Low	■ Two or more self-limited or minor problems ■ One stable chronic illness ■ Acute uncomplicated illness	■ Physiological tests without stress ■ Noncardiovascular imaging with continued ■ Superficial needle/skin biopsy ■ Laboratory tests requiring arterial puncture	■ Over-the-counter drugs ■ Minor surgery—no identified risk ■ Physical or occupational therapy ■ IV fluids without additives
Moderate	■ One or more chronic illnesses with mild exacerbation ■ Two or more stable chronic illnesses ■ Acute complicated injury ■ Acute illness with systemic symptoms ■ Undiagnosed new problem with uncertain prognosis	■ Physiological tests under stress ■ Diagnostic endoscopies ■ Deep needle or incisional biopsy ■ Cardiac imaging with contrasts ■ Obtain fluid from body cavity	■ Minor surgery with identified risks ■ Elective major surgery ■ Endoscopy (no risk) ■ Prescription drug management ■ IV fluids with additives ■ Closed treatment fracture/dislocation
High	■ One or more chronic illnesses with severe exacerbation ■ Acute or chronic illness or injury that poses threat ■ Abrupt change in neurological status	■ Cardiac imaging with contract and risks ■ Cardiac electrophysiological test ■ Diagnostic endoscopy with identified risks ■ Discography	■ Emergency major surgery with risks ■ Emergency major surgery ■ Parenteral controlled substance ■ Drug therapy with intensive monitoring ■ Decision not to resuscitate

Source: U.S. Department of Health and Human Services, Centers for Medicare and Medicaid Services. *KOH*, Potassium hydroxide.

R E M I N D E R

Choosing the level of decision-making requires any two out of the three factors of diagnosis, complexity, or risk.

 R E M I N D E R

To choose the level of risk, review the three columns; the highest of any of the three becomes the level of risk.

E X A M P L E

Selecting Risk Factors

A patient with a stable chronic condition has a chest x-ray and obtains a refill for a prescription. The level of diagnosis is *low*, diagnostic procedures are *minimal*, and the management option is *moderate*. Judging from these three factors, you would choose the highest category (management options), making the risk factor for this patient *moderate*.

Exploring the Three Contributing Factors

The three contributing factors are counseling, nature of presenting problem, and time.

Counseling is a discussion with the patient or family. Discussion areas include diagnosis, test results, and recommended studies; prognosis; risks or benefits and instructions for the management of care; and education of the patient or family assisting the patient.

Nature of the presenting problem is categorized as minimal; self-limited or minor; or low, moderate, or high severity. "Minimal" is used to code services provided by ancillary personnel.

E X A M P L E

A patient presents to the office for an injection based on orders charted by the physician. Services are provided by the nurse.

Self-limited or *minor* is used when a problem runs a definite and/or prescribed course and is transient in nature. A self-limited or minor condition is not likely to permanently alter health status.

E X A M P L E

Examination of a patient with acute tonsillitis.

A low-severity problem has a low risk of morbidity without treatment and little or no risk of mortality without treatment. Full recovery without functional impairment is expected.

> ### EXAMPLE
> A teenage patient presents for the treatment of severe acne.

A moderate-severity problem carries a moderate risk of morbidity or mortality without treatment and increased probability of prolonged functional impairment without treatment.

> ### EXAMPLE
> Initial evaluation of a 40-year-old man with a 7-month history of recurrent frontal headaches.

A high-severity problem has a high risk of morbidity or mortality without treatment or a high probability of severe, prolonged functional impairment without treatment.

> ### EXAMPLE
> Initial visit of a 10-year-old girl with daily coughing and sneezing that interfere with sleep and other activities.

Time

Time is an exception to the rule. When a visit consists predominately of counseling or coordination of care, time may be the key or controlling factor in coding a particular level of E&M service, provided certain conditions have been met. Time becomes the key factor when *50% or more* of the visit is spent face to face with the patient in activities involving counseling or coordination of care. To report time, the record must indicate how much time the physician actually spent with the patient, the reason for counseling, and any other notations regarding the encounter. The necessary criteria are as follows:
- 50% or more of the visit must be spent counseling the patient.
- Time includes only the *physician's* face to face time with the patient—not the time of ancillary personnel or a resident.
- The record must clearly indicate the reason for counseling.
- The record must clearly indicate the total physician face to face time with the patient.
- In the hospital setting, time is based on face to face time with the patient and floor time.

> ### EXAMPLE
> **Time**
> An established patient was seen for problem-focused history, with an expanded problem-focused examination and moderate-complexity decision-making. The patient and doctor spent 30 minutes face to face, of which 20 minutes were spent discussing diabetic care and treatment. Because time dominated the visit, the level of service can be chosen based on the time factor alone. The correct code would be 99214, Established patient visit.

TEST YOUR KNOWLEDGE   Contributing Factors

1. An established patient with minimal history, a problem-focused examination, and low-complexity decision-making spent 40 minutes face to face with the doctor. During this time, 20 minutes had been spent discussing diet and exercise management of a medical condition.

    Answer: _____

OUTPATIENT SERVICE CODES (99201 TO 99215)

These codes are generally used to report services provided in the physician's office, but they may also be applied to services provided in an outpatient or other location as long as it is not in an inpatient setting. Code selection is based on the level of history, examination, or decision-making documented in the record. If counseling dominates the visit, then time can be used for code selection provided the record indicates the total face to face time of the visit, the total time spent counseling, and the reason or medical necessity for counseling.

New Patient versus Established Patient

Now that we have explored the various components for choosing a level of service and the importance of time, the next step is to understand selections based on patient category. Some codes make a distinction in the selection based on whether the patient is a *new patient* or an *established patient*. The following definitions should clarify the difference between new and established patients.

New Patient

A new patient is one who has not received professional services from the same physician within the past 3 years, or from another physician of the same specialty within a group practice. This one sentence is loaded with information for correct code selection. Definitions for the highlighted items are as follows:

- Professional services: Face to face services rendered by a physician and reported by a specific CPT code(s).
- 3 years: Time frame for treatments to define new versus established patients.
- Same specialty: In a group practice, different physicians may have different specialties. However, when a patient is seen by another physician within the group and that physician practices the same type of specialty as the original physician, the patient would still be considered an established patient.
- Group practice: Group practice is defined as a group of physicians who have the same tax identification number for billing purposes.

Established Patient

An established patient is one who received services by the same physician or physician of the same specialty in a group practice within a 3-year period.

The following activity provides situations to assist you in determining new patient versus established patient status.

Directions: Read the following examples to determine if the patient is new or established for the practice. Circle the correct answer.

1.   Jane was seen by Dr. Jones at the hospital for a consultation. Two weeks later she is scheduled to see Dr. Jones in his office to begin a treatment program for her condition.

New Patient   Established Patient

2.   While Dr. X was on vacation, her partner, Dr. Z, saw Dr. X's patient for a sore throat. Both physicians specialize in family practice.

New Patient   Established Patient

3.   John and his family have just moved into town. John has asthma and requires medication to control the condition. He has an appointment with Dr. Y on April 4th. John had his records from his previous physician transferred to Dr. Y's office before the appointment.

New Patient   Established Patient

4.   Tom was in the Army for 2 years. During that time he did not see his hometown doctor. The office has a policy to place any inactive files on microfilm after 18 months of inactivity. After finishing his tour of duty, Tom returns home and makes an appointment to see his family physician regarding his foot pain.

New Patient   Established Patient

OBSERVATION UNIT CODES (99217 TO 99220)

Observation unit codes may be used to report services for patients designated as "observation status" in a hospital setting. Services include initiation of observation status, supervision of the care plan, and performance of periodic reassessments.

Guidelines for Use

All three elements of history, examination, and decision-making must meet or exceed the criteria for the code. Typical times have not been established for these codes.

Only one code may be reported per date of service. Should a patient in observation status be admitted to the hospital, the only charge for that day would be the hospital admission. Observation status may occur over several days. Subsequent care after the initial admission should be reported using established patient, outpatient services (99211 to 99215).

Based on hospital policies regarding subsequent days, the patient may be considered an inpatient. When this occurs, use subsequent hospital daily care codes (99231 to 99233) and hospital discharge codes (99238 to 99239), as applicable.

Discharge from Observation (99217)

This code may be used, provided it is a separate date of service. It may be used if another service has not been billed that day.

E X A M P L E

After a fall down a flight of stairs, a patient is admitted for observation to ascertain if there are any complications or if there is a concussion.

HOSPITAL CODES (99221 TO 99239)

Hospital services include the admission of a patient and the daily care visits necessary for the treatment of a patient during a hospital stay. When care is performed in another location (e.g., the physician's office or the emergency room) before admission, these areas and places of care should be incorporated into the level of service for the hospital admission.

In the hospital setting, *time* is defined as unit or floor time. This includes the following:

- Time spent on the hospital unit or floor reviewing records, writing notes, or communicating with other medical staff regarding care and management of the patient.
- Time spent with the patient for examination or treatment.

Time spent off the floor to perform such tasks as collecting laboratory or radiology test results is not part of the total visit time and should not be incorporated in these codes.

Observation or Inpatient Care (99234 to 99236)

These codes are used to report observation or inpatient hospital care services provided to patients who are admitted and discharged on the same date of service. For patients admitted and discharged on separate dates of service, use observation unit codes 99218 to 99220 (admit) and 99217 (discharge) and inpatient codes 99221 to 99223 (admit) and 99238 to 99239 (discharge).

E X A M P L E

A patient was admitted for observation of a possible appendicitis at 3 PM Monday afternoon. After test results and observation, the patient was discharged at 7 PM Monday evening.

Correct coding: Observation unit codes 99218 to 99220 (admit) and 99217 (discharge)

Hospital Discharge (99238 to 99239)

Hospital discharge codes are time-based codes. The record should indicate the time spent in patient discharge. Discharge codes may be used to report discharge planning, provided another service has not been provided to the patient on the same date of service. Services include the following:

- Final examination of the patient
- Discussion of the hospital stay with the patient and/or family
- Instructions for continuing care
- Preparation of the discharge record
- Preparation of prescriptions and referral forms

Hospital discharge codes may be used to report services for the discharge of a deceased patient even if the physician did not see the patient that day.

 CODING TIP

If time is not documented, you cannot code higher than 99238.

CPT CODING EXERCISE 3   E&M Services

Directions: Read the following descriptions to determine the level of history, examination, and decision-making. Then select the appropriate code based on the code classification (e.g., new versus established patient). Write the answer in the space provided.

1.   A new patient, a 10-year-old girl, presents with acute contact dermatitis. The history is problem-focused, as is the examination. Decision-making is straightforward. The patient is given a prescription for the dermatitis with instructions to return to the office if the condition does not improve in a few days.

Answer: _____

2.   An established patient with a history of allergic rhinitis (expanded problem-focused) presents to the office with acute exacerbation of coughing and wheezing, which is thought to be secondary to an upper respiratory infection. A problem-focused examination of the affected body area was performed, with limited diagnoses and management problems. Currently, the patient has low-complexity decision-making.

Answer: _____

3.   An 18-month-old toddler was admitted to the hospital with a third episode of wheezing and respiratory distress. The patient has had decreased appetite and has a low-grade fever. A comprehensive history is taken with a complete multisystem examination. There are extensive diagnoses and management options and an extensive amount of data to be reviewed. Decision-making is high complexity.

Answer: _____

4.   An initial evaluation of a 35-year-old woman with a 6-day history of nasal congestion, postnasal drip, halitosis, and frontal headache was performed. History is detailed with a detailed examination of the patient. There are limited diagnoses and management options and a low risk of complication. Decision-making is low complexity.

Answer: _____

5.   A follow-up examination of a 40-year-old man who is insulin-dependent reveals rectal bleeding after using the bathroom and pain from prolonged sitting. The patient is to have a fasting blood sugar test and stool culture. History is expanded problem-focused with a detailed examination. The patient has multiple symptoms with a moderate risk of complications and moderate-complexity decision-making.

Answer: _____

6.   A 45-year-old woman with pneumonia is admitted to the hospital. A comprehensive history and examination were completed with minimal diagnoses or management options and minimal risk of complications. Decision-making is straightforward.

Answer: _____

7. A follow-up visit is provided on the third day after admission for a 45-year-old woman receiving medication for uncomplicated pneumonia. History is problem-focused with a problem-focused examination and straightforward decision-making.

Answer: _____

CONSULTATION CODES (99241 TO 99255)

Consults differ in definition from outpatient codes or hospital services, because these codes are used only when a physician is asked to give advice to another physician on how to treat a patient.

Types of Consultation Services

Office/outpatient services	99241 to 99245
Hospital	99251 to 99255

When Does A Visit Become A Consult?

This is one of the more difficult aspects of coding because the interpretation of the term *consult* has been distorted and misused by many practices. To have a consult, several factors must be part of the documentation.

Documentation in the requesting physician's medical record must include the request for a consultation from the attending or other appropriate source and must state the need for the consultation. Documentation in the consulting physician's medical record must include who requested the opinion and why it was requested, the consultant's examination or review of the condition, any services ordered or performed, and a written report to the requesting physician detailing findings and recommendations for care.

The consulting physician may initiate **diagnostic services** or **therapeutic services**; however, he or she does not perform follow-up on the patient to determine the effectiveness of the treatment. The patient is told to return to the requesting physician for follow-up. When a consulting physician assumes any portion of the patient's care or establishes a plan of treatment, he or she is no longer considered to be consulting on the case. Rather, that physician becomes a rendering care physician and must code from the appropriate level of E&M services based on the place of service.

Consult Defined

A consult is a request for advice or opinion. The request may come from another physician or other appropriate source (e.g., physician's assistant, nurse practitioner, doctor of chiropractic, physical therapist, occupational therapist, speech pathologist, psychologist, social worker, lawyer, insurance company). It is a service provided by a physician whose opinion or advice regarding the evaluation and/or management of a specific problem is requested by an appropriate source. The name and **UPIN** of the referring physician must be present on the CMS-1500 claim form in items 17a and 17b.

When a patient or a patient's family requests a second opinion or consultation, this service should be billed as an office or outpatient service.

Referral Defined

A referral is a service provided by a physician when all or a portion of patient care has been transferred from one physician to another physician. Services are then reported with appropriate codes based on the location of the service (e.g., outpatient, inpatient, nursing home).

Understanding the Consult Code Types

Office or Other Outpatient Consultation

An outpatient consult does not allow you to distinguish between a new patient and an established patient. It may be used in an outpatient or ambulatory facility. Any follow-up visits must be reported with the appropriate level of established patient code.

Initial Inpatient Consultation

An initial inpatient code is used to report services provided in the inpatient setting of a hospital or nursing facility. Only one initial consultation may be billed per admission.

CPT CODING EXERCISE 4   Consultations and Referrals

Directions: Circle the appropriate answer.

1.   Dr. Kay, a primary care physician, has been treating a patient for a rash on the wrist; a medicated cream has not provided relief of the problem. Because the problem is growing worse each day, Dr. Kay has suggested that the patient make an appointment with a dermatologist for continued treatment of the problem.

    Consult   Referral

2.   Dr. Lee, an orthopedic surgeon, has been treating a patient after surgery. The patient has not responded to treatment and shows no sign of improvement. Dr. Lee asks Dr. Moe, a psychiatrist, to evaluate the patient to determine if the problem is more psychosomatic than physical in nature.

    Consult   Referral

3.   Dr. Cee has been asked to examine a patient and provide a second opinion before surgery to remove a kidney stone.

    Consult   Referral

4.   Dr. No, an internist, asked Dr. Yes, a cardiologist, to assist in caring for a hospitalized patient with a known cardiac condition.

    Consult   Referral

5.   Dr. Adams, an emergency room physician, called Dr. Bee, an orthopedic surgeon, to evaluate a patient concerning the need for surgery following an automobile accident. Upon examination of the patient, Dr. Bee determines that the situation is critical and orders the patient to be taken directly to surgery.

    Consult   Referral

MISCELLANEOUS E&M SERVICES

Emergency Department Services (99281 to 99285)

Emergency department codes may be used by any physician. These codes may be used to report services in a hospital emergency department. However, they are primarily used for physicians assigned to the emergency department.

Critical Care Services (99291 to 99292)

Critical care services include specific services delivered by the physician in constant attendance to a critically ill patient. Services are usually, but not always, delivered in a critical care unit (CCU) or an emergency care facility. Notes define specific emergency services that are included under the critical care codes. Services not listed in the notes but provided by the physician during the critical care period should be reported separately. Codes are selected by the amount of time the physician spends providing these services. Time for critical care includes the physician's face to face time with the patient as well as time outside the room when the physician is reviewing tests or reports or discussing patient care with other health care providers.

Pediatric and Neonatal Critical Care (99293 to 99296)

Neonatal critical care codes are used to report services provided by physicians directing the care of a neonate or infant in a neonatal intensive care unit (NICU) in an inpatient setting. Care begins with the date of admission and may be reported only once per day.

Neonatal codes pertain to an infant who is 28 days of age or younger. Pediatric care is defined for the treatment of a patient who is 29 days of age through 24 months of age.

Nursing Facility Services Codes (99304 to 99318)

Nursing facility codes are used to report E&M services delivered in nursing facilities and in psychiatric residential treatment centers. There are two categories of nursing facility services—comprehensive nursing facility assessment and subsequent nursing facility care. Use of these codes does not require that patient status be defined.

Domiciliary, Rest Home, or Custodial Care Services (99324 to 99337)

Use these codes to report E&M services in a facility that provides room, board, and other personal assistance services, generally on a long-term basis.

Home Service Codes (99341 to 99350)

Use home service codes to report services delivered in a private residence to new patients or to established patients.

Prolonged Services with or without Face to Face Contact (99354 to 99359)

Prolonged-service codes are used when the physician provides prolonged service that is beyond the usual service in inpatient or outpatient settings. It is important to distinguish between services *with* direct patient contact and those *without* direct patient contact; it is equally necessary to notate the location of service (e.g., office versus hospital).

Prolonged-service codes are add-on codes, meaning that they are used in addition to another code that has a typical time listed (e.g., outpatient visit, hospital). These codes may only be used when the time spent on patient care exceeds the typical time of an E&M code by at least 30 minutes.

Physician Standby Service (99360)

The physician standby service is at the request of another physician and involves prolonged physician attendance without face to face patient contact.

Case Management Service Codes (99361 to 99373)

Use case management codes to report services delivered by a physician responsible for direct care to a patient and for conducting and controlling access, initiating, or supervising other health care services needed by the patient. Subcategories for these codes are team conferences and telephone calls.

Care Plan Oversight Service (99374 to 99380)

Only one physician may report services for a given period of time spent in a predominantly supervisory role overseeing the care of a particular patient. The service must be 30 minutes or more during a 30-day period.

Preventive Medicine Codes (99381 to 99429)

Preventive medicine codes are used to report the routine evaluation and management of adults and children when these services are performed in the absence of patient complaints.

Newborn Care Service Codes (99431 to 99440)

Newborn care codes are used to report services provided to normal or high-risk neonates in several different settings.

SURGERY

Surgical coding is very complex and involves multiple procedures and variations. The primary purpose of this text is to teach the reader the necessary skills for proper coding; you must use these skills to adapt to complicated or unusual coding situations. Because coding for surgery is complex, it is not possible to discuss each code in detail, but some of the basic or more common areas are highlighted to provide a basis from which to work and obtain knowledge of the principles of surgical coding.

Physicians may use their own jargon or version of terms in the documentation of a service. It is always a good policy to have the correct terminology listed for insurance filing with a list of the physician's "slang" next to the codes for ready reference and easy translation.

Surgical Packages

One of the unusual aspects of surgery is that the services are packaged. The surgical package includes the operation or procedure; local infiltration, metacarpal/digital block, or topical anesthesia when used; and normal, uncomplicated follow-up care. It does not include follow-up care for complications, exacerbations, recurrence, or coexisting disorders. It does not include supplies that are additional to those required to perform the procedure. It also does not include preoperative diagnostic services and procedures.

Section

The CPT surgical section is organized first by body system and body part and then by procedure.

Body System and Body Part

■ Integumentary System	(10021 to 19499)
■ Musculoskeletal System	(20000 to 29999)
■ Respiratory System	(30000 to 32999)
■ Cardiovascular System	(33010 to 37799)
■ Hematologic and Lymphatic System	(38100 to 38999)
■ Mediastinum and Diaphragm	(39000 to 39599)
■ Digestive System	(40490 to 49999)
■ Urinary System	(50010 to 53899)
■ Male Genital System	(54000 to 55899)
■ Female Genital System	(56405 to 58999)
■ Endocrine System	(60000 to 60699)
■ Nervous System	(61000 to 64999)
■ Eye and Adnexa	(65091 to 68899)
■ Auditory System	(69000 to 69979)

Procedure

■ Incision

■ Excision

■ Introduction (of a prosthesis or other foreign material)

■ Removal (of a prosthesis or foreign body)

■ Repair

■ Miscellaneous

Separate Procedures

Only use separate procedure codes when the procedure is performed independently and is not considered part of the major service. You may also use these codes for procedures that are commonly performed as part of another service but might be performed independently. When a procedure is performed with another service, do not bill these designated codes in addition to the main procedure or service. **Minor procedures** performed during the course of surgery, such as excision of a normal appendix during abdominal surgery or simple lysis of adhesions during a hysterectomy, are not coded separately.

EXAMPLE	
51570	Cystectomy, complete (separate procedure)

Integral Procedures

Integral procedures are procedures that must be performed to complete the major procedure; they are not coded separately. For example, closing the incision is integral to a splenectomy; cystoscopy is integral to a transurethral resection of the prostate; and thromboendarterectomy is integral to a coronary artery bypass with autogenous graft.

Unlisted Procedure Codes

Unlisted procedure codes should be used to report procedures when a service or procedure is not described in CPT or in HCPCS level II. Each section of CPT has its own set of unlisted codes. When you use an unlisted procedure code, you must include a written report or explanatory letter with the claim to explain the service.

The following items should be included in the report:

- Detailed description of the procedure
- Documentation of medical necessity for the procedure
- Time, effort, and equipment required to perform the procedure
- Patient diagnosis and/or symptoms
- Any concurrent problems or conditions requiring treatment or management
- Appropriate follow-up care and prognosis

E X A M P L E
28899   Unlisted procedure, foot or toes

Steps to Coding Surgical Procedures

1. Review operative room reports, emergency room records, progress notes, and any other documentation to select the procedures to be coded.
2. Identify main terms and subterms of each procedure. These could be abbreviations, anatomical sites, conditions, eponyms, procedures, or synonyms.
3. Locate the main term in the Index.
4. Review any notes that appear at the beginning of the anatomical section and instructions that appear in parentheses under the code description.
5. After verifying the procedure description with the selected code's description, assign the CPT code.
6. When applicable, apply a two-digit modifier to complete the code description.

Multiple Procedure Codes

In surgery it is not unusual to code a variety of services during one operative session. The important factor is to list the surgeries in the order of their importance or significance for payment. Payments for subsequent procedures are usually reduced by carriers by at least 50% of the allowed amount for subsequent procedures performed on the same date of service. In some cases, the third through sixth procedures may be reduced by as much as 75% of the allowed amount. Each carrier makes a determination of the importance of the procedure and the ruling order for payment allocations. Correct priority listing of surgeries may have a direct impact on reimbursement.

When selecting the primary surgery, coders predominantly list the most time-consuming procedure. This is not always the most accurate method of determining the primary selection. Insurance companies make their own decisions regarding the reimbursement amounts for each procedure by use of a relative value study (RVS). A relative value is a means to set fees based on the work component, overhead expense, and malpractice insurance costs for that procedure. RVS will be discussed in more detail in the chapter on reimbursement. It is important that coders monitor reimbursements to be aware of the carrier's policy for each code.

EXAMPLE

Importance of Ranking Codes Appropriately

The insurance company allows 100% of the usual customary rate (UCR) for the primary procedure and reimburses subsequent procedures at 50% of the UCR. A claim was submitted to the carrier for two procedures performed on the same date of service at the same operative session.

The physician's charge for Procedure A is **$700**; the charge for Procedure B is **$500**. The allowed amount from the insurance company for Procedure A is **$350** and for Procedure B is **$450**.

The office, by knowing the carrier's payment policy, can maximize reimbursement through application of the basic principles of ranking codes by order of relative value and by monitoring the explanation of benefits from the insurance company.

Scenario 1

Using the charges of the physician in ranking the codes (Procedure A, primary; Procedure B, secondary), payment by the insurance company would be as follows:

    Procedure A = $350
    Procedure B = $225
    (Paid at 100% UCR)
    (Paid at 50% UCR)
    Total reimbursement = $575

Scenario 2

If the office is aware of the allowance by the insurance carrier and submits the codes differently (Procedure B as the primary service; Procedure A as the secondary service), the payment would be as follows:

    Procedure B = $450
    Procedure A = $175
    (Paid at 100% UCR)
    (Paid at 50% UCR)
    Total reimbursement = $625

By not monitoring reimbursement or using a relative value system, the office lost $50 by incorrectly sequencing the surgical procedures.

For multiple procedures, it is crucial to use appropriate modifiers to indicate any reductions in fees. It is also in the best interest of the practice to state on the form that the fees have been reduced based on multiple surgical procedures. Using modifiers to show multiple procedures and reduced rates will serve to protect profile and charge history data.

A common practice in billing multiple procedures is to charge the full fee for the primary surgery and reduce fees for the other procedures by 50%. Many offices, on the other hand, elect to have insurance carriers reduce the fees based on allowed amounts. Reduction of the fee on the part of the physician is a courtesy based on carrier payments allocated for surgical procedures. As an example of carrier determination, it is helpful to examine Medicare's stance on this issue.

Billing Multiple Surgeries

Insurance companies have varying payment schedules and guidelines for payments. When you are billing procedures in which separate incisions are made to perform the surgery, a general rule of thumb is to bill the service as separate procedures.

Medicare guidelines are to pay 100% of the allowed amount for the primary procedure, 50% for the secondary procedure, and 50% for subsequent procedures. Commercial carriers generally reimburse multiple procedures at a rate of 100% of the **allowed amount** for the first or primary procedure, 50% for the secondary procedure, and 25% for each subsequent procedure. To maximize reimbursement, practices should bill all procedures at 100% of their fee schedule amounts and allow the carriers to make the necessary adjustments on the explanation of benefits. The office would then write off the difference between the billed amount and the allowed amount after receiving a copy of the payment advisory.

Assistance Fees

Assistance fees may be allowed for many complicated procedures requiring the assistance of another physician. Use of modifier -80 identifies a service as being reduced for assistance fee. The formula used to determine an assistance fee is usually 16% of the actual charge.

If the full fee for code 12007, Simple repair of superficial wounds, is $150, then the assistance fee would be $24.

Bilateral Procedure

Bilateral procedures differ from multiple or separate procedure codes. A bilateral procedure involves similar anatomical sites on both sides of the body (e.g., right arm, left arm).

Bilateral procedures, as a general rule, are not subject to the reductions applied to multiple procedure codes. Do not reduce charges for bilateral procedures when billing a carrier without consulting the carrier for determination of benefit payments for a specific procedure.

When coding bilateral procedures, the carrier should be contacted to determine if the modifier -50 or the code followed by RT (right) and LT (left) should be used to distinguish between the service areas. This will aid reimbursement and help ensure correct payment of the claim. In the case of Medicare, reducing the charge for a second area for a bilateral procedure could result in incorrect profile data.

EXAMPLE				
Bilateral Surgery				
Correct coding			Fee	Unit Count
10-10-03	28292	McBride procedure-RT	$500	1
10-10-03	28292-50	McBride procedure-LT	$500	1
Alternate Method				
04-28-2011	28292-50	McBride procedure	$1000	1

Additional Codes

In our discussion of surgical coding, we must review a small select number of codes that indicate the number count of an item for surgical removal. These codes are found primarily in the integumentary section of the CPT manual. In the following example, the 17000 code series will be used to demonstrate additional count codes.

E X A M P L E

A patient presented to the office for removal of 13 premalignant lesions from the face. The correct way to code this service is as follows:

Correct Coding

17000	First lesion = one unit
17001	Second through 13th lesion = 12 units

Total lesions = 13 lesions removed

To correctly file this with the insurance carrier, the coder must record the number of lesions in the unit section count of the claim form (item 24-G). It is also advisable to list the count in the descriptive part of the claim. By doing this, the coder ensures that the person processing the claim will obtain the correct count. In the descriptive area for ICD-9-CM, the total number of lesions should be listed to help the claims processor correctly adjudicate or process the claim.

Surgical Terms and Definitions

In discussing surgery, we must review each section of the surgical codes both to learn what they are and to alert you to the special conditions within the language of the codes. The wording of the description plays a key role in the correct method for coding. If the coder does not understand the wording within the phrase, the service will be incorrectly coded. This results in delayed or denied payments.

Each indicates that each item may be billed as a separate unit.

E X A M P L E

26060	Tenotomy, percutaneous, single, each digit

Each additional indicates a block or series.

E X A M P L E

15786	Abrasion; single lesion (e.g., keratosis, scar)
15787	. . . each additional four lesions or less

(s) indicates one or more factors as described by the code.

E X A M P L E

11720	Debridement of nail(s) by any method(s); one to five

With or without means that both parts of the procedure do not have to be performed to qualify for correct code use.

E X A M P L E

23515	Open treatment of clavicular fracture, with or without internal or external fixation

And means both parts of the description must be performed.

E X A M P L E
25900   Amputation, forearm, through radius and ulna

Or means one or the other part of the description must be performed.

E X A M P L E
26034   Incision, bone cortex, hand or finger (e.g., osteomyelitis or bone abscess)

It should be noted that the examples in this text are for the purpose of practice coding exercises only. Codes and service descriptions are not given as examples of correct medical treatment or patient care. The examples are provided to serve as an instrument to practice various coding techniques.

Integumentary Section (10021 to 19499)

The integumentary system is the first section of the surgical category. It refers to the covering of the skin and its many layers, such as the hair, nails, sebaceous glands, and sweat glands.

This section includes the following categories:
- Debridement (cleansing of wounds)
- Skin excision and repairs
- Reconstruction of skin parts

Debridement

Under debridement, the thickness of the skin must be identified to properly code from this section. The skin definition will be examined so that we may determine the levels for coding.
- Full thickness: Includes removal of damaged skin from both layers
- Subcutaneous tissue: The layer below the skin, includes removal of full thickness into the subcutaneous area
- Subcutaneous tissue/muscle: Removal of skin, subcutaneous layer, and into the muscle
- Subcutaneous tissue, muscle, bone: Includes removal to a depth past skin, tissue, and muscle and into the bone
- Debridement: The cleansing of the wound or incision. In most cases it is considered part of the surgical global package. CPT guidelines allow for coding debridement or cleaning a wound as a separate code when prolonged cleansing or treatment is needed, usually without intermediate or prompt closure. When coding for debridement, it is important to document time spent on actual debridement. Based on the duration of the procedure, insurance companies will make payment after reviewing the procedures.

Skin Excision and Repairs and Reconstruction of Skin Parts

- Incision: The division of the soft parts of the body with a knife. It is a surgical wound.
- Excision: The operative removal of a portion of a structure or organ. In most cases an incision has to occur before an excision can be performed.
- Partial thickness: Damaged skin to a depth of the epidermis or upper skin and part of the dermis, the second layer.

Wound Repair Codes (12001 to 13160)

The main classifications of wound closures are as follows:

Simple Closure

- A superficial wound generally involving primary epidermis or dermis or subcutaneous tissue
- Generally closed with simple, one-layer suturing

Intermediate Closure

- Single-layer closure of a profusely contaminated wound requiring extensive cleaning or debris removal
- Wounds or lacerations involving a superficial wound and at least one of the layers of tissue under the skin

Complex Closure

- Repairs requiring more than layered closure or the creation of a defect
- Revision of a scar
- Repairs requiring extensive undermining, placement of stents to support or maintain surgical correction of the wound, or retention sutures
- Repair with extensive stellate, irregular wound with a number of flaps
- Repair of deep wounds requiring exploration to rule out damage to tendons, nerves, blood vessels, or other underlying structures

Instructions for Assigning a Wound Repair Code

The repaired wound should be measured in centimeters. For repairs of multiple wounds, add wounds of the same type and anatomical site. When more than one classification is involved, report each as a separate code. Simple ligation of vessels is considered part of the wound closure. Simple explorations of nerves, blood vessels, or tendons exposed in an open wound are part of the closure procedure. Do not use repair codes for closures with butterfly or other adhesive bandages.

Lesions (11400 to 11772)

To code a lesion, several factors should be reviewed based on the documentation in the medical record. Before choosing a code you must consider the method of removal (e.g., excision, cryosurgery, shaved) and the morphology of the lesion (malignant or benign). Code selection is determined by the excised diameter of the actual lesion and the excised margin, *not* by the specimen size obtained from the pathology report. In reporting lesions, each lesion is separately billable. You would need to append modifier -59 to each subsequent lesion after the first lesion is removed.

Determining the Size of the Lesion

- Obtain size from the operative report, not from the pathology report.
- The excised diameter is determined by measuring the greatest clinical diameter of the lesion plus the narrowest margin required for complete excision.
- The measure of the lesion plus the margin should be made before excision.
- The size should be listed in centimeters (1 inch = 2.5 cm).

The record should state the number of lesions removed. You may also code for the type of closure of the defect, provided the required repair is an intermediate or complex repair. A simple closure is always considered to be part of the lesion excision.

Coding Reexcisions Based on Pathology Findings

- Only one code may be used to report the additional excision.
- Size is based on the final widest excised diameter.
- Append modifier -58 when the reexcision is performed in the postoperative period.

E X A M P L E

Excision of 0.6 cm X 0.4 cm benign lesion of the cheek with 0.2-cm margins.

Obtaining size: Add the longest clinical lesion diameter (0.6 cm) plus the sum of both margins (0.2 cm + 0.2 cm) = 0.6 cm + 0.4 cm = 1 cm total size.

Correct coding: 11441

 CODING TIP

When coding a lesion removal, a simple wound repair is considered part of the procedures and cannot be billed separately. However, for closure requiring an intermediate or complex repair, the repair can be billed in addition to the removal of the lesion.

CPT CODING EXERCISE 5   Integumentary System

Directions: Locate the correct code and underline the key word.

Example: Description: Incision and drainage of abscess, simple

Code: 10060

DESCRIPTION	CODE
1. Destruction by any method, flat wart	_____
2. Suction-assisted lipectomy, lower extremity	_____
3. Layer closure of skin wound over 30 cm, trunk	_____
4. Repair of nail bed	_____
5. Incision and drainage, hematoma, skin, simple	_____
6. Tattoo removal, dermabrasion	_____
7. Cryotherapy, skin	_____
8. Mastectomy, partial	_____
9. Excision, benign lesion, skin, arm over 4 cm	_____

Musculoskeletal System (20000 to 29999)

The musculoskeletal section of the CPT manual is the largest and perhaps most complicated portion of the book. As previously stated, this section is based on the anatomical part or location. When using this section, it is wise to determine the anatomical site and refer to that section only. In other words, when coding a problem pertaining to the arm, review codes in the section that pertains to the arm. By not carefully reading each section, you could accidentally code a revision or repair to the foot instead of the arm. Should this happen, the claim would be denied because the diagnosis code (ICD-9-CM) would not relate to the procedure.

Musculoskeletal system refers to the muscles and skeletal parts of the body. This section covers the muscles, bones, and joints; tendons, ligaments, and cartilage; and fracture care and casting.

This section includes the following procedures:
- Incision and excision
- Introduction, removal, and repair
- Revision and reconstruction
- Fracture care and casting

Each section in this heading is divided by body parts beginning at the top of the skull and progressing to the feet.

Fracture Care

Fracture care is a global package. Services include the following:
- History and physical examinations
- Hospital admissions
- Treatment or stabilization of the fracture or dislocation
- Inpatient hospital follow-up
- Discharge from the hospital
- Follow-up care for a predetermined number of days
- Application and removal of the first cast

Replacement Casts

Should a patient require cast replacement, you may charge for the additional casting application. The code for application of a cast includes the cost or charge for cast removal. Insurance carriers will generally pay for only one casting application and removal per fracture. In coding the second application, check the codes for casting and strapping applications in the CPT book (codes 29000 to 29799). If the correct code cannot be found in this list, the miscellaneous supply code 99070 may be used, listing the type of material or device.

For Medicare patients, you may need to use the appropriate HCPCS level II codes—for example, A4580 for regular casting supplies or A4590 for large casting materials.

E X A M P L E
A patient comes to the office after sustaining a fall in a grocery store. X-rays reveal a closed Colles' fracture of the right wrist.

Correct coding:	25600	Colles' fracture
	73100	X-ray wrist; AP and lateral views

CODING TIP

Fracture care does not include ancillary services (e.g., casting materials, windowing/wedging a cast). These services may be billed in addition to the fracture codes.

Arthroscopy

This service is usually performed in an outpatient setting at an ambulatory surgical center or hospital. This may be either a diagnostic process or a surgical procedure. The determining factors for course of care are as follows:

1. Level of service rendered to a patient
2. Condition(s) encountered upon entry into the affected area

When you code surgical arthroscopy, diagnostic arthroscopy is included in the surgical code and should not be billed separately. This type of procedure may have more than one applicable code.

EXAMPLE

Mary played volleyball in college. During a game, she sustained an injury to her left knee. Five years later, Mary was playing tennis and injured her left knee.

When Mary went to the physician, the physician scheduled diagnostic arthroscopy. During the study of the knee, the physician discovered Mary had a torn meniscus and that the old injury from volleyball had caused additional damage to the knee. The physician performed a limited synovectomy, a medial and lateral meniscus repair, and an anterior cruciate ligament repair.

Correct billing sequence:

29883   Medial and lateral meniscus repair
29888-51   Anterior cruciate ligament repair
29875-51   Synovectomy, limited

By correctly documenting the service, the physician was able to substantiate the need for the synovectomy and ligament repair based on an old injury. The physician should not have a problem obtaining reimbursement from the insurance company for the services rendered to the patient.

CPT CODING EXERCISE 6   Musculoskeletal System

Directions: Underline the keyword(s) and locate the correct code.

Example: Description: Colles' fracture, closed without manipulation; code: 25600

DESCRIPTION	CODE
1. Total hip replacement	_____
2. Bunion correction, McBride type	_____
3. Injection of ganglion cyst	_____
4. Release of trigger finger	_____
5. Hammertoe operation, one toe	_____
6. Application of body cast, Minerva type	_____
7. Treatment of closed patella dislocation without anesthesia	_____
8. Amputation of foot (Chopart type)	_____
9. Injection of small joint bursa	_____
10. Biopsy bone trocar or needle superficial	_____

Female Genital System

KEY TERMS

Term	Definition
Cervical canal	Opening or canal within the cervix that extends from the uterine cavity.
Fallopian tubes	Consist of two tubes, one on each side of the uterus, that serve as passages for ejection of nonfertile eggs (ova).
Ovaries	Small, almond-shaped organs on either side of the uterus to develop and nurture egg cells (ova).
Perineum	A skin-covered muscular area between the vaginal opening and the opening to the rectum (anus).
Trimester	One of three periods into which a pregnancy is divided. Each period is usually of 3 months' duration.
Uterus	A pear-shaped organ between the bladder and the rectum. This organ serves as the holding area for a developing fetus.
Vagina	A collapsible tube between the bladder and urethra that functions as the organ for intercourse, the birth canal, and the passage of menstruation products.
Vulva	The region including the group of structures that form the external female genital organs. This includes the mons pubis, labia majora, labia minora, clitoris, urethral meatus, and vaginal orifice.

The female genital system includes the following areas: perineum, vagina, vulva, uterus, oviducts, and ovaries.

Working with the female genital system and obstetrics and gynecology may involve codes from several different areas of CPT based on the services offered by an individual practice. The coder may use codes from the surgical section, the E&M section, the laboratory section, or the medical section.

Each office has a unique structure based on its geographic locality, the needs of the patients, and the skills of the physicians and technicians of the office. Therefore, we will focus our discussion for this section on the surgical codes as they pertain to obstetrics and gynecology.

Obstetrics and Gynecology

Obstetric (OB) care is a global service when providing uncomplicated care during pregnancy. Services include antepartum care, the delivery, and postpartum care (code 59400).

The following items include services that are **not** considered part of the global OB package. These services may be billed as separate services in addition to the global OB package:

- Laboratory procedures such as a Pap smear or OB panel (routine chemical urinalysis is part of the OB package)
- Medically indicated evaluation procedures (e.g., fetal nonstress tests, amniocentesis, ultrasound, biophysical profiles)
- Treatment of other medical conditions (e.g., vaginitis, sinusitis, urinary tract infection)
- Treatment of complications (e.g., gestational diabetes, preeclampsia, hyperemesis, observation for preterm labor)
- Other procedures during labor and delivery (e.g., induction of labor, intensive fetal monitoring, management of intravenous tocolysis, or other services requiring the constant attendance of a physician)

An admission and any daily hospital care visits pertaining to the admission may be charged in addition to the delivery. This is billable when a patient is admitted for another problem or condition up to the day of delivery.

Antepartum Care

Antepartum describes the period between conception and the beginning of labor. Antepartum care includes the following prenatal services and procedures:

- Initial and subsequent patient history
- Physician examinations
- Recording weight and blood pressure
- Listening to fetal heart tones
- Routine urinalysis
- Office visits (generally includes 12 to 14 routine visits)

The following code sets should be used to report antepartum visits when the global rules do not apply:

E&M codes	One to three antepartum visits only, any trimester
59425	Four to six antepartum visits only, any trimester
59426	Seven or more antepartum visits, any trimester

If the physician sees a patient for three or fewer visits, such as one initial visit and up to two subsequent visits, these should be billed using the appropriate level of E&M service based on new patient or established patient guidelines.

Labor and Delivery

According to CPT guidelines, the delivery includes the following items:

- Hospital admission
- An admission history and physical examination

- Management of an uncomplicated pregnancy
- Vaginal or cesarean delivery

Should the patient require an episiotomy or forceps delivery, these services are also included in the vaginal delivery and should not be billed as a separate item. The entire service is reported with one CPT code and a single fee for the service.

Delivery (59409 to 59515)

The delivering physician may not be the same physician who saw the patient in the antepartum period. If this occurs, there are specific codes that should be used to report these services. They are as follows:

59409	Vaginal delivery only
59410	Vaginal delivery and postpartum care only
59515	Cesarean delivery and postpartum care

Delivery after Previous Cesarean Section (59610 to 59622)

This code series is used for patients who had a previous cesarean section delivery but now present with the expectation of a vaginal delivery. These codes are based on global pregnancy care or divisions of care as determined by the type of delivery.

59610	Routine OB package including antepartum care, vaginal delivery, and postpartum care
59612	Vaginal delivery only
59614	Vaginal delivery with postpartum care
59618	Routine OB care including antepartum care, cesarean delivery, and postpartum care
59620	Cesarean delivery only
59622	Cesarean delivery with postpartum care

Postpartum Care

Postpartum refers to a specific period, usually 6 weeks, for continued care following a vaginal or cesarean delivery. Items included in postpartum services are as follows:

- Daily care visits in the hospital
- Discharge from the hospital
- Office visits for approximately 6 weeks after delivery

The physician providing the postpartum care might not be the same physician who delivered the baby or saw the patient during antepartum care. If this is the case, the services for the postpartum care should be reported using CPT code 59430, Postpartum care only.

Occasionally, the same physician does not treat a patient for the entire pregnancy or provide complete antepartum care—for example, because of a change in insurance or the patient left the vicinity. When this occurs, the complete package must be divided in component billing.

High-Risk Pregnancy

High-risk pregnancy is generally not considered part of the global concept. When a patient has a high-risk pregnancy, it is necessary to document cause and factors relative to the high-risk condition and list them on the superbill (a form designed by a medical practice listing the most frequently used diagnoses and procedure codes) or insurance form.

During the course of a normal pregnancy, a patient may be seen 10 to 14 times. In the case of a high-risk pregnancy, a patient may be seen twice that many times to monitor or observe conditions or problems associated with the pregnancy. Accurate and correct documentation is the key to reimbursement for high-risk pregnancies.

Coding High-Risk Visits

Show the dates of service included under the regular code 59400. Use appropriate levels of E&M codes (99201 to 99215) to report additional office visits associated with a high-risk pregnancy. Be sure to state on the claim form that the visits were related to the high-risk nature of the pregnancy.

Summary of Surgical Section

In many surgical specialties, coding should be based on the documentation found in the operative reports or medical chart. In some circumstances, repeat procedures or services may be listed on a super-bill or encounter form to make the job of coding a little easier.

It should be noted that the superbill or encounter form used in an office may have been designed by regular office personnel who do not have a medical terminology background or an understanding of the various terms used in coding. It is possible that the responsibility to review or set up a superbill may become one of the coder's responsibilities.

In addition to finding correct codes, the coder may be called upon to help set prices for services or procedures. Setting fees is a very misunderstood area within most practices. Because most offices do not have a guide to assist in establishing fees, other than the Medicare profile, fees are generally too low for the services rendered. Medicare reimbursement is often much lower than the amount allowed by other carriers. One method to determine fees is to monitor the explanation of benefits from the various commercial insurance carriers regarding what they allow for a service. A second alternative is to purchase an RVS to develop fees.

RADIOLOGY

Radiology encompasses several areas of study and has multiple factors that need to be considered for correct coding. The codes used for x-ray give a description of the procedures performed.

X-rays can be broken into the two following categories for charges:
- Technical component (TC): Person who takes the x-ray
- Professional component (PC): Person who reads the x-ray

When using the TC, use the letters "TC" and adjust the charge accordingly. For the PC, use the modifier -26. X-rays are considered global when the physician owns the equipment and provides a report of the results.

E X A M P L E

Dr. J purchased some x-ray equipment for his office and employed a full-time x-ray technician. Therefore, based on the guidelines in the CPT manual for global testing, any x-rays taken at his office would include the cost of the TC and the PC. To bill for the service, the practice would use the correct CPT code describing the service without any modifiers (71010, Chest x-ray, single view). Had the doctor not owned the equipment, but just read the x-ray, the office would have billed the code as 71010-26, Chest x-ray, single view, PC only.

Radiology has the following subsections: Diagnostic Ultrasound, Therapeutic Radiology, and Nuclear Medicine.

PATHOLOGY

Pathology and laboratory codes are used for a variety of services in the office or lab setting. These studies may be for diagnostic or therapeutic purposes.

CODING TIP

Routine venipuncture is not found in the Pathology section. It is under Surgery (36400 to 36425) because it is a puncture into the skin. Most carriers allow routine blood withdrawal to be billed in addition to any other laboratory tests performed.

Medicare and Pathology/Lab

To obtain reimbursement on all laboratory procedures, the practice must accept what Medicare allows for the service. This is called accepting assignment. Currently laboratories and practices are not allowed to ask the Medicare patient for payment for these services unless Medicare denies the service as being a routine procedure. The practice may seek payment from the patient for laboratory services only after Medicare has denied payment based on routine service.

EXAMPLE

A patient with diabetes comes to the office for a urinalysis as a precautionary measure. Without a diagnosis to show the diabetes was out of control or there was a problem, Medicare would deny the claim as a routine procedure. The office could then collect for the service from the patient.

In another situation, a patient comes to the office complaining of burning and frequent urination. In this case, the test is diagnostic in nature; therefore, Medicare would pay for the service, and the patient could not be billed for any portion of the urinalysis.

To qualify for Medicare payments on laboratory services, the practice must have a Clinical Laboratory Improvement Amendments (CLIA) number. Effective September 1, 1992, Medicare established the Clinical Laboratory Improvement Act to monitor testing and services provided to Medicare patients. This act was established to prevent misuse of laboratory services and overuse of the system.

Practices may obtain a CLIA number from their local Medicare carrier. Offices that do not have a CLIA number will not be eligible to provide laboratory services to Medicare recipients.

INJECTIONS

When billing an injection, you should know the carrier's rules for billing if you are to maximize reimbursement. There are at least five different methods to bill an injection based on carrier specifics.

Billing for immunizations has specific rules based on carrier guidelines. Generally these codes are given in conjunction with a medical service. According to AMA guidelines, it may be appropriate to bill a minimal service code (99211) in addition to the injection code when an immunization is the only service provided. To ensure correct billing of an injection, you must be carrier-specific when making your code selections.

Table 3-18 represents correct billing applications based on AMA guidelines. It should be remembered that each carrier has its own particular rules and guidelines when it comes to billing an injection.

Immunizations (90281 to 90749)

This category consists of immune globulins, administration, and vaccines and toxoids.

TABLE 3-18   Correct Billing Applications

Code Series	Vaccine Descriptions	Administration
90281-90399	Immune globulins	96365-96368, 96372, 96374-96375
90476-90748	Vaccines, toxoids	90471-90474
95120-95170	Allergen immunotherapy	95115-95117
Other injectable substances (e.g., J codes)	Therapeutic, prophylactic, or diagnostic injections	96370-96376 96360-96361
	Therapeutic or diagnostic infusions	96365-96369

Immune Globulins (90281 to 90399)

To code immune globulins correctly, you must identify the immune globulin products. Furthermore, you must report these codes in addition to the administration codes (96365-96368, 96372, 96374, 96375). This code series includes broad-spectrum and anti-infective immune globulins, antitoxins, and erythrocytic isoantibodies.

Administration Codes (90460 to 90474)

The administration codes must be reported in addition to vaccine and toxoid codes (90476 to 90749).

90470	Use this code to report H1N1.
90471	Use this code to report a single immunization administration of vaccine or a combination vaccine (e.g., 90720).
90472	Use this code to report each additional administration. This code is reported **in addition to** 90471 for multiple administrations.
90473	Use this code to report administration by an intranasal or oral route, one vaccine (single or combination vaccine).
90474	Use this code for each additional administration. (Report **in addition** to 90473.)

Vaccines and Toxoids (90476 to 90749)

These codes identify the vaccine only. Codes are reported based on the chemical formulation, dosage, or route of administration (need to know supplier). Report combination codes for purchased combination vaccines, not individual codes.

Therapeutic or Diagnostic Injections (96365 to 96379)

To bill this series correctly, you must pay close attention to each carrier's guidelines. Each company differs in what it will allow based on the codes required to report the service. According to AMA guidelines, it is appropriate to bill an office visit in addition to the injection procedures if you need to evaluate the patient for a reason other than to give the injection. The supply of the injected material is not included with these codes. Supplies may be separately billed using the AMA miscellaneous code (99070) or an HCPCS J code to identify the injected substance.

EXAMPLE

A patient comes to the office for a penicillin injection (600,000 units) for an infection.

Correct coding:	99213-25	Office visit
	96372	Injection
	J0530/99070	600,000 units penicillin

Medicare guidelines require you to use a J code to report the injected material. J codes are HCPCS codes to describe injectable substances not listed in the CPT book (e.g., J0530, Penicillin). Medicare will not pay an office visit and an administration fee on the same day of service. Some commercial insurance carriers follow AMA guidelines and some follow Medicare rules. To maximize reimbursement, always check carrier guidelines before coding.

E X A M P L E

A Medicare patient comes to the office for a penicillin injection (600,000 units) for an infection.

Correct coding:	99213	Office visit
	J0530/99070	Injection, penicillin, up to 600,000 units
Alternate coding:	96372	Intramuscular injection of antibiotic (specify)
	J0530/99070	Injection, penicillin G benzathine and penicillin G procaine, up to 600,000 units

---

The types of injections listed in Table 3-19 are exceptions to the usual Medicare rule. Medicare will allow an office visit in addition to these three types of injections, provided there is documentation to support billing an office visit.

CPT CODING EXERCISE 7   Injections

Directions: Review the following statements to determine correct code selection(s). Place the answer(s) in the space provided.

1.   A patient with Blue Shield is given an injection of 25 mL fast-acting insulin by the nurse. The patient did not see the physician.

   Answer: _____

2.   A patient with Aetna sees a physician for a limited office visit for a sore throat. The physician instructs the nurse to give the patient an intramuscular injection of 10 mL of penicillin.

   Answer: _____

3.   The patient is given a routine immunization by the nurse for measles, mumps, and rubella.

   Answer: _____

TABLE 3-19   Types of Injections That Are Exceptions to Medicare Guidelines

| | | ADMINISTRATION | |
Type	Vaccine	Medicare	AMA
Influenza	90656	G0008	96372
Pneumonia	90732	G0009	96372
Hepatitis B	90744-90747	G0010	96372

Allergy Injections (95115 to 95180)

You will find that the rules for coding allergy injections are vastly different from the guidelines pertaining to codes in the immunization and therapeutic or diagnostic sections.

According to CPT guidelines, an office visit should not be charged if the patient's only reason for the visit is to have an allergy injection. However, if the patient is seen and evaluated by the physician, then an office visit may be billed in addition to the administration fee and the injectable substance fee subject to medical necessity and individual carrier guidelines.

To clarify allergy injection codes, the AMA has changed the description of several codes. These codes now indicate that a unit count of one (1) must be used to report the service regardless of the actual number of injections given. The following list identifies administration codes for allergy injections:

95115	Professional services for allergen immunotherapy not including the provision of allergenic extracts; single injection
95117	Professional services for allergen immunotherapy not including the provision of allergen extracts; two or more injections
95125	Professional services for allergen immunotherapy in the prescribing physician's office or institution, including the provision of allergenic extracts; two or more injections

The following two codes may apply in reporting allergy injections, the administration code and the code(s) for the allergen. When billing for the antigen, the coder must first determine who will be providing the antigen and administering the injection.

95115 to 95117	Administration of the antigen (the injection)
95125 to 95134	Provision **and** administration of the antigen (treatment board). Whereas Medicare no longer pays these codes, other carriers do.
95144 to 95170	Provision of the antigen only

CPT CODING EXERCISE 8   Allergy Injections

Directions: Code the following injections using the appropriate code for the services provided.

PROCEDURE	CODE
1. Professional services including provision of allergenic extract, five stinging venoms	_____
2. Rapid desensitization procedure, each hour	_____
3. Photo tests	_____
4. Scratch test with allergenic extracts	_____
5. Direct nasal mucous membrane test	_____

TESTS AND DIAGNOSTIC STUDIES

Within CPT, coders will find a variety of tests based on anatomical sites and the nature of the services. Some tests have both a PC and a TC. To bill for both the technical and the professional service, the following apply:

- The office owns the equipment.
- The technician is employed by the office.
- The physician interprets the tests and provides a written report of the findings.

In cases in which tests are performed outside of the office, tests may need to be broken into two categories, technical and professional services. The TC consists of the technician who performs the test, the cost of the equipment, operational expenses, and the materials required to perform the test. The PC consists of ordering the test, supervising the test or study being provided, reading and interpreting the test or study results, and providing the written report.

Cardiology (92950 to 93799)

In this section, procedures represent treatments or diagnostic studies. Services may be invasive (incision or puncture of the skin) or noninvasive (does not require the skin to be broken). To code correctly from this section, the coder must carefully read the complete code text, descriptors, and references before selecting the appropriate code. Typically several codes may apply to report one service or procedure.

93000	Routine ECG with at least 12 leads; with interpretation and report (global service when an office owns the equipment and does the work).
93005	ECG, 12 leads, tracing only (TC only; this is generally used when work is completed outside the physician's office.)
93010	ECG, 12 leads, interpretation and report only (PC is used when the physician does only interpretation of the test)

Otorhinolaryngology (92502 to 92598)

Examination is based on the level of E&M supported by the documentation. It is inappropriate to bill for component procedures such as otoscopy, rhinoscopy, or the tuning fork test.

For audiological function tests, codes imply the use of calibrated electronic equipment. Codes refer to the testing of both ears. When only one ear is tested, use modifier -52 to indicate a price reduction. All descriptions apply to individual testing; use code 92559 to report group testing.

Pulmonary Tests (94010 to 94799)

Codes in this series are used to report tests to measure lung function, services to aid in the diagnosis of a lung condition, and services to provide treatment for lung diseases or conditions. Codes in this section are broken into two distinct categories for reporting. Codes include physician services, interpretation of results, and baseline assessments.

94010 to 94610	Used to report assessments or diagnostic studies
94620 to 94640	Used to report therapeutic studies
94680 to 94799	Used to report therapeutic service

PSYCHIATRY (90801 TO 90899)

It is important to remember that psychiatric services are not paid by the same methods applied to regular medical services. Many carriers have special riders or agreements regarding how psychiatric services will be reimbursed. If you work for a psychiatric office, you should be familiar with the various carrier rules and determinations for the reimbursement of this specialty. Some insurance programs do not have or offer provisions for psychiatric services.

Medicare has a special rule for paying psychiatric services. Instead of the normal 80% payment on the allowed charge, Medicare pays outpatient psychiatric services at a rate of 62.5% of the allowed amount payable at 80%. The bottom line concerning Medicare reimbursement for outpatient psychiatric services is that Medicare pays 50% of the allowed amount and the practice collects the remaining 50% of the allowed amount from the patient. Therefore, for psychiatric services, when the physician accepts assignment on a claim, the patient is liable for the amount up to the allowed amount under the Medicare contract. When the practice does not accept assignment, the patient is liable for the charge limit amount of the contract.

OPHTHALMOLOGY (92002 TO 92499)

In the matter of ophthalmology, it should be noted that the office has a choice of using the level of service codes for visits or the special eye examination codes.

The AMA has devised some special codes based on new patient and established patient status for eye examinations. These higher levels of examination are to be used primarily once every 6 months. They follow the same guidelines as the higher levels of service found in the medical codes.

Intermediate ophthalmological services include the level of service pertaining to the evaluation of the problem or condition. This includes the history and general medical observation and external ocular and adnexal examination. It may include the use of mydriasis (i.e., dilating the pupils).

Comprehensive ophthalmological services include a general evaluation of the complete visual system with patient history, general medical observation, and an external and ophthalmoscopic examination. The examination includes gross visual fields and basic sensorimotor examination. Other tests may be included in the service and should not be coded separately. These include biomicroscopy, examination with cycloplegia or mydriasis, and tonometry.

Special Service Codes (99000 to 99091)

The special service codes were designed for use as **adjunct codes**—codes used in addition to other service codes that enable the identification of extra time or unusual circumstances for a service. Most of the codes in this section are not reimbursable by insurance carriers. They are, rather, a means by which a physician may report time or services in addition to the regular care of a patient.

Special service codes cover a variety of events, from specimen handling to after-hours services. These codes may also be used to indicate follow-up visits when the physician does not charge the patient, such as in global fees for surgery (code 99024).

The function of the special service codes is to provide the physician with a means to report services that are in addition to basic services and to obtain supplemental payment in addition to regular service payments. As stated previously, the main function of CPT coding is to be a time use chart for the physician. When using special service codes, the coder must have complete accurate documentation in the chart to justify the special circumstances. The coder should check with local insurance carriers to determine correct use and payment guidelines. Many of these codes might not be reimbursed by insurance carriers.

The following list of codes is presented to give the coder a clearer definition of some of the more controversial codes used in practices and to understand their correct applications.

Codes Used in Addition to Other Services

99050	Services provided after office hours
99052	Services requested between 10 PM and 8 AM that are in addition to basic services
99054	Services requested on Sundays and holidays
99056	Services at the request of the patient in a location other than the office
99058	Office services provided on an emergency basis (some carriers use this as a primary or stand-alone code instead of as an adjunct code).

CPT CODING EXERCISE 9   Medical Services/Special Service Codes

Directions: Code the following services.

DESCRIPTION   CODE

1.   Supplies or materials provided by the physician (e.g., surgical tray)   _____

2.   Handling and conveyance of specimen from the physician's office   _____
     to a laboratory

3.   Office services provided on an emergency basis   _____

4.   Postoperative follow-up visit in a postoperative period   _____

Having finished your review of the CPT manual, you can now take all the information you have learned at this point and put the coding principles into practice. As with all the exercises provided in this book, the purpose is to learn and train. Take your time, and code to the best of your ability.

You have been coding simple exercises with the codes completed and given as listed in the CPT manual. To provide practice with actual coding, the following exercises are based on written documentation formats.

CPT CODING EXERCISE 10   Written Summaries

Directions: Read the following situations. Locate all the billable codes applicable to the problem.

Problem 1

Mrs. Smith has been experiencing pain in her right knee for the past 2 weeks every time she climbs stairs or bends her knee. She has taken various over-the-counter pain relief medications and has soaked the knee in hot water without obtaining relief. On the advice of her family physician, she made an appointment with an orthopedic surgeon.

After an expanded problem-focused review of her condition and history, the orthopedist determines that she is suffering from an inflammation of the bursa. The surgeon injects the knee with 2 mL of cortisone. Mrs. Smith also mentioned to the physician that she is having similar pain in her shoulder. Upon further evaluation, the orthopedist determines she has a slight strain of the shoulder and prescribes a muscle relaxant to help with the pain. He recommends that she return to her family physician for monitoring of the condition. The orthopedist then sends a written report of the findings, recommendations, and treatment to the family physician.

Code the services of the orthopedist.

_____
_____
_____
_____
_____
_____
_____
_____
_____

Problem 2

Ann, a new patient, saw a urologist for bladder pain. An initial, expanded, problem-focused history and detailed examination were performed with a qualitative urinalysis. Decision-making is low complexity. The urine sample revealed a bladder tumor. Ann was scheduled for a cystourethroscopy. During the procedure a biopsy was performed on the tumor. The pathology report indicated a benign tumor. Ann was scheduled for hospital admission in 3 days for the removal of the tumor.

The physician performed a cystotomy for excision of the tumor. After 5 days, Ann was released from the hospital for follow-up in the office.

Code all billable services of the urologist.

_____
_____
_____
_____
_____
_____
_____
_____
_____

Problem 3

Mary, a Medicare patient, has been having a problem with her eyes. She scheduled an appointment with an ophthalmologist. She has a comprehensive eye examination and history. The examination reveals that the patient has a retinal detachment of the left eye. The physician explains that she will need surgery to correct the condition. Surgery is scheduled for next week at the outpatient clinic of the hospital. Decision-making is moderate complexity.

The physician performed a repair of the retinal detachment with scleral buckling, vitrectomy, and an injection of air. The operation is successful. Mary is released and is to return to the office for follow-up care.

Code all billable services of the ophthalmologist.

_____
_____
_____
_____
_____
_____
_____
_____
_____
_____

Problem 4

Sue has an appointment with her primary care physician. She has low energy levels and headaches, and she tires easily. The physician performed an examination of the affected body area and other related problems with a brief history and moderate-complexity decision-making. While she was in the office, Sue had a complete CBC via venipuncture. The results of the test indicated Sue was anemic. Based on her age and history, the physician ruled out the possibility of a menstrual condition. She suggested that Sue have an upper and lower gastrointestinal (GI) series. Testing was performed by a member of the radiology department of the hospital. The results of the GI study revealed a suspicious mass in the colon. Sue was then scheduled for a diagnostic colonoscopy, which was provided by her family physician. During the colonoscopy, three large polypoid lesions were removed and sent for pathological evaluation. Sue was released with instructions to the call the office next week for the pathology results.

Code for all billable services of the primary care physician.

_____
_____
_____
_____
_____
_____
_____
_____
_____

Problem 5

Martha was a patient of Dr. Jay, a psychiatrist. Martha had been seeing Dr. Jay for a period of time for major depression. She was scheduled for a 50-minute session on Monday. When Martha arrived at the office, she was extremely agitated and upset. The physician tried to calm her during the session, but she became incoherent and hysterical. After 20 minutes, the physician decided to admit her to the hospital. A staff member accompanied Martha to the hospital. The psychiatrist completed a detailed history and examination with low-complexity decision-making. Martha was in the hospital for 5 days. Dr. Jay saw her Tuesday for a 50-minute session. On Wednesday, she spoke with her briefly and changed her medications. On Thursday, they had a 25-minute session. Friday involved a 50-minute session with the patient followed by a 30-minute conference with the family to discuss the possibility of discharge. Martha was discharged on Saturday.

Code all the billable services of the psychiatrist.

Problem 6

Jamie was brought to the emergency department (ED) by ambulance after being injured in an automobile accident. The ED physician performed a detailed history and examination. He ordered x-rays that revealed a dislocated left shoulder, three broken ribs (uncomplicated), and a fractured ulna and radius. Jamie was coherent and alert during the initial assessment.

The ED physician then called an orthopedic surgeon to complete the treatment. The orthopedist completed a detailed examination with brief history and moderate-complexity decision-making. After the orthopedic surgeon had reviewed the x-rays and other information from the ED physician, Jamie was taken to the operating room and was administered anesthesia.

The orthopedist manipulated the closed shoulder dislocation, treated the ribs with taping, and manipulated the closed radius and ulna shaft fracture. Jamie was taken to the recovery room in satisfactory condition.

Code the services of the ED physician.

Code the services of the orthopedist.

Problem 7

John was scheduled for outpatient surgery to correct bunion problems on both feet. The physician completed a right and left bunion correction using a Mayo procedure.

Code for the surgery.

Problem 8

While at work on a construction site, Jake received second-degree burns on the arm and wrist when his welding torch became entangled in his glove. He was taken to the offices of the company physician.

The arm and wrist sustained medium second-degree burns. While in the office, the physician debrided the area without anesthesia. A dressing was applied. Jake was given pain medication and told to stay home and rest the arm for the next 3 days, after which he was to return to the office for follow-up care of the burn.

Code all billable services.

Problem 9

Sam, a long-time patient of Dr. Stone, a dermatologist, was seen in the office because of lesions on the chin, cheek, and nose. After taking a brief history and expanded problem-focused examination, the physician determined that the lesions were caused by keratoses and suggested they be removed at this time. Sam agreed, and the physician removed 10 lesions from the facial area.

Code for all billable services.

REVIEW QUESTIONS   CPT CODING

1. Name the organization responsible for creating and maintaining the CPT manual.

    _____

2. Name the two-digit numerical system used to explain special circumstances or conditions.

    _____

3. Match the correct modifier to the description.

    ____ 1. -26   A. Two surgeons

    ____ 2. -57   B. Multiple procedures

    ____ 3. -62   C. Assistant surgeon

    ____ 4. -80   D. Professional component

    ____ 5. -51   E. Decision for surgery

4. List all billable services used to report an injection when the patient presents only for the purpose of receiving an injection.

    _____

5. A _____ is the transfer of a patient's care from one physician to another.

    _____

6. _____ codes provide the physician with a means to obtain supplemental payment in addition to regular services.

7. _____ refers to the covering of the skin, and _____ refers to skeletal parts and muscle.

8. Which section of the CPT manual lists the code for routine venipuncture?

    _____

9. The following statements are true or false. Circle the correct answer.

    A. There are eight ways to locate a code in the Index.   T   F

    B. A black triangle before a code indicates a description change.   T   F

    C. When a carrier does not recognize a code, the claim will not be paid.   T   F

D. Coding takes expertise and practice. It is an art, not an exact science.   T   F

E. Outpatient services may be rendered only in the physician's office.   T   F

10.   Match the term to the definition.

_____ 1. Add-on codes   A. Involves similar anatomical sites

_____ 2. Separate procedure   B. Operative removal of organ

_____ 3. Bilateral procedure   C. Division of soft parts of body

_____ 4. Incision   D. Normal cleansing of a wound

_____ 5. Debridement   E. Codes billed in addition to another service

_____ 6. Excision   F. Service performed independent of other services

11.   List the three **key** factors used to determine E&M codes.

_____

_____

_____

12.   What are the three elements required to support the use of time as a key factor in selecting a code?

_____

_____

_____

4

HCPCS Coding System

CHAPTER OUTLINE

HCPCS Background Information
    HealthCare Common
      Procedure Coding
      System
Levels of Codes
HCPCS Format

Types of HCPCS Level II Codes
Correct Code Selection
    Types of Level II Codes
Permanent National Codes
    Dental Codes
    Miscellaneous Codes

Temporary National Codes
    Types of Temporary HCPCS
      Codes
Modifiers
Drug Table

KEY TERMS

Term	Definition
ADA	American Dental Association
AMA	American Medical Association
CDT	Current Dental Terminology
CMS	Centers for Medicare & Medicaid Services
CPT	Current Procedural Terminology
DME	Durable Medical Equipment
HCFA	Health Care Financing Administration; former name of CMS
HCPCS	Healthcare Common Procedure Coding System
HHS	Department of Health and Human Services
HIPAA	Health Insurance Portability and Accountability Act of 1996
MAC	Medicare Administrative Contractors
NDC	National Drug Code
PDAC	The pricing, data analysis, and coding, contractor to CMS
PDR	Physician's Desk Reference

OBJECTIVES

After reviewing this chapter, readers should be able to:

- Understand the importance of the HCPCS system.
- Discover that the coding system is for all insurance companies, not just Medicare.
- Identify main terms.
- Choose a main term.
- Understand the application of HCPCS modifiers.

HCPCS BACKGROUND INFORMATION

Each year in the United States health care insurers process over 5 billion claims for payment. For Medicare and other health insurance programs to ensure that these claims are processed in an orderly and consistent manner, standardized coding systems are essential. The **Healthcare Common Procedure Coding System (HCPCS)** Level II Code Set is one of the standard code sets used for this purpose. The HCPCS is divided into two principal subsystems, referred to as level I and level II of the HCPCS. Level I of the HCPCS is comprised of **CPT** (Current Procedural Terminology), a numerical coding system maintained by the American Medical Association **(AMA).** The CPT is a uniform coding system consisting of descriptive terms and identifying codes that are used primarily to identify medical services and procedures furnished by physicians and other health care professionals. These health care professionals use the CPT to identify services and procedures for which they bill public or private health insurance programs. Decisions regarding the addition, deletion, or revision of CPT codes are made by the AMA. The CPT codes are republished and updated annually by the AMA. Level I of the HCPCS, the CPT codes, does not include codes needed to separately report medical items or services that are regularly billed by suppliers other than physicians.

Level II of the HCPCS is a standardized coding system that is used primarily to identify products, supplies, and services not included in the CPT codes, such as ambulance services and durable medical equipment, prosthetics, orthotics, and supplies (DMEPOS) when used outside a physician's office. Because Medicare and other insurers cover a variety of services, supplies, and equipment that are not identified by CPT codes, the level II HCPCS codes were established for submitting claims for these items. The development and use of level II of the HCPCS began in the 1980s. Level II codes are also referred to as alphanumeric codes because they consist of a single alphabetical letter followed by four numerical digits, whereas CPT codes are identified using five numerical digits. HCPCS level II codes are not only used by Medicare to report services, they are also used by almost all insurance companies to report services not described in the CPT coding system.

In October of 2003, the Secretary of the U.S. Department of Health and Human Services **(HHS)** delegated authority under the Health Insurance Portability and Accountability Act of 1996 **(HIPAA)** legislation to the Centers for Medicare & Medicaid Services **(CMS)** to maintain and distribute HCPCS level II codes. As stated in 42 CFR Sect. 414.40 (a), CMS establishes uniform national definitions of services, codes to represent services, and payment modifiers to the codes. Within CMS there is a CMS HCPCS Workgroup, which is an internal work group composed of representatives of the major components of CMS, as well as other consultants from pertinent federal agencies. Prior to December 31, 2003, level III HCPCS were developed and used by Medicaid state agencies, Medicare contractors, and private insurers in their specific programs or local areas of jurisdiction. For purposes of Medicare, level III codes were also referred to as local codes. Local codes were established when an insurer preferred that suppliers use a local code to identify a service, for which there is no level I or level II code, rather than use a "miscellaneous or not otherwise classified code."

HIPAA required CMS to adopt standards for coding systems that are used for reporting health care transactions. CMS published, in the Federal Register on August 17, 2000 (65 FR 50312), regulations to implement this part of the HIPAA legislation.

These regulations provided for the elimination of level III local codes by October 2002, at which time the level I and level II code sets could be used. The elimination of local codes was postponed, as a result of section 532(a) of HIPAA, which continued the use of local codes through December 31, 2003.

HealthCare Common Procedure Coding System

HCPCS is a set of health care procedure codes based on the AMA's CPT.

History

The acronym HCPCS originally stood for HCFA Common Procedure Coding System, as the Centers for Medicare & Medicaid (CMS) was previously (before 2001) known as the Health Care Financing Administration **(HCFA).** HCPCS was established in 1978 to provide a standardized coding system for describing the specific items and services provided in the delivery of health care. Such coding is necessary for Medicare, Medicaid, and other health insurance programs to ensure that insurance claims are processed in an orderly and consistent manner. Initially, use of the codes was voluntary, but with the implementation of HIPAA, use of HCPCS for transactions involving health care information became mandatory.

LEVELS OF CODES

HCPCS includes two levels of codes:

- **Level I** consists of the AMA's CPT and is numerical.
- **Level II** codes are alphanumeric and primarily include nonphysician services, such as ambulance services and prosthetic devices, and represent items and supplies and nonphysician services not covered by CPT-5 codes (level I). Level II alphanumeric procedure and modifier codes are a single alphabetical letter followed by four numerical digits; the first alphabetical letter is in the A to V range. Level II codes are maintained by CMS. There is some overlap between HCPCS codes and National Drug Code (**NDC**) codes, with a subset of NDC codes also in HCPCS, and vice-versa. The CMS maintains a crosswalk from NDC to HCPCS in the form of an Excel file. The crosswalk is updated quarterly.

The HCPCS level II coding system is a comprehensive and standardized system that classifies similar products that are medical in nature into categories for the purpose of efficient claims processing. For each alphanumeric HCPCS code, there is descriptive terminology that identifies a category of like items. These codes are used primarily for billing purposes. For example, suppliers use HCPCS level II codes to identify items on claim forms that are being billed to a private or public health insurer.

HCPCS is a system for identifying items and services. It is not a methodology or system for making coverage or payment determinations, and the existence of a code does not, of itself, determine coverage or noncoverage for an item or service. Although these codes are used for billing purposes, decisions regarding the addition, deletion, or revision of HCPCS codes are made independent of the process for making determinations regarding coverage and payment.

Currently, there are national HCPCS codes representing over 4000 separate categories of like items or services that encompass millions of products from different manufacturers. When submitting claims, suppliers are required to use one of these codes to identify the items they are billing. The descriptor that is assigned to a code represents the definition of the items and services that can be billed using that code.

In summary, the HCPCS level II coding system has the following characteristics:

- This system ensures uniform reporting on claims forms of items or services that are medical in nature. Such a standardized coding system is needed by public and private insurance programs to ensure the uniform reporting of services on claims forms by suppliers and for meaningful data collection.
- The descriptors of the codes identify a category of like items or services and typically do not identify specific products or brand or trade names.
- The coding system is not a methodology for making coverage or payment determinations. Each payer makes determinations on coverage and payment outside this coding process.

Information Symbols of HCPCS Level II

☯ Special coverage instructions apply to these codes. This symbol means there are instructions included in the Internet-only manuals or in Appendix A.

◆ Not covered or valid for Medicare.

✳ Carrier discretion. This symbol is an indication that the coder should contact the individual insurance company to determine payment availability.

Indications for New, Revised, or Additional Codes

▲ NEW. New code added that was not in a previous edition.

← REVISED. Changes have been made in the line or code since the last edition.

✓ REINSTATED: Indicates a code that was previously deleted has been reactivated.

✖ DELETED: Wording has been removed from the current edition.

HCPCS FORMAT

- The manual includes guidelines on how to use the national codes
- A list of modifiers
- The HCPCS codes
- A table of drugs
- The index

TYPES OF HCPCS LEVEL II CODES

There are several types of HCPCS level II codes depending on the purpose for the codes and who is responsible for establishing and maintaining them. HCPCS is published by several different companies. Therefore, each publisher adds their own bells and whistles to assist a coder in correct use and application of a HCPCS code.

In order to locate a HCPCS code, the first step is to understand how the index works. Main terms in the index identify items such as tests, services, supplies, orthotics, prostheses, medical equipment, drugs, therapies, and various medical and surgical procedures. You will also find subterms listed under a main term.

E X A M P L E

Extremity

| Belt/harness, | E0945 |
| *traction*, | *E0870-E0880* |

CORRECT CODE SELECTION

- Start with the index.
  - Locate the main term or applicable subterm.
  - Review the code information provided.
- Go to the alphanumeric code listed.
  - You will be taken to a single code or a range of codes.
  - Review each service in the range to make correct selection.

E X A M P L E
*E0945   Extremity belt/harness

For purposes of review, the following pages provide a breakdown of HCPCS level II codes for easy identification. By having an idea of what is represented in each section, the coder will have an easier time locating the code at a future date.

Types of Level II Codes

The letters at the beginning of HCPCS level II codes have the following meanings:

A0000-A0999	Transportation services
A4000-A9999	Medical and surgical supplies
A9000-A9999	Miscellaneous and experimental

B4000-B9999	Enteral and parenteral therapy
C1000-C9999	OPPS
D0000-D9999	Dental procedures
E0100-E9999	Durable Medical Equipment (DME)
G0000-G9999	Temporary procedures/professional services
H0001-H9999	Behavioral health and/or alcohol and drug abuse treatment
J0100-J9999	Drugs other than chemotherapy
J9000-J9999	Chemotherapy drugs
K000-K9999	Temporary codes assigned to DME regional carriers
L0100-L4999	Orthotics
L5000-L9999	Prosthetics
M0000-M0301	Other medical services (make sure information is in alignment)
P0000-P9999	Laboratory services
Q0000-Q9999	Temporary codes assigned by CMS
R0000-R9999	Diagnostic radiology services
S0000-S9999	Temporary national codes
T1000-T9999	National T codes established by Medicaid
V0000-V2999	Vision services
V5000-V5999	Hearing services

PERMANENT NATIONAL CODES

National permanent HCPCS level II codes are maintained by the CMS HCPCS Workgroup. The Workgroup is responsible for making decisions about additions, revisions, and deletions to the permanent national alphanumeric codes. These codes are for the use of all private and public health insurers. Because HCPCS is a national coding system, all payers will be represented in the Workgroup including representatives from private insurance agencies. The **PDAC** and Medicaid will participate in the Workgroup meetings and provide input as to what is necessary to meet each party's program operating needs.

The permanent national codes serve the important function of providing a standardized coding system that is managed jointly by private and public insurers. This standardized approach to developing a set of uniform codes provides a stable environment for claims submission and processing.

Dental Codes

The dental codes are a separate category of national codes. The Current Dental Terminology (**CDT**) is a publication copyrighted by the American Dental Association (**ADA**) that lists codes for billing for dental procedures and supplies. The CDT is included in HCPCS level II. Decisions regarding the revision, deletion, or addition of CDT codes are made by the ADA and not by the CMS HCPCS Workgroup.

Because HHS has an agreement with the AMA pertaining to the use of the CPT codes for physician services, it also has an agreement with the ADA to include CDT codes as a set of HCPCS level II codes for use in billing for dental services.

Miscellaneous Codes

National codes also include "miscellaneous/not otherwise classified" codes. These codes are used when a supplier is submitting a bill for an item or service and there is no existing national code that adequately describes the item or service being billed. The importance of miscellaneous codes is that they allow suppliers to begin billing immediately for a service or item as soon as it is allowed to be marketed by the U.S. Food and Drug Administration (FDA), even though there is no distinct code that describes the service or item. A miscellaneous code can be used during the period of time a request for a new code is being considered under the HCPCS review process. The use of miscellaneous codes also helps us to avoid the inefficiency and administrative burden of assigning distinct codes for items or services that are rarely furnished and for which we expect to receive payment.

Because of miscellaneous codes, the absence of a specific code for a distinct category of products does not affect a supplier's ability to submit claims to private or public insurers and does not affect patient access to products. Claims with miscellaneous codes are manually reviewed, the item or service being billed must be clearly described, and pricing information must be provided along with documentation to explain why the item or service is needed by the beneficiary.

Ordinarily, before using a miscellaneous code on a claim form, a supplier should check with the entity that will receive the claim for payment to determine whether there is a specific code that should be used rather than a miscellaneous code. In the case of claims that are to be submitted to one of the four Durable Medical Equipment Medicare Administrative Contractors (DME **MAC**s), suppliers that have coding questions should check with the PDAC contractor to CMS.

The PDAC is responsible for providing suppliers and manufacturers with assistance in determining which HCPCS code should be used to describe DMEPOS items for the purpose of billing Medicare.

 REMINDER

Based on publishers, the HCPCS manuals will greatly vary in the layout and design.

The PDAC has a toll free helpline for this purpose: (877) 735-1326. In addition, the PDAC publishes a product classification list on its web site that lists individual items to code categories. More information about the PDAC and the PDAC's product classification list can be found at http://www.dmepdac.com.

If no code exists that describes the product category to which the item belongs, and if the item fits a Medicare benefit category, then the PDAC may instruct the supplier to submit claims using a "miscellaneous/not otherwise classified" code. If an item does not fit a Medicare benefit category, then the PDAC might assign a code that indicates that the product is not covered by Medicare, for example, code A9270, Non-covered item or service. If an item is included or bundled into another code and not separately reimbursed by Medicare, then the PDAC may assign the code that includes the item or a code that indicates that the item is included as a component of another code. In those cases in which a supplier or manufacturer has been advised to use a miscellaneous code because there is no existing code that describes a given product, and the supplier or manufacturer believes that the code is needed, it should submit a request to modify the HCPCS in accordance with the established process. The process for requesting a revision to the HCPCS level II codes is explained later.

TEMPORARY NATIONAL CODES

Temporary codes are for the purpose of meeting, within a short time frame, the national program operational needs of a particular insurer that are not addressed by an already existing national code. The CMS HCPCS Workgroup has set aside certain sections of the HCPCS code set to allow the Workgroup to develop temporary codes. Decisions regarding the number and type of temporary codes and how they are used are also made by the CMS HCPCS Workgroup. These codes are used at the discretion of CMS.

This means that if, before the next scheduled annual update for permanent codes, the CMS HCPCS Workgroup needs a code in order to meet specific operating needs that pertain to its particular programs, it may establish a national temporary code. In the case of Medicare, decisions regarding temporary codes are made by the CMS HCPCS workgroup.

For example, Medicare may need additional codes before the next scheduled annual HCPCS update to implement newly issued coverage policies or legislative requirements. Although we establish temporary codes to meet our specific operational needs, the temporary codes we establish can be used by other insurers. Temporary codes allow insurers the flexibility to establish codes that are needed before the next January 1 annual update for permanent national codes or until consensus can be achieved on a permanent national code. Permanent national codes are only updated once a year on January 1.

The CMS HCPCS Workgroup may decide to replace temporary codes with permanent codes. However, temporary codes do not have established expiration dates. Whenever a permanent code is established by the CMS HCPCS Workgroup to replace a temporary code, the temporary code is deleted and cross-referenced to the new permanent code.

Types of Temporary HCPCS Codes

C Codes

C codes are used to report drugs, biologicals, and devices eligible for transitional pass-through payments and for items classified in new technology ambulatory payment classifications under the **Outpatient Prospective Payment System.**

G Codes

G codes are used to identify professional heath care procedures and services that would otherwise be coded in CPT but for which there are no CPT codes that meet the requirements of CMS.

H Codes

H codes are used by state Medicaid agencies that are mandated by state law to establish separate codes for identifying mental health services such as alcohol and drug treatment services.

K Codes

K codes are used by durable equipment companies. These codes are used when the existing permanent national codes for supplies and certain product categories for supplies and products do not include the codes required for a medical review policy.

Q Codes

Q codes are temporary codes to used to bill for supplies: screenings, drugs, devices, hospice care, contrast agents, and cast supplies. These codes are billed in addition to established procedure codes.

S Codes

S codes are used to report drugs, services, and supplies for which there are currently no national codes available. They were established to meet the needs of the private sector and by some Medicaid programs. These codes are not payable by Medicare.

T Codes

T codes are used by state Medicaid agencies to establish codes for items that are not included in the permanent national use codes. These are codes that are necessary to administer the Medicaid program. These codes can be used by private insurers but are not payable under the Medicare program.

MODIFIERS

As part of HCPCS coding, Medicare has also developed its own modifiers in addition to the modifiers found in the CPT manual. It is important for a practice to know and use these modifiers whenever applicable because they could help prevent revenue loss.

HCPCS modifiers are two-position codes with descriptors. The purpose of the modifiers is to indicate that a service or procedure has in some way been altered by a specific circumstance without changing the purpose or definition of the code. HCPCS modifiers may be two alpha indicators or alphanumeric characters.

E X A M P L E
-AF: Identifies a specialty physician.
-GA: Indicates the office has a waiver of liability statement on file

DRUG TABLE

J codes identify the type of drug given and the dosage amount

J codes typically identify drugs by a generic name. (Occasionally a drug will be known only by its brand or trade name) The *Physicians' Desk Reference* (**PDR**) is a publication containing information on prescription drugs and lists both the generic and the brand names.

E X A M P L E			
Drug Name	Dosage	Method Of Administration	HCPCS Code
Penicillin G potassium	up to 600,000 units	IM, IV	J2515, J2540
Penicillin G procaine, aqueous	up to 600,000 units	IM, IV	J2510

As you can see, the drug table provides the name of the drug, dosage, method of administration and associated HCPCS code or J code. At the very beginning of the table, a chart is provided to identify the method of administration.

IA	Intra-arterial administration
IV	Intravenous administration
IM	Intramuscular administration
IT	Intrathecal
SC	Subcutaneous administration
INH	Administration by inhaled solution
VAR	Various routes of administration
OTH	Other routes of administration
ORAL	Administered orally

CODING EXERCISE 1   HCPCS Level II Coding

1. Injection of tolazoline, 20 mg
2. Automatic blood pressure monitor

3. Replacement walker

4. Gradient compression stocking, below right knee, 18 to 30 mm Hg for treatment of open venous stasis ulcer

5. Placement of endorectal intracavity applicator for high intensity brachytherapy

6. One manual wheelchair antitipping device

7. Portable oxygen concentrator, rental

8. Colorectal cancer screening for patient not meeting high-risk criteria

9. Mental health assessment by nonphysician

10. Digoxin injection, 0.5 mg

11. Thoracic-lumbar-sacral orthosis (TLSO), inclusive of furnishing initial orthosis only

12. Implantable neurostimulator radiofrequency receiver

13. Influenza vaccine, administration only

14. Gynecological examination, annual, established patient

15. Screening Papanicolaou smear

16. Prostate cancer screening, digital rectal examination

17. Screening mammography

18. Oxygen mask

19. Nasal application device

20. Wound closure adhesive

CODING EXERCISE 2

Directions: Match the statement with the correct modifier by placing the single alphabetic letter in the space provided.

Example: Had you been given a definition of substance abuse program (Z), the correct modifier would have been HF. The letter Z would have been placed beside the correct modifier.

MATCH the Description to the Correct Modifier

Modifier	Answers	Letter	DESCRIPTION
1.	P2	A	Medicare Secondary Payer (MSP)
2.	V8	B	Lower right eyelid
3.	TF	C	Technical component
4.	A5	D	Clinical psychologist
5.	M2	E	"Opt out" physician or practitioner emergency or urgent service
6.	Q6	F	Infection present
7.	GO	G	Intermediate level of care
8.	AH	H	Services provided by a locum tenens physician
9.	TC	I	Patient with mild systemic disease
10.	E4	J	Dressing for five wounds

Understanding Insurance Policies

5

CHAPTER OUTLINE

SECTION 1
Insurance Carriers and Policies

KEY TERMS

Term	Definition
Actual Charge	The amount charged by the practice when providing services.
Adjudicate	A term for processing payment of a claim.
Adjudicator	Person who reviews the claim to determine payments.
Allowed Charge	The amount set by the carrier for reimbursement of services.
Assignment of Benefits	Request that money be paid directly to the physician for services rendered on a given claim. In some instances, accepting assignment may result in adjustments or write-offs.
BR	By Report. Based on the codes submitted, the claim may need to have a report sent explaining the charges.
Capitation	A form of prepayment in which a provider agrees to furnish services to members of a particular insurance program for a fixed fee. Capitations mostly affect monthly payments to primary care physicians in HMO groups.
CF	Conversation Factor. Dollar value multiplier for fee calculation.
COB	Coordination of Benefits. A clause that has been written into a health insurance policy stating the primary insurance will take into account benefits payable by a secondary insurance. Prevents overpayment of the charges billed to the patient.
Co-payment	The amount the insured has to pay toward the amount allowed by the insurance company for services.
CPT	Current Procedural Terminology. Nomenclature published by the American Medical Association as a means to describe services rendered to a patient using numerical codes.
Customary Charge	The amount representing the charge most frequently used by a physician in a given period of time.
Deductible	The dollar amount that must be paid by the patient before insurance will pay a claim based on coverage plans and benefits.
DOS	Date of Service.

DRG	Diagnosis-Related Group. Patient classification system to categorize patients who are medically related with respect to diagnosis, treatment, or statistically similar with regard to length of hospital stay.
EOB	Explanation of Benefits. Form accompanying an insurance remittance with a breakdown and explanation of payments for a claim; also referred to as a Remittance Advisory (RA).
HCPCS	Healthcare Common Procedure Coding System. More commonly referred to as "HCPCS" (sometimes pronounced *hick pix*). A coding system designed by the CMS to report patient services utilizing codes from CPT and other alphanumeric codes.
ICD-9-CM	*International Classification of Diseases, 9th edition, Clinical Modification.* The source of diagnosis coding required by insurance carriers and government agencies.
Indemnity Insurance	Traditional insurance programs referred to as "Fee for Service" programs.
PC	Professional Component. Defines services provided by a physician or other health care professional.
Percentile	The ranking of fees from all providers in a given area to develop a reimbursement base.
POS	Place Service Codes. Codes used on insurance claim forms to specify the location where services were provided. A complete list is found in the introduction section of the Professional Version of the CPT manual.
Precertification	A method for preapproving all elective admissions, surgeries, and other services as required by insurance carriers. Approval is essential before receiving payment for services.
Prevailing Charge	The charge most frequently used, in a specific area by physicians, based on specialty. The highest charge in the prevailing range establishes the absolute maximum limitation, or the highest amount a carrier will pay for a service.
PRO	Professional Review Organization. An organization of physicians that reviews services to determine medical necessity.
RBRVS	Resource-Based Relative Value Scale. A system of assigning values to CPT codes developed for Medicare to determine reimbursement amounts for services.
Relative Value Unit (RVU)	A method to calculate fees for services. A unit is translated into a dollar value using a conversion factor or dollar multiplier. The assigned value is generally based on three factors: physician work component, overhead practice expense, and malpractice insurance.
Remittance Advisory	Statement sent by an insurance company detailing how submitted claims were processed for payment along with payment amounts.
RVS	Relative Value Scale. The unit value attached to a code used to determine payment for services.
TC	Technical Component. The portion of a test or study that pertains to the use of equipment or technicians.
Third-Party Payer	A carrier that has an agreement with an individual or organization to provide heath care benefits.
Timely Filing Clause	The amount of time allowed by an insurance company for a claim to be submitted for payment from the date of the service.
UCR	Usual, Customary, and Reasonable. The reimbursement method that establishes a maximum fee an insurance company will pay for services.
Utilization Review	The process of assessing medical care services to ensure quality, medical necessity, and appropriateness of treatment.
Withhold Incentive	The percentage of payment held back for a risk account in the HMO program. Withhold arrangements are used to share potential losses or profits with providers of service.

OBJECTIVES

After completing this section, readers should be able to:

- Describe carrier reimbursement systems.
- Describe insurance carrier policy.
- Understand how to use a relative value study.
- Determine allowed amounts under a UCR method.

INTRODUCTION

Before obtaining an understanding of accounts receivable or how to file an insurance claim, it is imperative that the coder understands the various insurance companies' rules, regulations, and policy guidelines. A coder will need to understand the physician's responsibilities and obligations to the patients, as well as any agreements he or she may have with insurance companies regarding:

- Adjustments
- Charges
- Coding basics

Without this basic knowledge, a coder will find it difficult to address the common problems of claims submission.

Before beginning this section, the coder should take a few minutes to examine some of the basic terms used by commercial insurance companies, HMOs, PPOs, and federal and state programs.

In reviewing various insurance carriers, one needs to recognize the various ways in which a patient may obtain insurance coverage.

There are three ways a person may obtain insurance coverage:

- Group Health Plan: A plan arranged by an employer or special interest group for the benefit of members and their eligible dependents. This plan provides maximum benefit packages based on desired coverage and cost factors.
- Individual or Personal Plan: A plan issued to an individual. This type of coverage has a high premium with benefits based on the needs and financial factors of the individual policy holder.
- Prepaid Health Care Program: A plan whereby services are rendered by physicians or facilities that elect to participate in a set program for services.

DEFINING PAYMENT METHODOLOGIES

Private insurance companies, federal programs, and state programs use a variety of methods to determine the amount they will pay for services based on the submitted claim information. Methods vary based on the policy of the individual insurance company. However, some of the more commonly used methods include fee schedules, **relative value studies (RVS); usual, customary, and reasonable plans (UCR);** and **diagnosis-related groups (DRGs).** Another form of payment is ambulatory payment classification (APC), which pertains to outpatient hospital services.

To better understand payment policies, let's review some basic information used by insurance companies to determine payment allowances.

TEST YOUR KNOWLEDGE

1. Define the following abbreviations.

    UCR: _____   COB: _____

    PRO: _____   POS: _____

2. Define the term *deductible.*

    _____

3.   What is a timely filing clause?

_____

4.   What are the three factors used to determine a relative unit value of a code?

_____

5.   Define DRGs.

_____

Fee Schedules

A fee schedule is simply a listing of CPT and HCPCS codes that have been assigned a specific dollar value payable by the insurance company. A fee schedule designates the maximum amount or level of payment to be made by a carrier for a specific service. The physician's payment is based on the lower of either the submitted charge or the fee schedule. Most HMO and PPO programs have established fee schedules to reimburse the physician for services he or she renders to patients.

EXAMPLE	
Code	Allowed Amount
99201	$25
99215	$60
11040	$30

The patient's **co-payment** may be a percentage or a set dollar amount (e.g., $5 or $10) based on the allowed amount for the submitted code and the insurance company's contract with the patient.

Relative Value Study

The Relative Value Study (RVS) is the most popular method used to determine fees because it is the simplest. This system uses three factors to determine payment allowances, which then become a value or unit worth for a code. That unit worth or weight is then multiplied by a dollar amount (conversion factor) to determine payment allowances. Although there are several relative value studies available, the most widely accepted study is the Medicare **RBRVS**. Currently there are over 45 relative value studies available in the United States. Relative value studies incorporate the use of unit counts applied to a specific code in order to determine payment factors. This system takes into account the time, skill, and overhead expense of the physician as required by each service.

Conversion factors (CFs) or multipliers are used with the unit counts to arrive at a fee or reimbursement value for each procedure. By multiplying the conversion factor by the unit value the figures are translated into a dollar figure for use in calculating charges for services and payment allocable by insurance carriers.

Many insurance companies have developed relative value studies to use as reimbursement tables because they offer the most effective and efficient method to calculate pricing factors.

An RVS is based on the physician work component (the usual time it takes to complete the service), overhead practice expense, and the cost of malpractice insurance.

EXAMPLE

Code:	Description:	Physician work RVU:	Fully implemented nonfacility RVU:	Malpractice RVU:	Total RVU:
99201	Office/op visit/new	0.45	0.81	0.02	1.28
99241	Outpatient Consult	1.73	1.33	0.09	3.15

Payment calculation formula (RVU X CF = allowed amount)

Total RVU		CF		Allowed amount
1.28	X	$35.71	=	$ 45.71
3.15	X	$35.71	=	$112.49

Usual, Customary, and Reasonable Payment Plans

Usual, Customary, and Reasonable (UCR) plans have become one of the least used methods for payment determination because it is a complex system that compares three sets of fees per each provider. However, a few carriers such as **indemnity** providers may use this method to calculate reimbursement for a given population or geographic region.

When a carrier uses UCR as a basis for payment, three payment factors are taken into consideration in order for the carrier to establish a payment base for the allowed or covered amount of a service. Essentially, UCR means that payment is determined by: (1) ascertaining the usual fee a doctor charges to the majority of his patients for a particular service; (2) reviewing the geographic location of the practice and the specialty of the physician; and (3) reviewing complications or unusual circumstances or services. In the UCR method, reimbursement is based on the lowest of the usual, customary, or reasonable fees charged by a physician.

Usual Fee: The fee most often charged by a physician for a service or procedure.
Customary Fee: The fee most often charged by other physicians of similar training and experience within a geographic region for the same service or procedure.
Reasonable Fee: The fee the insurance company considers appropriate reimbursement based on the criteria of usual or customary fees.

The following scenario is an example of the usual, customary, and reasonable reimbursement method applied by insurance companies.

EXAMPLE

Four general surgeons in St. Louis, Missouri, submitted charges for hernia repairs with a mesh insert. Each patient has Blue Cross Blue Shield of Missouri through Chrysler Corporation, which pays 100% of the allowed amount for outpatient surgery. For this geographic region, Blue Shield allows a customary amount of $500.

Physician Charges:

Dr. Adams: $425 (Usual charge is $475—today she gave the patient a discount)
Dr. Brown: $500 (Usual fee)
Dr. Clark: $535 (Usual fee)
Dr. Dean: $500 (Usual fee was $450—the office had a rate increase)

Based on the UCR method, what would be the allowed amount for each physician?

Physician	Billed Amount	Usual Charge	Customary Charge	Allowed Amount
Dr. Adams:				
Dr. Brown:				
Dr. Clark:				
Dr. Dean:				

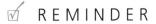 R E M I N D E R

Payment is based on the lower of the three factors: usual, reasonable, or customary charge.

Ambulatory Payment Classification

This is an outpatient classification system developed by Health Systems International based on patient classifications (diagnosis codes, CPT and HCPCS procedures, age, and gender) rather than disease classification. For Medicare patients, payments for specific services or procedures are bundled in the APC reimbursement.

APC payments are expected to be calculated on a prospective basis using sample survey and similar techniques to establish allowances for each listed procedure. The result is substantially lower Medicare payments than the cost of malpractice insurance that would have been paid had the same services been provided on an inpatient basis in a hospital.

TEST YOUR KNOWLEDGE   Payment Factors

1. What are the three factors that determine a relative value unit for a code?

   _____

   _____

   _____

2. List the four methods typically used by insurance companies to determine payments.

   _____

   _____

   _____

3. Define a conversion factor and how it is used.

   _____

   _____

   _____

4. List the three ways a patient can obtain insurance coverage.

   _____

   _____

   _____

5.   How is payment determined in a UCR scenario?

_____

_____

_____

SECTION 2
Insurance Health Plans

KEY TERMS

Term	Definition
Blue Cross Blue Shield	An independent, not-for-profit membership corporation providing coverage for hospital and physician services.
Carrier	Another name for an insurance company that covers health care services.
Case Management	The coordination and integration of a plan design through a patient care coordinator (e.g., Utilization Review or Second Opinion).
Claim	The format used to submit a claim to an insurance company.
COB	Coordination of Benefits, between insurance companies for claim payment.
Co-Insurance	A plan where the insured and the carrier share hospital and medical expenses resulting from illness or injury.
Concurrent Review	The method to monitor or control use by evaluation of patient needs and care during a hospital stay.
Crossover claim	Billing term for a patient who is simultaneously receiving benefits from Medicare and another payer (e.g., Medicaid). Medicare processes the claim for payment and then sends the balance due portion to the other insurance company.
Disability Income Insurance	An insurance plan to provide periodic payments for income replacement when the patient is unable to work.
Health Insurance	A generic term for all types of insurance coverage and reimbursement.
HMO	Health Maintenance Organization. A health care program providing services for its members by contract agreement with specific physicians, hospitals, and laboratories.
Life Insurance	Insurance that pays a specific dollar amount to a beneficiary when the insured expires.
Managed Care System (MCS)	A self-administered, self-insured program agreement between an employer and employee.
Medicaid	A state assistance program to provide quality care to low-income individuals with coverage varying based on individual state guidelines.
Preferred Provider Organization (PPO)	A special insurance program offering patients higher reimbursement by using physicians, hospitals, and laboratories within the PPO network. This form of insurance usually allows the patient more freedom of choice for providers of service than HMOs.
Primary Care Physician	The physician in charge of a patient's case within an HMO group; "primary" refers to physicians who are in family practice or internal medicine.
Prior Authorization	Evaluation of a provider's request for a specific service by an insurance company to determine medical necessity and appropriateness of care on behalf of a patient before a service can be provided.
Provider	One who supplies health care services.

Specialist	A physician in a specialty area other than primary care who provides specialized care to the patient (e.g., surgeons, radiologists, or anesthesiologists).
Spend Down	The amount a Medicaid recipient must pay out of pocket each month before becoming eligible for Medicaid financial requirements.
Third-Party Payer	A carrier that has an agreement with an individual or organization to provide heath care benefits.
TRICARE	Civilian Health and Medical Program of the Uniformed Services. A government-sponsored program providing hospital and medical services to active duty, retired personnel, and their eligible dependents.
Workers' Compensation (WC)	A contract that insures a person against on-the-job injuries paid for by the employer.

OBJECTIVES

After reviewing this section, readers should be able to:

- Identify various insurance plans.
- Obtain information from patient's identification (ID) cards.
- Describe the Medicaid system.
- Compare and contrast TRICARE (Medical Program for Uniformed Services) and CHAMPVA (Civilian Health and Medical Program of the Veterans Administration).
- Define who is eligible for TRICARE and CHAMPVA.
- Note differences between group insurance plans and Workers' Compensation insurance.

COMMERCIAL INSURANCE CARRIERS

Because most patients are in some type of health care plan, physicians now have multiple participation agreements and plans when providing services to patients. Because each plan is different based on covered services and payment calculations, billing clerks have the added responsibility of knowing each plan in order to bill correctly and within that carrier's payment guidelines.

It is important to note that not every service rendered by the physician will be covered by the insurance carrier. Covered services are part of the contract between the insurance company and the patient or employer. When a CPT code has been deemed a noncovered service by the insurance company, it is not a reflection on the physician nor is it intended to diminish the need for the service. Many physicians do not understand this fact and take it as a personal affront to their integrity.

It is not the responsibility of the physician to ensure that patients receive reimbursement from the insurance company for services rendered. However, it is the responsibility of physicians to accurately report the level or type of service they performed on behalf of patients according to the rules and regulations set forth by the American Medical Association. Insurance was not designed to relieve the patient of the financial burden of care. Insurance was designed to assist the patient with expenses incurred for medical treatment.

A good insurance file clerk is one who understands and uses the codes preferred by the individual carrier and any variations they have made to CPT codes. By understanding how the carrier wants the charge filed, the coder has won half of the battle of reimbursement.

☑ REMINDER

Coding is insurance company–specific.

Although coding is based on the information contained in the medical record, you must understand carrier rules in order to correctly apply the information to a claim form.

Blue Cross Blue Shield

Blue Cross pertains to inpatient hospital services, nursing homes, and home health care services. Because the primary focus of this text is outpatient and physician services, Blue Cross will not be discussed in this book.

Blue Shield is the portion of a patient's insurance providing financial assistance with outpatient costs for services, physician charges, and so forth. Blue Shield has many different programs within its system. A review of a few of the programs most common to the coder's area will help the coder become more familiar with the groups with whom that office may participate.

Blue Shield has provision for two types of providers:

- Indemnity providers
- UCR providers

Although the *indemnity provider* has a contract to see Blue Shield patients, the physician is not obligated to file insurance or to write off the difference of the **actual charge** and the **allowed charge**. The office may collect in full from the patient at the time service is rendered.

The *UCR provider* has a special contract with Blue Shield whereby the physician agrees to see Blue Shield patients, file the insurance to Blue Shield on behalf of the patient, and wait for payment from Blue Shield before collecting from the patient. In addition, the physician agrees to write off the difference between the actual charge or billed amount and the amount allowed by the carrier.

Blue Shield generally writes contracts with medical doctors (MDs) and Doctors of Osteopathy (DOs). Although the patient's contract or benefit package may allow for services by other health care practitioners (e.g., psychologists), Blue Shield will send the money directly to the patient unless the practitioner files the insurance and accepts assignment. Any practitioner who accepts assignment on a Blue Shield claim automatically agrees to write off the difference of the actual charge, billed charge, and the amount allowed by the carrier (UCR).

Central Certification Programs

Central certification is a special contract by Blue Shield for major corporations that have plants and employees all across the United States. The central certification program allows the patient to receive the benefits of their contract regardless of the state where the service is performed based on the rules and regulations of UCR providers.

Under this type of networking umbrella, workers have quick access to an insurance carrier and coverage information. The physician treats the patient the same as though he or she were treating a patient with Blue Shield coverage from the state with which the physician has a contract agreement.

An actual member's insurance card will have an emblem or map of the United States in the upper right-hand corner in order to identify members of the central certification program (Fig. 5-1 is only an example of a central certification ID card). However, you should be aware that this emblem may have a different meaning and interpretation from state to state. For example, the state of Alabama does not recognize central certification for outpatient services. The central certification portion of the program only pertains to inpatient services for hospital and physician care. This means the coder would only bill hospital care and visits to the local Blue Shield office. The coder should check with the individual state to determine the extent the central certification program is honored or practiced.

The physician must accept as payment the amount allowed under the UCR portion of his or her state contract, must file all insurance to Blue Shield, and collect from the patient any co-payments and deductibles as warranted by the individual policy. The physician's office should file the insurance and write off the difference between the allowed amount or UCR and the actual charge.

EFFECTIVE
DATE

SUBSCRIBER'S NAME

IDENTIFICATION CODE & NUMBER

GROUP NUMBER | BLUE SHIELD PLAN CODE | BLUE CROSS PLAN CODE

GROUP NAME

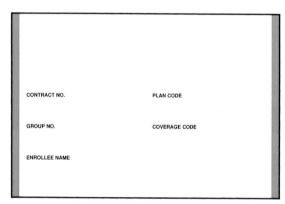

CONTRACT NO.   PLAN CODE

GROUP NO.   COVERAGE CODE

ENROLLEE NAME

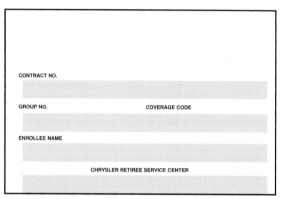

CONTRACT NO.

GROUP NO.   COVERAGE CODE

ENROLLEE NAME

CHRYSLER RETIREE SERVICE CENTER

FIGURE 5-1 Central certification identification cards.

Tricare

The Civilian Health and Medical Program of the Uniformed Services (TRICARE) is a federal program to assist active duty members and eligible dependents, as well as retirees and their eligible members, with the high cost of medical expenses. Eligibility is proven with a military identification (ID) card (Figs. 5-2 and 5-3). Always check the expiration date on the back of the card to determine if the member has eligibility. The military tracks eligibility through the Defense Enrollment Eligibility Reporting System (DEERS) program; however, this information is not available to a service provider because of the Privacy Act. Only the ID card will prove eligibility.

TRICARE is a packaged benefit program offering three types of coverage. The following charts provide costs for families using TRICARE health benefits at military treatment facilities. TRICARE also has a program called TRICARE for Life for individuals age 65 and older who are eligible for both Medicare and TRICARE. This program enables the participant to continue to receive health care at a military treatment facility, whereas before, under Medicare, they were not given a priority at a military treatment facility. TRICARE for Life is a secondary payer to Medicare with claims being transferred automatically to TRICARE for secondary payment processing.

TRICARE operates on a fiscal year instead of a calendar year. The fiscal year runs from October to October. This means that beginning each October, the deductible amounts must be met before TRICARE will begin paying claims.

Rules for Providers

Providers of service have to be approved by TRICARE in order for the patient to receive benefits for services. When a claim is filed against a provider, TRICARE will send the necessary documentation so the provider of service may be placed in the TRICARE computer for future reference and payment allowance.

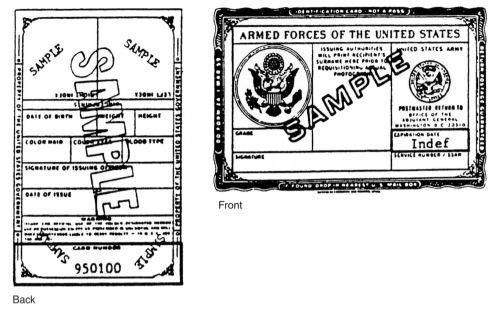

Back

FIGURE 5-2 Retired service member card.

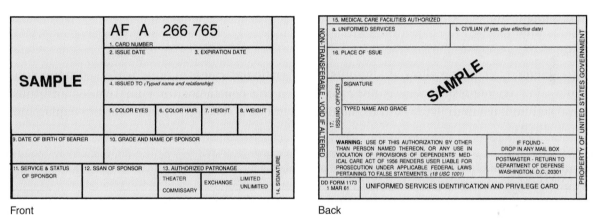

Front   Back

FIGURE 5-3 Active/retiree dependent member card. *(Source: Office of the Assistant Secretary of Defense [Health Affairs] and the TRICARE Management Activity.)*

As with any federal program, the provider is given the choice of becoming a participating provider of service or a nonparticipating provider of service. When the physician is a nonparticipating provider, he or she has the option to accept assignment for services rendered to the patient on a case-by-case or treatment-by-treatment basis.

When the provider elects to accept assignment on a claim, he or she agrees to accept as payment the amount allowed by TRICARE, to write off the difference of the actual charge and the amount allowed by TRICARE, and to file the claim for the patient. The provider must collect any co-payment amounts, noncovered items, or deductibles from the patient.

When the provider does not accept assignment, the practice may collect the full fee from the patient at the time service is rendered, is not bound by UCR agreements, and is not required to file claim forms.

All civilian hospital admissions require a nonavailability statement from the military facility before admission to a civilian hospital for members who live within a catchment area surrounding a military medical facility. The catchment area is defined by zip codes and is based on an approximately 40-mile radius surrounding the military medical facility. The obtainment of this waiver is the responsibility of the patient. Without the waiver, services could be denied for payment by TRICARE.

Claims

Claims are to be submitted to the regional contractor based on the patient's home address—not according to the location of the treatment facility.

Covered Benefits

TRICARE provides coverage for most medical and surgical conditions, contagious diseases, and nervous, mental, and chronic disorders, such as alcoholism and some obesity surgeries. The program pays for drugs prescribed by physicians or dentists when they are filled at a pharmacy by written prescription.

Any service considered to be experimental in nature is not a covered benefit of the program. However, a few organ transplant operations are allowed, such as cornea, kidney, liver, and bone marrow with some limitations imposed. Only active-duty dependents are eligible to receive one eye examination per year and well-child care from birth up to 17 years of age.

As for psychiatric services, the provider should be aware that after a certain number of visits (e.g., 33 for Missouri, 22 for Illinois), regardless of the number of times the provider actually saw the patient, an Ongoing Treatment Report (OTR) must be completed before the patient will receive further benefits or reimbursement from TRICARE.

Appeals

Disagreements concerning allowed amounts for a particular claim may be reviewed upon submission of a written request. Requests must be sent to the contractor for your regions and must be postmarked no later than 90 days from the date payment is received as listed on the explanation of benefits (EOB).

CHAMPVA

The Civilian Health and Medical Program of the Veterans Administration (CHAMPVA) was created in 1973 to provide a medical benefits program for spouses and children of veterans with total, permanent, service-related disabilities or for the surviving dependents of veterans who die as a result of service-related disabilities. Veterans are required to be enrolled in this program before dependents have eligibility. Members who receive TRICARE benefits do not qualify for coverage under CHAMPVA.

Dependent eligibility for benefits is determined by the Veterans Administration (VA). The prospective recipient must go to the nearest VA hospital or clinic to be reviewed for eligibility in the program. If the person is eligible for CHAMPVA benefits, the VA will issue the recipient a CHAMPVA identification card (Fig. 5-4).

Cost Sharing

In the CHAMPVA program, there is an annual deductible of $50 per individual and $100 deductible per family. In most cases, CHAMPVA pays 75% of the cost for care with the beneficiary having a 25% co-pay. The catastrophic cap is $3000 per calendar year.

CHAMPVA has developed a new program for spouses or dependents who are 65 and over and enrolled in Medicare Parts A and B. This program is CHAMPVA for Life. This program is a secondary payer after Medicare and other **third-party payers.**

Claims should be submitted to CHAMPVA's main office in Denver, Colorado, either electronically or on a UB-92 form for hospital billing and the CMS-1500 form for physician services.

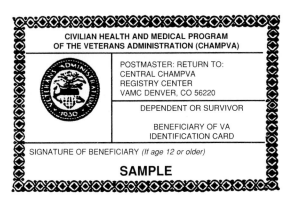

1. NAME OF BENEFICIARY	
2. DATE OF BIRTH	3. SEX
SAMPLE	
4. EXP. DATE	5. I.D. NUMBER

Use the identification number in block 5 when submitting CHAMPVA claims to the Fiscal Intermediary. If you have any questions regarding use of this card, call the CHAMPVA Center at 1-800-331-9935.

6. ISSUE DATE	

CIVILIAN HEALTH AND MEDICAL PROGRAM OF THE VETERANS ADMINISTRATION (CHAMPVA)

POSTMASTER: RETURN TO:
CENTRAL CHAMPVA
REGISTRY CENTER
VAMC DENVER, CO 56220

DEPENDENT OR SURVIVOR

BENEFICIARY OF VA IDENTIFICATION CARD

SIGNATURE OF BENEFICIARY *(If age 12 or older)*

SAMPLE

Front

Back

FIGURE 5-4 CHAMPVA identification card. *(Source: Office of the Assistant Secretary of Defense [Health Affairs] and the TRICARE Management Activity.)*

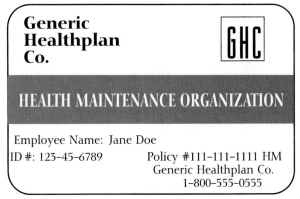

Generic Healthplan Co.

GHC

HEALTH MAINTENANCE ORGANIZATION

Employee Name: Jane Doe
ID #: 123–45–6789   Policy #111–111–1111 HM
                          Generic Healthplan Co.
                          1–800–555–0555

FIGURE 5-5 HMO identification card. *(Source: Department of Veterans Affairs Health Administration Center.)*

HEALTH MAINTENANCE ORGANIZATION

A Health Maintenance Organization (HMO) is generally referred to by its abbreviation "HMO." HMOs are special insurance contracts developed by insurance carriers to provide medical services to employers for their employees and eligible dependents at a lower fee than commercial or comprehensive programs (Fig. 5-5). These programs are mostly capitated. **Capitation** is a form of prepayment in which a provider agrees to furnish services to members of a particular insurance program for a fixed fee. Capitations mostly affect monthly payments to primary care physicians in HMO groups.

In an HMO program, the patient is usually responsible for a small co-payment, ranging from $5 to $25, for visits to the physician. The patient has a select group of physicians from which he or she may seek care. Should a patient elect to see a physician who does not participate in the HMO network, the patient may forfeit all benefits for those services. If the patient is not admitted to an HMO hospital, the patient may not receive any benefits for the hospital bill nor will the physician receive payment even though he or she is an HMO provider of service. However, in an emergency situation, the patient will usually have 24 hours in which to be transferred to an HMO facility unless it is a life-threatening situation.

Providers with HMO groups have special contract agreements to treat HMO patients. The provider of service must file insurance claim forms, collect any deductible or co-payment amounts, and write off the difference of the actual billed charge and the allowed amount.

In the HMO network, all patient care is under the direction of a primary care physician. The patient must go to the primary care physician before seeking treatment with another doctor or specialty group. It is the responsibility of the patient or primary care physician to receive correct authorization before seeing another physician. It is also the responsibility of the consulting or specialty physician to assist the patient in obtaining authorization because it is in the best interests of both parties to observe the rules and regulations. In some cases, the authorization may be arranged by a phone call or email to the insurance company from the primary care physician. Other carriers require the primary care physician to send a written request before the patient may seek service from another physician.

The primary care physician is generally held to a monthly *capitation* for the care and services rendered to the HMO patient. A primary care physician generally receives a fixed amount (e.g., $5 to $6) per month per HMO patient regardless of whether the patient has been in the office or not. In some instances, the primary care physician may not collect a co-payment from the patient for the office visit. The primary care physician is not eligible to receive any reimbursement other than the capitation amount each month except in special circumstances. The coder will need to check with individual HMO carriers to determine which services may be eligible for reimbursement or co-payments.

Specialty groups belonging to the HMO network must work with the primary physician to coordinate patient care. He or she must file insurance claims for all visits, and collect co-payments and any deductibles. Each visit could be subject to an incentive withhold amount that must be written off by the physician based on carrier and contract agreement. This incentive withhold amount penalty cannot be passed along to the patient as a payment responsibility. Offices are restricted from collecting this amount from the patient. However, should the HMO make a profit at the end of the year, each participating physician will receive a portion of monies within the incentive withhold pool.

HMO groups have many regulations regarding reimbursement that could cost the practice valuable revenue. The coder should be aware of some of the special conditions involved with the HMO participation agreement.

Timely Filing Clauses

HMOs have set time periods in which one may submit a claim for payment. The usual allowed time to file is 60 days. There are a few HMOs that have a 30-day time clause for claims submission. Timely filing is based on the date the patient was seen by the physician, not by the date the office submits the claim. If the claim is not filed with the set parameters of the **timely filing clause**, the office will forfeit reimbursement for the entire visit. In some instances, the office is required to refund any collected co-payment amounts. Additionally, the patient cannot be billed for any unpaid services when the office did not follow the timely billing guidelines defined in the insurance participation agreement.

Authorization for Service

If the patient is presented for service without proper authorization for the visit, the claim will be denied for payment by the insurance company. Again, the office could forfeit valuable revenue. In most cases, offices are not allowed to keep the co-payment collected from the patient. Authorizations may be based on time frames or number of visits. (See Figure 5-6 for an example of a prior approval authorization form.) Examples to demonstrate this principle follow.

PRIOR APPROVAL
AUTHORIZATION FORM

PATIENT INFORMATION

Patient Name __DOUGH, JANE__ Date of Birth __00–00–00__ ID Number __121212121__ Group # _____

Address __12 HOPE__ City __ANYTOWN__ State __USA__ Zip __12345__

Home Phone __123–4567__ Work Phone _____

Diagnosis / History __296.34 Major depression, recurrent, severe, w/psychotic features__

REFERRAL INFORMATION

Primary Care Physician __I. Am Physician, MD__ Phone __123–7777__ Date of Request __00–00–00__

Referring Specialist _____ Phone _____ Specialist Name __B. A. Doctor, MD__

Hospital _____ Phone _____ Address _____

CALL MADE TO SPECIALIST

Time: _____ Date: _____

To Whom: _____ Phone: _____ Tax ID # _____

[ ] Ambulance [ ] BLS [ ] ALS [ ] Round trip [ ] One Way From _____ to _____
[ ] DME [ ] Purchase [ ] Rental Specify Equipment: _____

[ ] Fertility services / sexual dysfunction: _____
  [ ] Continued Treatment: Testing _____ Medication: _____
[ ] Home Health Nursing: Service or Treatment Requested _____

Frequency: _____
[ ] Home IV Services -- Physician Orders: _____

[ ] Occupational / Speech Therapy: [ ] Initial Assessment [ ] Follow-up Visits _____ [ ] Quantity Used _____
[ ] Nonparticipating Provider -- Type of Service: _____ Negotiated Rate: _____
[ ] Nutritional Counseling: _____
[ ] Podiatry: [ ] Initial Assessment [ ] Follow-up Visits _____ [ ] x-rays [ ] PCP x-ray Location _____ (see below)
[ ] TMJ: [ ] Initial Assessment [ ] Follow-up Visits _____ [ ] x-rays [ ] PCP x-ray Location _____ (see below)
[x] Mental Health: [ ] Initial Assessment [x] Follow-up Visits _____ YTD __1__
[ ] MRI: _____
[ ] Other: _____

RESPONSIBILITY

[ ] Denied   [ ] Hosp/Doc   [ ] Member   [X] Approved   [ ] COD   [ ] Worker's Comp

Reason if denied: _____   Spouse's SS# _____ Employer _____

                                                     Name of Other Insurance _____
Ref # __123__ Letter ID# _____   Ref # __000000000__ Letter ID# _____

X__I. Am Physician, M.D.__   __00–00–00__   __3__
        Signature   Date   *Authorized units

Services Authorized from __02–02–XX__ Through __03–30–XX__ Caller __REC__
                                                              [ ] Hospital [X] Physician

Referring Physician: Provide appropriate medical records to specialist.
*Specialist: Only the number of visits or units specified above are authorized and must be completed within the time period authorized. Visits or units exceeding the number and/or time period specified are not authorized. If x-rays are authorized, use this form to order studies from the PCP's selected radiology location. Clearly specify each study requested, its indications, and any special requirements for patient management or reporting.

FIGURE 5-6 Prior approval authorization form.

EXAMPLE

Case One

A patient was allowed two visits to see the doctor from January 1 until February 15. The patient came for the first visit on January 15. The criteria were met and benefits were available.

For the second visit the patient did not return to the office until February 20. While the office was within the guideline for the number of visits, the allowed date had expired. If the office had not been aware of this and caught the error before the patient was seen by the doctor, the office would not have been able to collect for the visit.

Case Two

A patient was authorized to see a physician for two visits from January 15 through February 28. The patient kept the first appointment on January 19. The second visit occurred on February 10, and a third visit was scheduled for March 1.

In this example, both visits were within the time factor and number limit. The third visit, however, was not approved under this authorization. The physician would not be able to collect for services for the third visit without appropriate authorization.

Appeals

There is a set time period in which to protest payment or adjustments to your account. The usual time is 60 to 90 days from the date of the **remittance advisory** or **EOB**. If one has not made the appeal in this time frame, there may be no other course of action available to obtain payment for services.

The appeal consists of a letter sent to the carrier asking that the payment or charge be reviewed based on additional information. One should send a copy of the EOB as well as a copy of the insurance claim form so the carrier will have all the necessary information to review the appeal.

PREFERRED PROVIDER ORGANIZATION

Preferred Provider Organizations (PPOs) are special insurance groups that allow the patient and the physician more freedom of choice within a treatment program and benefit plan (Fig. 5-7). In the PPO program, the patient has a choice of physicians. When the patient elects to see a physician who is not a PPO provider, the patient still retains benefits for the services, but at a reduced rate. Most PPOs will pay 90% of the allowed amount for the charge, with the patient having a co-payment of 10%. When the patient sees a physician who is not a PPO provider, the insurance usually pays 60% to 70%.

However, one should verify coverage with each PPO because some carriers have a larger decrease of benefits when the patient elects to go to an out-of-network physician. In addition to a reduction in benefits, the patient will have to meet a deductible in addition to any co-payment amounts resulting in higher out-of-pocket expense. This is a great disadvantage for the patient who elects to go out of network.

Special Conditions

When a patient needs to be hospitalized, the physician has to call the carrier to precertify elective hospital admissions. For emergency admissions, the physician is given 24 to 48 hours to notify the insurance carrier. Most inpatient care is subject to medical review in order to continue patient treatment for inpatient services.

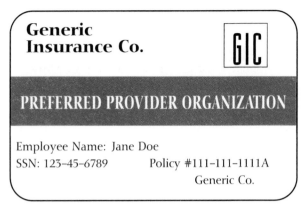

FIGURE 5-7 PPO identification card.

Appeals

To appeal a payment or problem with the PPO, you will need to send a request in writing advising the PPO of the problem. You should send a copy of the EOB and a copy of the insurance claim. Most appeals must be made within 60 to 90 days of the date of the explanation of benefits. Any additional information that will support the case should be included at that time.

TEST YOUR KNOWLEDGE

1.   What are the three types of TRICARE coverage?

   _____

   _____

   _____

2.   List the two types of providers for Blue Cross Blue Shield insurance plans.

   _____

   _____

3.   Who determines eligibility for the CHAMPVA program?

   _____

4.   What is an HMO?

   _____

5.   What is a timely filing clause?

   _____

SECTION 3
Workers' Compensation

KEY TERMS

Term	Definition
Arbitration	A method of settling a dispute with the judicial process involving an impartial third party to render a decision for settlement of a claim.
Deposition	The process of taking a witness's sworn testimony by an attorney outside of the courtroom setting.
Extraterritorial	A compensable injury to an employee hired in one state but is injured on the job outside of that state.
IME	Independent Medical Examiner. Appointed to review and report findings of work-related injuries who is appointed by the appeals board at the state's expense.
Impairment Rating	A payment percentage awarded to an employee based on a permanent work-related injury or illness.
Limited Duty	A work assignment given to a temporarily disabled employee limited in the scope of duties.
OSHA	Occupational Safety and Health Administration. A federal agency that regulates and investigates safety and health standards of a job site.
Permanent Disability	An injury or illness that prevents an employee from performing the duties associated with their job.
Second Injury Fund	A special fund that assumes all or part of the liability for benefits provided to a worker because of the combined effect of a work-related condition and a preexisting condition.
Temporary Disability	The recovery period following a work-related injury during which the employee is unable to work and the condition is not stabilized.
WC	Workers' Compensation insurance. An insurance program to provide cash benefits to workers who have become ill or injured as a result of a work-related injury.

OBJECTIVES

After reading this section, readers should be able to:

- Determine who is eligible for benefits.
- Understand the purpose of Workers' Compensation laws.
- Describe the types of compensation benefits.
- Define temporary disability versus permanent disability.
- Define terminology and abbreviations pertinent to Workers' Compensation cases.

PURPOSE OF WORKERS' COMPENSATION

Workers' Compensation insurance safeguards employees who experience job-related injuries. Except in cases of gross negligence, this coverage serves to relieve the employer of liability when an employee is injured on the job in the performance of his or her duty. This coverage enables the employee to receive compensation for loss of wages, medical expenses, and permanent disability.

Compensation Coverage

Premium or coverage payments, by law, are the responsibility of the employer. Coverage amounts are based on job descriptions and risks involved in job performance. In most cases, Workers' Compensation will cover the following services:

Medical Services

This includes treatment from an MD, DO, dentist, or chiropractor. Services may be performed in either outpatient or inpatient settings.

Temporary Disability Compensation

This is usually in the form of a weekly cash payment made directly to the patient.

Permanent Disability Compensation

Based on the rating of percent for permanent disability as ascertained by the physician, the patient may receive monthly, weekly, or lump sum payments for the injury. In a cash settlement award, the patient will not be eligible to receive payment coverage for the injury should a problem develop at a future date.

Survivor Death Benefits

This is a cash settlement to dependents when employees are fatally injured in the line of duty.

Rehabilitation Benefits

When the employee suffers severe disability due to a work-related injury, this coverage can be in the form of either medical or vocational rehabilitation. Several states, such as South Carolina and New Jersey, have structured Workers' Compensation Commissions that serve in place of insurance carriers for payment of claims.

Should the claim become delinquent or the carrier not pay the debt, a letter should be sent to the carrier as well as the employer advising that the office has yet to be paid for services. A copy of the letter should also be sent to the Workers' Compensation Commission of the state for their records.

Many states require a formal report or surgeon's report to be completed for the initial visit. (See Figure 5-8, Standard Form for Surgeon's Report.) Many insurance carriers will accept a CMS-1500 along with a copy of the office visit as necessary documentation to pay a claim. To ensure correct reimbursement, the coder should check with each Workers' Compensation carrier to determine the best way to file the claim to a particular carrier.

Purpose of Workers' Compensation

There are two kinds of statutes under Workers' Compensation: federal compensation laws and state compensation laws. Workers' compensation laws were established to protect employees for work-related injuries or illness.

The purpose of the program is to:

- Provide the best available medical care to achieve maximum recovery for the prompt return of the ill or injured party to the work force.
- Provide income for the worker or the worker's dependents regardless of fault of the injury or illness.
- Provide a single remedy to reduce costs, court delays, and increases of workloads arising from the litigation process.
- Prevent or relieve public and private charities of financial drains because of uncompensated industrial accidents.
- Eliminate costly payments to attorneys and witnesses due to time-consuming trials and appeal processes.
- Encourage employer interest in safety and rehabilitation through experience-rating mechanisms.
- Promote the study of causes of accidents and reduce human suffering by reducing preventable accidents from occurring in the workplace.

STANDARD FORM FOR
SURGEON'S REPORT
Issued by the
Division of Workmen's Compensation
Department of Labor and
Industrial Relations

State's Number For:	File #: _____
	Carrier #: _____
	Employer #: _____
Carrier's File No. _____	

The Patient

1. Name of Injured Person: _____ Age: _____ Sex: _____
2. Address: No. and St. _____ City or Town _____ State _____
3. Name and Address of Employer: _____

The Accident

4. Date of Accident: _____ Hour _____ Date disability began _____
5. State in patient's own words where and how accident occurred: _____
   _____
   _____
6. Give accurate description of nature and extent of injury and state your objective findings: _____
   _____
   _____
7. Will the injury result in (a) Permanent defect? _____ If so, what? _____
   (b) Disfigurement of normally exposed parts of body? _____
   (Permanent disability such as loss of whole or parts of fingers, disfigurement, etc., must be accurately marked on chart on reverse side of this report.)

The Injury

8. Is accident above referred to the only cause of patient's condition? _____ If not, state contributing causes: _____
9. Is patient suffering from any disease of the heart, lungs, brain, kidneys, blood, vascular system or any other disabling condition not due to this accident? _____ Give particulars: _____
   _____
10. Has patient any physical impairment due to previous accident or disease? _____ Give particulars: _____
    _____
11. Has normal recovery been delayed for any reason? _____ Give particulars: _____
    _____
12. Date of your first treatment: _____ Who engaged your services? _____

Treatment

13. Describe treatment given by you: _____
    _____
14. Were x-rays taken? _____ By whom? _____ When? _____
    (Name and Address)
15. Was patient hospitalized? _____ Name and address of hospital: _____
16. Date of admission to hospital: _____ Date of discharge: _____
17. Is further treatment needed? _____ For how long? _____

Disability

18. Patient was / will be able to resume regular work on: _____
19. Patient was / will be able to resume light work on: _____
20. If death ensued, give date: _____

REMARKS: (Give any information of value not included above) _____
_____

I am a duly licensed physician in the State of _____
I was graduated from _____ Medical School in _____ Year _____
Date of this report: _____ Signed: _____
This report must be signed personally by physician. Address: _____ Telephone _____
Cost of Medical aid: $_____

FIGURE 5-8 Standard form for surgeon's report.

State Compensation Benefits

In ordinary cases there are four principal types of state compensation benefits that may apply. They are:

Medical treatment: This benefit includes medical and surgical services, medications, and prosthetic devices.

Temporary disability indemnity: Assistance made in the form of weekly cash payments paid directly to the ill or injured employee.

Permanent disability indemnity: Either a weekly or monthly cash payment based on the percentage rating of the disability or a lump sum cash award.

Survivor death benefit: A cash payment to dependents of an employee who was fatally injured. Some states also include a burial allowance.

Claims

There are three types of state Workers' Compensation claims.

Nondisability Claim

The nondisability claim is the simplest type of claim that is easily adjusted. This category usually involves minor injuries in which the patient is seen by a doctor but is able to continue to work.

Temporary Disability Claim

In this type of claim, a reserve is established to cover medical bills and other related expenses. This can be a difficult task because the adjuster must predict in advance how much money may be needed in the course of the care or treatment. For example, an employee reports a minor back strain, which could escalate into a larger problem with the back that would require surgery or an extended period of hospital care. Usually these cases do not involve any permanent disability and the employee is able to return to work.

Permanent Disability Claim

With this type of injury, the employee is usually on temporary disability for a period of time and then is unable to return to his or her former occupation due to the severity of the injury. This type of claim usually results in a permanent disability rating for the employee because the residual disability would impede the patient's ability to compete in the open job market.

Factors that influence permanent disability ratings include:
- Severity of the injury
- Age of the injured person
- Patient's occupation at the time of the injury

Second Injury Fund

The **second injury fund** was established to handle problems that occur when an employee has a preexisting condition or injury and is subsequently injured on the job. When a preexisting condition is combined with a work-related injury, the disability is usually greater than the work-related injury would be alone. The functions of the second injury fund are: (1) to encourage hiring of the physically handicapped and (2) to allocate more equitable costs in providing benefits to the employee.

TEST YOUR KNOWLEDGE

1.   What are the four types of compensation benefits for Workers' Compensation?

_____

_____

_____

_____

2.   What is a second injury fund?

_____

3.   List the three types of state Workers' Compensation claims.

_____

_____

_____

4.   _____ is a method of settling a dispute with the judicial process involving an impartial third party to render a decision for settlement of a claim.

5.   What is indemnity insurance?

_____

REVIEW QUESTIONS: Insurance Companies

1.   Which prepaid health plan offers the best benefit package to the patient?

_____

2.   Match the term with the correct definition.

_____ 1. Primary Care Physician   A. Predetermined time limit to file

_____ 2. Assignment   B. Person who processes a claim

_____ 3. Adjudicator   C. Traditional insurance program

_____ 4. HCPCS Codes   D. Physician in charge of a case

_____ 5. Indemnity insurance   E. Usual, Customary, and Reasonable

_____ 6. UCR   F. Coding system developed by CMS

_____ 7. Time limit   G. Request that money be paid directly to the doctor

3. List the two types of providers of service in the Blue Cross Blue Shield program.

    _____

    _____

4. Explain the benefit of a Central Certification Policy.

    _____

5. What is the advantage of a PPO program over an HMO program?

    _____

6. What type of form should be used to report the initial visit for a Workers' Compensation claim?

    _____

7. Which program is an assistance program instead of an insurance program?

    _____

8. List the three components used to determine a Relative Value Unit.

    _____

    _____

    _____

9. _____ provides medical benefits for dependents of active duty or retired service members.

10. Which organization determines eligibility for dependents of deceased or disabled veterans?

    _____

6

Medicare and Medicaid

KEY TERMS

Term	Definition
Beneficiary	In the Medicare program, one who is eligible to receive Medicare benefits for medical coverage or illness or injury or for death benefits.
CMS	Centers for Medicare & Medicaid Services. The federal agency responsible for maintaining and monitoring the Medicare program, beneficiary services, and Medicaid and state operations.
Correct Coding Initiative (CCI)	Bundling edits created by CMS to combine various component items with a major service or procedure.
FI	Fiscal Intermediary. An insurance company under contract to the government that handles claims under Medicare Part A from hospitals, skilled nursing facilities, and home health agencies.
HCPCS	Healthcare Common Procedure Coding System; more commonly referred to as HCPCS (sometimes pronounced "*hick pix*"). A coding system designed by CMS to report patient services utilizing codes from CPT and other alphanumeric codes.
Hospice	An organization (private or public) that provides pain relief, symptom management, and support services to terminally ill patients and their families.
Inquiry Letters	Request from an insurance company for additional information required to process a claim for payment.
Limiting Charge	Typically applies to Medicare reimbursement. This is the absolute maximum fee a physician may charge a Medicare patient when not accepting assignment on the claim. This fee is set by the Centers for Medicare & Medicaid Services (CMS).
Locum Tenens	A physician who substitutes for another physician who is out of the office for an extended period of time.

Medicare	A national health insurance program for persons over the age of 65 and qualified disabled or blind persons regardless of income; administered by CMS.
Medicare Part A	A national health insurance program for persons over the age of 65 and qualified disabled or blind persons regardless of income; administered by CMS to cover the cost of hospitalizations and nursing facility charges.
Medicare Part B	An elective coverage program offered by CMS for aged and disabled patients to provide benefits for physician and other medical services as part of the Medicare program. This program has a monthly premium that must be paid by the beneficiary to keep the policy in good standing.
Medigap	A specialized insurance policy for Medicare beneficiaries that pays deductibles and co-payment amounts not covered by the Medicare program.
Medi-Medi	Insurance coverage by both Medicare and Medicaid.
PPS	Prospective Payment System. A payment method pertaining to hospital insurance based on a fixed dollar amount for a principal diagnosis.
SOF	Signature on File.

OBJECTIVES

After completing this chapter, readers should be able to:

- Define the two parts of the Medicare system.
- Define what is covered in the Medicare benefit program.
- Define who is eligible for Medicare benefits.
- Describe the Medicare payment system and payment formulas.
- Explain guidelines when Medicare is the secondary payer.
- Describe the types of providers in the Medicare system.
- Describe the Medicare provider identifying number system.
- Describe the rules and regulations of Medicare filing.
- Describe special filing instructions and forms.

INTRODUCTION

Medicare is a federal health care insurance program under the direction of the **Centers for Medicare & Medicaid Services (CMS)**. This program was established July l, 1966, by an act of Congress as a means to assist the elderly with the high cost of medical expenses. In later years, this program was expanded to include certain qualified disabled persons.

There are four divisions or programs within the **Medicare** system. Because each division or program has different policies regarding payment and coverage, separate organizations are responsible for the processing of claims as they pertain to each division.

Understanding the rules and regulations governing Medicare is essential to understanding the correct procedures for filing Medicare claims.

MEDICARE PART A

Medicare Part A provides coverage for inpatient care (hospitals, nursing homes, and skilled nursing facilities), **hospice**, and some home health services. Payments for Part A services are provided by a **fiscal intermediary** who is selected by CMS.

Part A does not require a monthly premium for coverage. Beneficiaries, although automatically eligible, must apply for the coverage. Individuals who are younger than the age of 65 but receive Social Security, Railroad Retirement, or disability benefits are automatically enrolled in the program the month they reach the age of 65. An enrollment package is sent to the individual 3 months prior to their 65th birthday or on the 24th month of disability.

For inpatient services, the patient has a cost share amount for each hospital stay. If the hospital visit extends beyond a certain amount of time, then the patient will be responsible for a daily co-payment in addition to the deductible.

MEDICARE PART B

Medicare Part B programs are under the direction of private insurance carriers who placed bids with the government to become intermediaries.

To participate in Medicare Part B, recipients have to pay a monthly premium for continued coverage. Part B covers physician services in both inpatient and outpatient settings; services of nonphysician professionals such as nurses, nurse midwives, and physician assistants; physical and occupational therapists, speech therapists, podiatrists, chiropractors, and clinical psychologists; diagnostic testing; radiology services and radioactive isotope therapy; ambulance services; durable medical equipment (DME) and supplies; and Prospective Payment System home health services.

With the Part B coverage package, the patient has a yearly deductible (e.g., $110), which applies to all covered outpatient services and a 20% co-payment on all assigned claims. For any items that are not covered under the Medicare program, the patient is responsible for the entire billed amount.

MEDICARE PART C

This is a Medicare Advantage program that combines Parts A and B, and sometimes Part D (prescription drug coverage). Medicare advantage plans are managed by private insurance companies approved by Medicare. These plans must cover medically necessary services. However, these plans can charge different co-payments, coinsurance, or deductibles for services.

MEDICARE PART D

This program helps pay for outpatient prescription drugs and may help lower the costs of prescription drugs and help protect against higher costs in the future.

ELIGIBILITY REQUIREMENTS

To qualify for coverage, the recipient must meet specific eligibility requirements. These requirements are determined by the Social Security Administration based on specific conditions and factors as listed below. General Medicare eligibility requirements are:

- Enrollee must have worked at least 10 years in Medicare-covered employment.
- Enrollee must be a minimum of 65 years of age.
- Enrollee must be a citizen or permanent resident of the United States.
- If an enrollee is younger than 65 years, he or she must be disabled or have permanent kidney failure.

MEDICARE IDENTIFICATION CARD

The Medicare identification card is red, white, and blue (Fig. 6-1). The letters following the patient's identification number signify the type of patient account. Most commonly used types are:

- A   Wage earner
- B   Husband's number used by wife 62 years of age or older

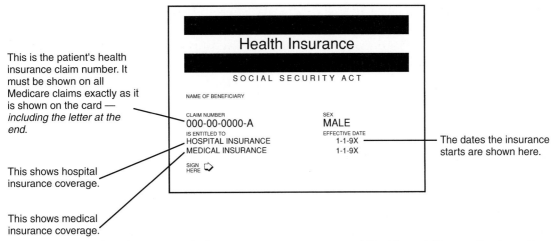

This is the patient's health insurance claim number. It must be shown on all Medicare claims exactly as it is shown on the card — *including the letter at the end.*

The dates the insurance starts are shown here.

This shows hospital insurance coverage.

This shows medical insurance coverage.

FIGURE 6-1 Medicare identification card. *(Source: U.S. Department of Health and Human Services, Centers for Medicare & Medicaid Services.)*

- ▪ D   Widow/widower
- ▪ HDA   Disabled adult
- ▪ C   Disabled child

This is a partial listing of the various identification letters used. A complete listing may be obtained from your local Social Security office.

The identification number is based on the Social Security number of the recipient or the husband's number in the case of a dependent wife. In addition to listing the gender of the patient, the card also provides the effective dates of coverage for hospital insurance (Part A) and medical insurance (Part B).

Assignment and Participation

Accepting *assignment* means the physician agrees to accept as payment the amount allowed by the fee schedule. Typically on an assigned claim, Medicare pays 80% of the allowed amount and the patient has a co-payment of 20%, provided the annual deductible has been met.

Types of Providers

A *participating provider* has a contract to see Medicare patients and agrees to accept as payment the dollar amount set by Medicare based on the relative value or worth of a procedure code or service.

A *nonparticipating provider (non par)* has a contract to see a Medicare patient but has the option of deciding on a case-by-case basis whether to accept assignment or have the patient pay the limiting charge. When a non par accepts assignment, reimbursement is based on a fee that is 5% less in value than the fee of the participating provider. Provided the patient has met the annual deductible, Medicare pays 80% of the allowed amount and the patient pays a 20% co-payment. If the non par does not accept assignment, the office may collect for services directly from the patient. Fees allowed by Medicare in this circumstance are the allowed amount of the participating provider plus an additional 15%. This fee is called a *limiting charge* amount.

EXAMPLE

Medicare Physician Fee Schedule

Code	Participating Fee	Nonparticipating Fee	Limiting Charge
99212	$36.42	$34.60	$39.79
99213	$51.13	$48.50	$75.83
99214	$79.82	$75.83	$87.20

*Fees shown are based on Medicare payment schedule for 2006.

MEDICARE PAYMENT SYSTEM

Medicare bases payments on a Relative Value Study. For covered items, after the patient has met the yearly deductible (e.g., $110), Medicare will pay 80% of the allowed amount. In the case of outpatient psychiatric services, Medicare multiplies the allowed amount by 62.5% and then pays the new calculation at a rate of 80%.

Patient Services Payment Formula

Allowed Amount × 80% = Medicare Payment
Allowed Amount × 20% = Patient Co-payment

Outpatient Psychiatric Coverage Formula

- Allowed Amount × 62.5% × 80% = Medicare Payment
- Allowed Amount × 62.5% × 20% = Patient Co-payment
- Allowed Amount × 62.5% × 37.5% = Additional Payment by Patient

  For outpatient psychiatric benefits, the physician is entitled to collect from the patient *up to* the amount allowed for the service under the Medicare profile. Therefore, in addition to the 20% co-payment, the patient will be responsible for the additional 37.5% of the allowed amount.

 REMINDER

The physician may collect up to the **allowed** amount for all covered services when accepting assignment on a Medicare claim. When not accepting assignment, the physician may collect only up to the "Limiting Charge" amount.

EXAMPLE

The patient was seen for a full session of psychotherapy in the office. The participating physician charged $125 for this service. The Medicare allowed amount for the service was $100. Under the payment formula, Medicare will pay $50 of the fee.

- ($100 × 62.5 payable at 80% = $50)
- The patient's co-payment is $12.50.
- ($100 × 62.5% × 20% = $12.50)
- The patient has an additional payment of $37.50.
- ($100 × 37.5% = $37.50).

LABORATORY FEES

In recent years, Medicare has made several changes to the way fees are collected for laboratory services. The laboratory providing the services must bill for the services and collect the money from Medicare. Medicare pays laboratory work at 100% of the fee schedule amounted for covered services. The patient does not have a co-payment or deductible for allowed services. The laboratory office must write off the difference of the allowed amount and the actual billed amount.

MEDICARE PAYMENT SCHEDULE

The Medicare payment schedule is the means devised by Medicare to advise an office how much is allowed for payment of specific CPT codes based on the participating status of the practice (par vs. non par), the place of service, and the limiting charge amount. The payment allocations are based on a relative value study or unit of worth for each code. This value is then multiplied by a conversion factor to develop the actual amount allowed for a service or procedure. In the Medicare fee schedule, the participating physician's payment is based on the par column, which is 100% of the allowed amount. The nonparticipating physician's payment is based on the non par column when that physician accepts assignment on a claim. This amount is 5% less in value than the participating's column.

When not accepting assignment, the non par is held to the **limiting charge** amount and cannot charge more than that value for services. The limited charge column is equal to 115% of the participating physician's charge column.

	E X A M P L E		
CPT Code	Fee Schedule Value: Participating Physician	Fee Schedule Value: Non Participating	Limiting Charge Amount
99201	$24.95	$23.70	$28.44
99202	$31.28	$29.72	$35.66
99203	$45.34	$43.07	$51.68
99204	$64.78	$61.54	$70.77*
99205	$102.24	$97.13	$116.56
99211	$18.87	$17.93	$21.52†
99212	$19.63	$18.65	$22.38
99213	$29.80	$28.31	$33.97†
99214	$52.50	$49.88	$59.86†
99215	$73.42	$69.75	$83.70†

CPT codes listed do not reflect actual values for services. They are provided for demonstration only.
*Denotes that limiting charge is less than 120% of the nonparticipants fee schedule.
†This fee amount and limiting charge apply when the place of service is the hospital's outpatient department.

INQUIRY LETTERS

When Medicare receives a claim with incomplete or incorrect information, the carrier will send a request to the provider of service for additional information required to process the claim. These requests are called "inquiry letters." The office may receive an inquiry letter for: (1) incorrect name or ID number, (2) more information is needed to process the claims such as type of medication or injection, or (3) additional information is required regarding the diagnosis.

After receiving the inquiry letter, the practice has 30 days to comply with the request for additional information. After that time, the claim is closed for payment due to incomplete information. The coder will then have to resubmit a corrected copy to the carrier in order to obtain reimbursement.

Although the primary purpose of the inquiry letter is to obtain additional information for the payment of a claim, the letters provide another service to Medicare carriers. They may be used as a tracking system by the carrier to report or review violations of: (1) inappropriate charges, (2) procedure coding, or (3) diagnostic coding.

EXPLANATION OF MEDICARE BENEFITS

Remittance Advisory

When a claim has been approved for payment, Medicare will send a remittance advisory with the check. This information is used to correctly credit the account with payments and adjustments based on the Medicare fee schedule. Information includes:

- The patient's name and ID number.
- The name and address of the person who provided the service.
- Date, place, and type of service.
- Procedure or service rendered to the patient.
- Amount allowed by Medicare for the service.
- Patient co-payment information.
- Claim action information (e.g., if claims crossed over to another agency or carrier).
- Reason(s) claim was paid or denied.
- Any additional adjustments/write-offs.

See Figure 6-2 for an example of a Medicare Remittance Advisory.

When payment is made on a claim, the patient also receives an explanation of benefits (EOB) from the Medicare carrier. The patient's EOB is generally easier to read than the remittance advisory received by the provider of services. The information provided to the patient includes:

- The date of service, the provider of the service, and how much was charged for the service.
- The amount Medicare allowed for the service and the expected payment amount.
- The amount that is the responsibility of the patient.

Secondary Payer Provision

There are occasions when Medicare is not the patient's primary insurance. Under the Social Security Act of 1966, certain criteria were established making Medicare a secondary payer to other insurance policies held by the patient. The following situations establish Medicare as the secondary insurance or secondary payer:

- When the patient has coverage under a group plan or has coverage through a working spouse's insurance program
- If illness or injury resulted from an automobile accident or third-party liability
- Black Lung victim
- Veterans with a Cash Card from the VA
- Work-related injuries that fall under Workers' Compensation insurance

When Medicare is the secondary payer, the supplier or provider of services is still restricted to the rules and regulations governing the billing and collecting for services based on the provider's contract agreement with Medicare. Under no circumstances may a provider collect more from the Medicare recipient than the Medicare profile allows for the service.

REMITTANCE NOTICE FOR HEALTH INSURANCE SOCIAL SECURITY ACT

PHYSICIAN OR SUPPLIED NUMBER	DATE OF STATEMENT MO. DAY YR.

GENERAL AMERICAN LIFE INS CO.
P. O. BOX 505
ST LOUIS, MO 63166

NAME OF PATIENT	HEALTH INSURANCE CLAIM NUMBER	PHYSICIAN OR SUPPLIER NAME	SERVICE DATES FROM TO MO DAY / MO DAY YR	TYPE PLACE	PROCEDURE CODE	TOTAL CHARGES	REMARKS CODES A B	NON-ALLOWED CHARGES	DEDUCTIBLE	CO-INSURANCE	PAYMENT TO PAITENT	PAYMENT TO PHYSICIAN OR SUPPLIER

GRAND TOTALS	TOTAL NO. OF CLAIMS	TOTAL CHARGES	TOTAL NON-ALLOWED CHARGES	TOTAL DEDUCTIBLE	TOTAL CO-INSURANCE	TOTAL INTEREST	TOTAL PAID TO PATIENTS	TOTAL PHYSICIAN OR SUPPLIER PAYMENT

FIGURE 6-2 Sample remittance notice.

However, there is one exception to this rule. When the provider accepts assignment for the service and the primary insurance *pays more* than the Medicare allowed amount, the provider may keep all monies paid by the primary insurance carrier provided he or she does not bill the Medicare recipient for any portion of the balance of the submitted bill.

Crossover Claims

There are several instances where Medicare will send a copy of the claim to another carrier on behalf of the patient. This is called a "crossover" claim. However, before a claim can be forwarded to another insurance company, the patient has to sign a release form. (See Signature on File form.)

When a claim is sent to another carrier, an explanation will appear in column B of the Remittance Advisory to advise the coder the claim has been sent to the secondary insurance company. When a claim is crossed over by Medicare to another carrier, it will save the practice the time, problems, and expense involved in filing secondary insurance.

Medicare will cross claims over to Blue Cross Blue Shield, Medicaid, and other carriers that participate in Medicare's specialty programs. However, the Remittance Advisory should always be reviewed to determine if the claim was actually forwarded. When a claim is not automatically crossed over to another designated carrier, the office will have to file a secondary insurance claim.

There may be an occasion when the claim did not cross over to Medicaid. When this occurs, the coder will need to inform the Medicaid carrier that the claim did not cross over so that Medicaid can send a corrected list of eligible recipients to the Medicare office.

MEDIGAP

Medigap is a special program available to Medicare recipients. The purpose of Medigap is to help the patient with costs incurred from medical expenditure over and above the Medicare allowed amount. This program pays more than the Medicare allowed amount based on individual contract agreement. For instance, when the patient receives care from a nonparticipating physician who does not accept assignment on the claim, Medigap pays any deductibles, co-payments, and portions over the allowed amount.

EXAMPLE

The office visit was $35. Medicare allowed $22.
   Medicare payment = $17.60
   Patient co-payment = $4.40
   Additional patient expense $13
   Medigap will pay the co-payment ($4.40) and the additional balance ($13.00) for a total payment of $17.40.

Currently, Medicare forwards the patient's claim to the Medigap carrier for participating offices when sufficient information has been provided on the claim form to allow Medicare to complete the information for secondary insurance and the Release of Information form has been signed.

The necessary information for Medigap should appear in Box 9 of the Medicare CMS-1500 claim form. The following information is required for the claim to be forwarded:
- The complete name and address of the secondary carrier
- The name and identification number of the insured
- The patient's signature, which should be on file in the office of the practice

SIGNATURE ON FILE FORMS

Because Medicare is a government-operated entity, the rules governing the Privacy Act are strictly enforced. Before an office may file a claim with Medicare on behalf of the recipient, the office must either have the actual signature of the patient on the claim form or be established in the Medicare system as a **Signature on File (SOF)** provider of service.

The SOF provision is a special contract agreement between the Medicare carrier and the provider of service. Medicare has to preapprove the terminology used in the SOF form before a practice is established as an SOF provider. To be an SOF provider, the patient must sign a one-time form containing specific language that complies with Medicare guidelines. Once a practice has been accepted into the SOF program, the office will only need to indicate "Signature on File" or "SOF" on the claim form in order to release medical information (diagnosis and procedures) and/or to obtain payment directly from the Medicare carrier.

Specific wording of an SOF form should include the following:

 Signature on File Information

Name of beneficiary:

HIC Number (Medicare ID Number):

   I authorize any holder of medical or other information about me to release to the Centers for Medicare & Medicaid Services or its intermediaries any information needed for completion of this or a related Medicare claim. I permit a copy of this authorization to be used in place of the original.

   I request payment of authorized Medicare benefits to be made either to me or on my behalf to (name of physician/supplier) for any services provided by that physician or supplier who accepts assignment. Regulations pertaining to Medicare assignment of benefits apply.

_____   _____

Patient Signature (Guardian)   Date

In order for Medicare to cross over or send a copy of the claim to another insurance company, with the exception of Medicaid, there has to be a signed release from the patient stating that Medicare can release this information.

This can be accomplished by use of an additional paragraph on the SOF form. The additional wording should include:

 Signed Release

Name of beneficiary:

HIC Number (Medicare ID Number):

Medigap policy number:

   I request that payment of authorized Medigap benefits be made either to me or on my behalf to _____ for any services furnished me by that physician or /supplier. I authorize any holder of medical information about me to release to (name of Medigap insurer) any information needed to determine these benefits or the benefits payable for related services.

Because this is lifetime authorization, the patient should sign the form. If the patient is physically or mentally unable to sign the form, the following person(s) may sign for the patient:

- Relative
- Legal guardian or representative

- Friend or neighbor
- Case worker
- Representative of a facility providing patient care (e.g., nursing home representative or charge nurse)

When this circumstance occurs, the person signing the form should write the patient's name, followed by his or her name, and a notation as to why the patient could not sign the form.

E X A M P L E

| Jane L. Brown | Mavis A. Brown (Daughter) | (Patient has crippling arthritis) |
| (Patient name) | (Person signing and relationship) | (Reason patient could not sign) |

If a patient does not know how to write but is otherwise physically able to sign the form, the physician or a staff member may witness the patient's mark on the form. The witness should write, in parenthesis, "his/her mark, witnessed by (his/her name with title)." No explanation is necessary concerning the reason why the patient cannot sign because the patient's mark is his or her signature.

E X A M P L E

XX (patient's mark), witnessed by Sally Secretary, Office Manager

---

 CODING TIP

Signatures obtained by the hospital and on file at the hospital do not cover the services provided by the physician. The office must obtain a signature from the patient before billing for physician services.

PROVIDERS OF SERVICE

Who can provide care or treatment to a Medicare recipient? Medicare writes contracts for service with the following providers of service:

- Medical doctors (MDs)
- Doctors of Osteopathy (DOs)
- Licensed Clinical Psychologists
- Accredited Clinical Social Workers
- Laboratories
- Outpatient Hospital Services
- Qualified Ambulatory Surgical Centers

In the Medicare program, there are two types of providers of service for a Medicare recipient: participating providers and nonparticipating providers of care.

The participating provider (par) has a special contract with Medicare to treat Medicare patients. Based on this type of contract, the provider of services: (1) must file all insurance claims to Medicare on behalf of the patient; (2) accept as payment the amount allowed by Medicare; (3) collect only co-payments and deductibles from the patient; and (4) write off the difference between the Medicare allowed amount and the actual billed amount.

When a service is not covered by Medicare, and when the provider knows the service to be a noncovered item, he or she does not have to bill Medicare. The provider may collect the fee at the time service is rendered. However, for the patient to collect for the service from a secondary insurance policy, not a supplementary policy, Medicare must be billed on behalf of the patient in order to obtain an explanation of benefits showing this to be a noncovered item. (Patients may not submit any claims to a Medicare carrier.)

The nonparticipating provider (non par) also has a contract to treat Medicare patients. Under this contract, like the par physician, the non par has to file all Medicare claim forms.

However, unlike the par provider, the non par may elect on a case by case basis to accept assignment or not to accept assignment. Billing and collection is based on which way he or she elects to handle the claim.

When accepting assignment on a claim, the non par is not held to the *limiting charge* factor. However, he or she must write off the difference of the actual billed amount and the allowed amount based on the Medicare profile. The provider must make a reasonable effort to collect all co-payments and deductibles.

When the provider elects not to accept assignment on a claim, he or she is held to the limiting charge set by the profile data. He or she should collect the fees for services at the time they are rendered. Although the provider must file insurance, the provider is not required to write off the difference between the allowed amount and the billed amount because the physician or provider of service is held to the limiting amount.

E X A M P L E

Non Par Physician

A nonparticipating physician saw a patient for a level 2 office visit. The limiting charge for this service is $35 with an allowed amount of $25.00. Because the physician did not accept assignment and was a nonparticipating physician, he was allowed to collect the full $35.00 (limiting charge) from the patient.

Par Physician

A participating physician saw a patient for a level 2 office visit. The office bills this service at a fee of $35. Medicare's allowed amount for the service is $25. The office must make an adjustment to the account by writing off the difference of the billed amount ($35) and the allowed amount ($25). The Medicare adjustment results in a write-off of $10.

Payment of the Claim is as Follows:

Medicare pays 80% of the allowed amount ($25), or $20.   ($25 × 80% = $20)

The patient pays 20% of the allowed amount, or $5.   ($25 × 20% = $5)

Perhaps the most frequently asked question is: "Why should a provider become a participating versus nonparticipating provider?" The answer is based on the reimbursement factor. Although participating and nonparticipating status both have advantages, there are some important factors to take into consideration when determining which role suits the needs of the office.

Par Advantage

Advantages for par providers include the following:
- Receive a 4% to 5% higher reimbursement on the allowed amount.
- Receive faster processing of claims.
- Do not have to complete Elective Surgery Letters.
- Notice increased patient flow because the practice is listed in the directory distributed to Medicare.
- Receive increased hospital referrals because hospitals are required to give the names of par providers to recipients.

Non Par Advantages and Disadvantage

When the non par does not accept assignment, he or she has a definite advantage over the par when it comes to payment because the limited charge amount may be billed and collected from the patient (a 15% increase in fees).

- The disadvantages: When the non par accepts assignment he or she cannot collect over the non par allowed amount. When accepting assignment on a high percentage of Medicare patients, the practice is losing 5% of its potential income.
- Fees are regulated by Medicare.
- Claim turnaround is longer than par processing.
- Non pars are required to complete Elective Surgery Letters for any surgery costing over $500.

MANDATORY ASSIGNMENT

The providers who must accept assignment on all Medicare covered services are nonphysician providers, which include physician assistants (PA), nurse practitioners (NP), nurse midwives, clinical nurse specialists (CNS), clinical psychologists, clinical social worker (CSW), and certified registered nurse anesthetists (CRNA). There are also Limited License Practitioners (LLPs), which include psychologists, clinical psychologists, and clinical social workers.

The following services are mandatory when paid by Medicare on an assignment basis only:

- Clinical diagnostic laboratory tests
- Physician services provided to Medicaid eligible recipients
- Ambulatory surgical centers (ASC) facility fees.

EXAMPLE

A patient was seen in the office by a nonparticipating physician who did not accept assignment for the level 3 visit and laboratory tests. In this case, two claims must be submitted, one for the office visit and an assigned claim for the laboratory services.

PROVIDER IDENTIFICATION NUMBERS

Medicare issues several numbers to each physician based on the type of practice wherein the physician operates. Medicare also issues identification numbers to suppliers and ambulance services as well. Suppliers and ambulance provider numbers are generally a six- to eight-digit number that may be followed by a special designated modifier. These numbers will vary from state to state in length and application. A provider number is used to identify the provider of service to a Medicare **beneficiary.**

Medicare Practice Provider Number

Physician provider numbers are usually comprised of nine digits. The first four to five digits are generally zeros.

Five-Digit Number

When five numbers are listed after the series of zeros, this generally indicates that the practice has been established as a clinical practice in the Medicare system. This type of practice usually has more than one specialist or physician.

21. DIAGNOSIS OR NATURE OF ILLNESS OR INJURY. (RELATE ITEMS 1,2,3 OR 4 TO ITEM 24E BY LINE)										22. MEDICAID RESUBMISSION CODE			ORIGINAL REF. NO.			

1. 250.91   3. |___.___

2. |___.___   4. |___.___

23. PRIOR AUTHORIZATION NUMBER

24.	A DATE(S) OF SERVICE						B Place of Service	C TYPE of Service	D PROCEDURES, SERVICES, OR SUPPLIES (Explain Unusual Circumstances) CPT/HCPCS MODIFIER		E DIAGNOSIS CODE	F $ CHARGES	G DAYS OR UNITS	H EPSDT Family Plan	I EMG	J COB	K RESERVED FOR LOCAL USE	
	From MM	DD	YY	To MM	DD	YY												
1	01	01	xx				21	1	99221		1	$100.00	1				010012345	DR. B
2	01	02	xx				21	1	99231		1	25.00	1				010012345	DR. B
3	01	03	xx				21	1	99231		1	25.00	1				020012345	DR. A
4	01	04	xx				21	1	99231		1	25.00	1				020012345	DR. A
5	01	05	xx				21	1	99238		1	60.00	1				010012345	DR. B
6																		

FIGURE 6-3 Placement of physician identification numbers on the CMS-1500 form. *(Source of CMS-1500 form: US Department of Health and Human Services, Centers for Medicare and Medicaid Services.)*

Four-Digit Number

When four digits are listed after the zero series, this generally indicates an individual or solo practice. The provider number must appear in Block 33 along with the address of the provider of services on the CMS-1500 claim form.

For an individual practice, the provider number should be placed by the letters "PIN #" in Block 33.

For a group/clinical practice, the provider number should be placed by the letters "GRP #" in Block 33 on the CMS-1500 claim form (Fig. 6-3).

Currently, Medicare requires physicians to report only the service(s) they provide to the patient. There are no provisions for trading days, covering physicians, or **Locum Tenens**. Each physician must report his or her actual service to the Medicare recipient.

Under the administrative simplification provision of HIPAA, a standard identification number must be established for third-party payers, Medicare, Medicaid, and providers of service. In accordance with this provision, Congress recently passed the National Provider Identifier (NPI) Act. This act requires the assignment to health care providers of an 8- to 10-character alphanumeric identification number. This new number will eliminate the need for the UPIN and CPIN numbers currently used in the Medicare system. Each provider will have only one number to be used on claim forms.

EXAMPLE

Dr. A saw Joe Smith for Dr. B on Saturday and Sunday at the hospital. According to Medicare guidelines:

- Dr. A's NPI number should appear on the claim to correspond to the services provided on Saturday and Sunday.
- Dr. B's NPI number would be used to correspond with the days he actually saw the patient at the hospital.

TEST YOUR KNOWLEDGE   Medicare

1. What are the rules for participation in the Medicare program?

_____

2. List the two types of Providers of Service in the Medicare program.

_____

3.   Which department of the federal government is responsible for the Medicare program?

   _____

4.   What is the purpose of a Medicare Inquiry Letter?

   _____

5.   List the five occasions when Medicare is not a primary payer.

   A.   _____

   B.   _____

   C.   _____

   D.   _____

   E.   _____

SPECIAL BILLING CONSIDERATIONS

In recent years, Medicare has discovered the advantage of providing preventive services care to patients to detect diseases during their beginning or early states.

   One type of preventative service is the "Welcome to Medicare" physical examination. This examination helps the patient and physician develop a personalized plan to prevent disease, to improve patient health, and to help the patient stay well. Some important factors regarding this examination are as follows:

- This examination is completely free to the patient. There are no co-payments and no deductibles to be met.
- This examination is available during the first 12 months you have Medicare. After the first 12 months the patient will then be eligible for a yearly wellness examination which is also free of charge to the patient. The advantage to the physician is that these types of examinations are paid at a higher rate than a regular office visit.

The following table has been provided to show what is included in the "Welcome to Medicare" and the yearly wellness examinations.

Medicare Covered Test/Screening/Service	Date You Got This Test/ Screening/Service	Next Test/Screening Service Due
Abdominal Aortic Aneurysm Screening	_____	_____
Bone Mass Measurement	_____	_____
Cardiovascular Screening	_____	_____
Colorectal Cancer Screening	_____	_____
Fecal Occult Blood Test	_____	_____
Flexible Sigmoidoscopy	_____	_____
Colonoscopy	_____	_____

Barium Enema	_____	_____
Diabetes Screening	_____	_____
Diabetes Self-Management Training	_____	_____
Flu Shot	_____	_____
Glaucoma Test	_____	_____
Hepatitis B Shot	_____	_____
HIV Screening	_____	_____
Mammogram	_____	_____
Medical Nutrition Therapy Services	_____	_____
Pap Test and Pelvic Examination (includes breast examination)	_____	_____
"Welcome to Medicare" Preventive Visit	_____	_____
Yearly Wellness Visit	_____	_____
Pneumococcal Shot	_____	_____
Prostate Cancer Screening	_____	_____
Smoking Cessation Counseling	_____	_____

Purchased Tests

When a physician purchases tests such as x-rays, Holter monitors, and so on, from a source outside of his or her office, this is termed *purchased tests*. Special handling is required for the billing of a purchased test.

When purchased tests are billed, special modifiers must be used with the procedure code to indicate this situation. Offices are required to give the name and address of the supplier and may only charge the patient the same rate that was charged to the office for the service. In other words, an office cannot make a profit on purchased tests.

SURGICAL PROCEDURES

Billing surgical procedures is not as easy as it may seem. There are several rules and regulations governing the billing of surgical procedures based on the nature and type of the procedure. One thing to keep in mind when billing a procedure is that all carriers, including Medicare, have the right to interpret use of codes as they deem applicable for the procedure and their payment guidelines.

As part of the CMS program's initiative to contain costs while maintaining quality care for its beneficiaries, offices must use a coding edit system for bundling of procedures. This program is the **Correct Coding Initiative (CCI)**. The CCI is an ongoing process to standardize bundled codes and control improper coding that would lead to inappropriate payment for Medicare claims for physician services. These edits make up the computerized screening system process used by Medicare to reject, return, or deny payment of a claim with improper coding. The CCI is revised every 3 months and may be obtained from a variety of sources. The updated information may be obtained for free from the Medicare website.

Elective Surgery Letters

When a **nonparticipating** provider performs a surgical procedure and the procedure is valued at $500 or more, the non par must complete an Elective Surgery Letter. This letter clarifies for the patient the amount the patient will owe for his or her portion of the bill as payment for the procedure. Failure by the nonparticipating office to comply could result in loss of revenue for the practice or fines and penalties being imposed on the practice.

This form will show the patient: (1) the actual amount the physician will bill for his or her service; (2) how much Medicare will actually pay for the service; and (3) the total amount that will be the responsibility of the patient.

☑ REMINDER

Supplementary policies to Medicare do not pay more than the amount allowed under the Medicare fee schedule for any physician. The purpose of a supplemental policy is to pay deductibles and co-payment amounts based on the provider's profile and Medicare's allowed amount.

Medicare's allowed amount is different from the limiting charge amount that the nonparticipating physician is entitled to bill under Medicare rules and regulations. However, all payment is based on the Medicare allowed amount, not what the physician bills the patient.

☑ *Elective Surgery Letter*

Dear Patient:

Because I do not take assignment for elective surgery, Medicare requires that I give you certain information before surgery when my charges exceed $500.00.

The following information concerns the surgery we have discussed.

These estimates assume you have already met your yearly deductible.

Type of surgery: _____

Estimated charge: _____ (Item 1)

Medicare estimated allowance: _____ (Item 2)

Your estimated payment: _____ (Item 5)

_____   _____

Date   Patient's Signature

☑ *Worksheet for Charges*

1. Actual charge: _____
2. Medicare allowed amount: (-) _____
3. Difference between the actual charge (Item 1)
   and the Medicare allowed amount (Item 2): _____
4. 20% of number 2: (+) _____
5. Patient's out-of-pocket expense: (Item 3 + Item 4) _____

SPECIAL FILING NOTICES

Frequently in the Medicare program, special forms are required to explain requests for payments or to enable the practice to collect money when Medicare denies payment of a claim.

The following are some special forms required by Medicare to obtain reimbursement either from the carrier or from the patient for specific services and items. Use of these forms will save coders problems in the future.

ADVANCE BENEFICIARY NOTICE (ABN)

This form is designed to allow the physician to collect from the patient when services are disallowed by Medicare based on frequency or the type of service. Medicare only pays a set number of office visits per month based on the diagnosis and the services provided to the patient. If this form has not been signed, the practice will not be able to collect from the patient if Medicare denies payment based on medical necessity.

If one is a nonparticipating provider of service, a copy of this form must be sent to Medicare when sending the claim form. However, participating providers may keep the form in their files and only be required to mail the form when payment is denied based on reasons of medical necessity. The signed statement must be mailed with a copy of the explanation of benefits to the Medicare carrier before collecting from the patient.

Offices who send claims electronically, regardless of participation status, must use the modifier "-GA" to indicate that a signed form is on file at the office. When the claim is denied for payment based on medical necessity, the coder then needs to send the letter to Medicare attached to the explanation of benefits.

Injections are excluded from medically unnecessary statement (MUS) letters. Payments for noncovered services or frequent services may be collected from the patient without the signed statement should the claim be denied by Medicare as a noncovered service or based on frequency. This rule also applies to laboratory services.

There are a few rules attached to the use of these statements. In order for the practice to collect for this condition, the letter or form must be signed before the doctor sees the patient. The coder cannot have the patient sign the form after Medicare denies the claim.

Also, one cannot "blanket" visits. Blanketing visits means having the patient sign one of these forms for each visit or keep a signed, but undated, form on file for use whenever the service is denied for payment by Medicare.

The ABN form requires the practice to do the following:
- Identify the test, service, or procedure for which Medicare is unlikely to reimburse.
- Document the reason for which you believe Medicare will deny payment.
- Estimate the amount the patient will have to pay out-of-pocket for the service.

The following list contains phrases most likely to be accepted by Medicare on an MUS. An example of the ABN form is shown in Figure 6-4.

Reasons for Denial

- Medicare does not usually pay for this many visits or treatments.
- Medicare usually does not pay for this service.
- Medicare usually pays for only one nursing home visit per month.
- Medicare usually does not pay for this injection.
- Medicare usually does not pay for this many injections.
- Medicare usually does not pay for this because it is a treatment that has yet to be proven effective.
- Medicare does not pay for this office visit unless it was needed because of an emergency.
- Medicare usually does not pay for like services by more than one physician during the same time period.
- Medicare usually does not pay for like services by more than one physician of the same specialty.
- Medicare usually does not pay this many services within this period of time.
- Medicare usually does not pay for more than one visit per day.
- Medicare usually does not pay for such an extensive procedure.

Patient's Name: Medicare # (HICN):

ADVANCE BENEFICIARY NOTICE (ABN)

NOTE: You need to make a choice about receiving these health care items or services.

We expect that Medicare will not pay for the item(s) or service(s) that are described below. Medicare does not pay for all of your health care costs. Medicare only pays for covered items and services when Medicare rules are met. The fact that Medicare may not pay for a particular item or service does not mean that you should not receive it. There may be a good reason your doctor recommended it. Right now, in your case, **Medicare probably will not pay for –**

Items or Services:
Because:

The purpose of this form is to help you make an informed choice about whether or not you want to receive these items or services, knowing that you might have to pay for them yourself. Before you make a decision about your options, you should **read this entire notice carefully.**
- Ask us to explain, if you don't understand why Medicare probably won't pay.
- Ask us how much these items or services will cost you (**Estimated Cost: $**_____), in case you have to pay for them yourself or through other insurance.

PLEASE CHOOSE **ONE** OPTION. CHECK **ONE** BOX.   **SIGN & DATE** YOUR CHOICE.

☐ **Option 1. YES.**   **I want to receive these items or services.**

I understand that Medicare will not decide whether to pay unless I receive these items or services. Please submit my claim to Medicare. I understand that you may bill me for items or services and that I may have to pay the bill while Medicare is making its decision. If Medicare does pay, you will refund to me any payments I made to you that are due to me. If Medicare denies payment, I agree to be personally and fully responsible for payment. That is, I will pay personally, either out of pocket or through any other insurance that I have. I understand I can appeal Medicare's decision.

☐ **Option 2. NO.**   **I have decided not to receive these items or services.**

I will not receive these items or services. I understand that you will not be able to submit a claim to Medicare and that I will not be able to appeal your opinion that Medicare won't pay.

_____   _____
Date   **Signature of patient or person acting on patient's behalf**

NOTE: Your health information will be kept confidential. Any information that we collect about you on this form will be kept confidential in our offices. If a claim is submitted to Medicare, your health information on this form may be shared with Medicare. Your health information which Medicare sees will be kept confidential by Medicare.

OMB Approval No. 0938-0566   Form No. CMS-R-131-G   (June 2002)

FIGURE 6-4 Advance beneficiary notice (CMS-R-131-G). *(Source: U.S. Department of Health and Human Services, Centers for Medicare & Medicaid Services.)*

- Medicare usually does not pay for this equipment.
- Medicare does not pay for this laboratory test.

HCPCS MODIFIER USED WITH ABN FORMS

-GA   Waiver of liability statement on file

Used when you believe a service will be denied by Medicare and you provided the patient with an advance beneficiary notice.

-GY   Item or service statutorily excluded or does not meet the definition of any Medicare benefit (not covered by Medicare)

Used when you believe a claim will denied because it is not a covered Medicare benefit or the service does not meet all of the requirements of the definition of a benefit or when a claim has to be submitted to obtain a denial from Medicare before billing to a secondary carrier.

-GZ   Item or service expected to be denied as not reasonable and necessary (not covered by Medicare)

Used when you believe the service will be denied because it does not meet Medicare program standards and you did not obtain a signed ABN form from the patient or you gave the patient an ABN form but the patient refused to sign the form.

PENALTIES AND FINES IMPOSED BY MEDICARE

Medicare Rules and Regulations

Medicare is governed by several rules relating to legal issues. This section will discuss some of the more common situations the medical office may face.

Civil Monetary Penalty Law

This law was established in 1983. It is applicable to Medicare and Medicaid cases involving fraud. This ruling gives the Secretary of Health and Human Services the right to impose civil money penalties against medical providers and supplies for incorrect billing practices. In 1994, CMS gave the responsibility of enforcing these rules to the Office of Inspector General (OIG).

COBRA

COBRA stands for Consolidated Omnibus Budget Reconciliation Act. It was established in 1986. This law allows recipients to maintain group insurance and rates from group insurance when an employee has left a job for any reason. COBRA may be used up to 18 months in order to provide a person with time to obtain new medical coverage.

Penalties

In addition to the many laws governing the Medicare program, there are several guidelines that should be followed. In the Medicare section of this chapter, Elective Surgery Letter, MUS, and some other items important in billing Medicare recipients were discussed. When these guidelines are not followed, the office can be fined or sanctioned by Medicare for noncompliance. The following is a brief review of the fines and penalties that can apply to a Medicare case for office noncompliance with Medicare rules and regulations.

☑ *Reasons for Penalties*

1. Noncompliance with ICD-9-CM Ruling 1989
2. Noncompliance with CPT-4 Ruling 1986
3. Violation of special charge limits
4. Incorrect collection of fees
5. Incorrect write-off or adjusted amounts
6. Upcoding levels of service

Penalties imposed are based on the problem and frequency of the violation. Penalties include loss of income for incorrect coding (the practice must refund money to the patient, or Medicare withholds payment of the claim); loss of provider number; and lowering of fee schedule amounts for offices that do not collect payments or deductibles. The practice can also be fined up to $10,000 per claim for infractions of the rules. If there is cause, Medicare will audit all of the practice's Medicare accounts; if it finds evidence of fraud, the provider could face federal prosecution, loss of his or her medical license, and possibly imprisonment.

Because the law cannot look into the heart, mind, or soul of the physician, the law cannot make a distinction between outright fraud and negligence or errors in billing. Therefore, it is extremely important for all personnel involved in coding and claims submission to be aware of all the rules and regulations as they pertain to specific carriers.

Audits

Medicare conducts many types of audits for claims to uncover fraud or incorrect billing procedures. These investigations are generally conducted by the OIG as part of the Department of Health and Human Services, the agency responsible for the Medicare program.

Should the office ever be involved in an audit situation, following a few simple guidelines could mean the difference between disaster and a satisfactory outcome. When the office is notified that an audit is underway, the first step is to notify the attorney for the practice. The attorney can advise the practice regarding the steps necessary to get through the audit process.

Only information that was requested by the carrier should be released. Photocopies of the information you sent to the investigative team should be retained. The attorney should be notified regarding the information sent and the date it was sent.

Some audits occur without the office even being aware of the problem. Only when the carrier discovers an inconsistency or problem will the office be notified and directed to a course of action.

☑ *Ways to Avoid Audit Situations*

- Keep current on billing rules and regulations.
- Keep current on CPT codes and applications.
- Obtain and read update bulletins from Medicare.
- Maintain accurate records and documentation.

The following are some suggestions to help offices avoid problems. Like the old saying, an ounce of prevention is worth a pound of cure.

- If a record is lost or destroyed, make a note in the chart explaining the situation. This will avoid interpretations that information was deliberately lost or destroyed.

- Avoid using correction fluid on a ledger. When an error occurs, cross out the error and then add a notation to explain the reasons for the error. Always date and initial changes. Then, list the correct entry on another line.
- Notify Medicare immediately of billing errors or overpayments.
- Document any meetings and conversations with Medicare representatives. Always include as part of the documentation the date of the meeting, where it took place, the name of person to whom you spoke, and the topics discussed.
- Whenever possible, obtain any information you receive in writing.
- Many problems can be avoided or simplified when documentation supports your actions or deeds.

MEDICARE APPEAL PROCESS

Although Medicare has many rules and regulations, it also has designed an appeal process. Some of the levels are very easy steps to help with reimbursement or coding errors.

Informal Review

An informal review must occur within 6 months of date of the Medicare EOB. Items to be addressed should be in the form of a written request and should include a copy of the EOB, a copy of the claim form, and a letter or statement explaining the reason for the review. The local Medicare carrier may have a simplified form to assist with this first level of appeal. When sending in this level of appeal, sign the request or have the physician sign the request.

Fair Hearing Review

If the practice is not satisfied with the findings of the informal review, it may request a fair hearing review. To qualify for this level, contested amounts must be at least $100 in cumulative value.

The request for the review should be submitted in writing on a special Medicare form, CMS-1965, within 6 months from the date of the findings of the informal review.

This can be either a written request, or the claimant may elect to meet with the carrier to present the reasons for dissatisfaction with the previous ruling of the claim. Written notification from the fair hearing office will be sent to the office to notify the physician of the findings and actions to be taken.

COBRA Appeal Level

Administrative Law Judge Hearing

To qualify for this level of review, the claim must total $500 or more. Claims must be similar or related services must be grouped into the $500 requirement for this level of appeal.

Judicial Review

To qualify for this level of review, claims must be $1000 or more. As with the previous level, claims must be similar or related services in order to qualify for this hearing.

RAILROAD MEDICARE

Railroad Medicare is currently the only other program recognized by the federal system. Federal carriers send copies of profile data to the carrier (Travelers) for Railroad Medicare to be used as payment guidelines.

Railroad Medicare follows most of the guidelines for reimbursement as defined by federal standards.

- Medically unnecessary letters
- Elective surgery disclosure
- Appeals
- Fines and penalties

Some coding for Railroad Medicare claims may differ slightly from the federal program, although Railroad Medicare uses coding guidelines established by the AMA and CMS.

It is easy to recognize a Railroad Medicare recipient from a federal Medicare recipient because the ID numbers are written differently. Railroad Medicare ID numbers list the alphabetical letter(s) first, followed by the Social Security number of the recipient (e.g., A123456789 or WA123456789).

Coders should not be alarmed if Railroad Medicare recipients only have a six-digit number following the alphabetical letter. In the early 1900s, the railroad used a six-digit number to identify recipients.

MEDICAID

It is important to know and understand that Medicaid *is not* an insurance program. Medicaid is a state-funded assistance program created to help ease the burden and expense of quality medical care for qualified recipients. Please remember that Medicaid policies, reimbursement rates, and medical insurance cards will vary due to state requirements (Fig. 6-5).

Eligibility

Medicaid is available to certain needy and low-income families. Some of those who may be eligible include older adults (65 years of age or older), the blind, the disabled, and families with dependent children who have been deprived of the support of at least one parent and who are financially eligible on the basis of income.

Eligibility for Medicaid is typically a month-to-month requirement based on the income of the recipient. Therefore, it is vital for office staff to check the patient's benefit status at the time of a service each month to ascertain the patient's eligibility (e.g., a patient may have benefits for January, not have benefits for February, and then be eligible again in March).

Physician's Agreement

A physician must sign a special contract with Medicaid in order to treat Medicaid patients and receive reimbursement. Medicaid writes contracts with MDs and DOs. In most states, Medicaid will not pay for services rendered by any professional other than an MD or DO. This rule may vary from state to state. Check with your local Medicaid office for a list of covered entities.

The physician's agreement with Medicaid states that he or she will treat the patient, file the claim form, and accept as payment in full the amount allowed by Medicaid. The physician may not bill the patient for any portion of the charge. However, if a patient is seen in an outpatient clinic or an emergency room there is typically a co-payment (e.g., $1 to $5) for the facility that may be collected by the hospital. When a service is not covered under the Medicaid program, the physician may then collect for the services from the patient.

Medicaid will not pay a claim unless the doctor accepts assignment and is a contracted Medicaid physician. Should a physician elect not to accept a patient's Medicaid, the patient will not receive any benefit for that visit. Physicians do not have to accept Medicaid for every visit. If the patient is willing to sign a waiver of benefits before seeing the physician, then the physician does not have to file for Medicaid benefits and the patient is responsible for the entire bill.

Expiration Date	Start Date	MISSOURI MEDICAID CARD		Pay Co.	Caseload No.
04-04-92	03-01-92			050	001
Recipient's Name		Birthdate S/R Medicaid Number	Program Restriction	MEDI-CARE	Pharmacy Limit
		06-91 FW 2222222	A B	EPSDT MEDICAL	1 2 3 4 5

A

COVERAGE	EXPLANATION
A	All available benefits (co-payment <u>not</u> required)
B	All available benefits (co-payment is required) for specified services
C	Client is eligible for outpatient care only, must reach spenddown for inpatient care
X	Client is eligible only for inpatient care, emergency room, and clinic services
Z	Limited benefits as explained in the shaded area on the face of this card

B

FIGURE 6-5 A, Medicaid Identification card; B, designates code explanations. *(Source: U.S. Department of Health and Human Services, Centers for Medicare & Medicaid Services.)*

Medicaid receives funding from state and federal agencies. Because federal programs assist in the funding of the state program, Medicaid is governed by many of Medicare's guidelines. Most Medicaid carriers have adopted the HCPCS codes published by Medicare. The coder will need to verify with the local agency which sections of the HCPCS codes are currently being used for reimbursement purposes.

Claims

Medicaid requires that claims be submitted with the diagnosis code taken to the highest levels of specificity. In other words, offices should submit claims using fourth- and fifth-digit subclassifications when applicable. Failure to comply with this ruling will result in the claim being denied for payment due to an invalid diagnosis code.

Filing and coding Medicaid claim forms can be difficult because of the various policies, rules, and regulations. The coder will need to check with the local Medicaid carrier to ascertain the specific guidelines for the state. Because the funding is regulated by the individual state, each state directs the handling of Medicaid claims differently.

In most states, Medicaid carriers will not develop or research a claim. If the claim is not in their specific format, the claim will be rejected for payment. The only notice the office will receive is the code listed on the explanation of benefits defining the reason for nonpayment.

E X A M P L E

Some Unusual Features of Medicaid Coding
- If a patient is still in the hospital at the time the claim is filed, the staff must write "Still In Hospital" in the area designed for the discharge date. Stating "In House" or "In Hospital" is not sufficient for Medicaid claims.
- Medicaid does not accept consecutive care dates when a psychotherapy or psychiatric diagnosis is involved. Each service must appear as a separate line item.
- In most states, for obstetrical (OB) care, you do not bill the global OB package. Each visit is separately reported with an E&M code followed by the code for the delivery.

Typically Medicaid will pay for the following: inpatient hospital care; outpatient services; laboratory and x-ray services; skilled nursing facility services; physician services; screening, diagnosis, and treatment of children under the age of 21; immunization programs; home health care services; and family planning services.

Based on individual state guidelines and fund availability, some additional services may be covered such as dental care, eye glasses, ambulance services, optometric services, psychiatric care, podiatry, chiropractic care, and prescription drugs.

MEDI-MEDI

The term **Medi-Medi** is not a misprint. It is important to understand the rules when the patient has both Medicare and Medicaid benefits. Recipients of the Medi-Medi programs are usually persons who qualify under the old age security assistance benefits (patients over the age of 65), the severely disabled, and the blind.

Because the beneficiary or patient enjoys the benefits of Medicare and Medicaid, assignment on the CMS-1500 form must always be accepted. Medicaid will not pay a claim unless the office accepts assignment on the Medicare portion of the claim regardless of the physician's participation status in the Medicare system. Also, the physician must be an approved Medicaid provider for Medicaid to make payment on a claim.

After Medicare processes the claim form, the claim will automatically cross over to the Medicaid carrier for payment. You will need to check the EOB to verify that the claim did cross over for payment because new recipients may not be on the Medicare list of qualified Medicaid crossover claims.

REVIEW QUESTIONS   Medicare

1. _____ _____ _____ were designed to allow physicians to collect for visits that have been disallowed by Medicare based on frequency of service or diagnosis.

2. _____ _____ _____ must be completed by nonparticipating physicians for surgeries over $500.

3. _____ _____ is the only other Medicare program currently recognized by the federal government.

4. List the two factors used by Medicare to determine the allowable amount used for reimbursement of Medicare claims.

     _____

     _____

5. What is the significance of "SOF"?

     _____

6. _____ _____ covers hospital charges and _____ _____ provides for outpatient and physician services.

     _____

7. Which agency determines a patient's eligibility for Medicare benefits?

     _____

8. What percentage of the allowed amount is paid by Medicare for medical services?

     _____

9. What is the formula for psychiatric benefit payments for outpatient services?

     _____

10. What is Medi-Medi?

     _____

7

Insurance Claim Forms

CHAPTER OUTLINE

Introduction
HIPAA and Electronic Claim Submission
Standards for Code Sets
Standards for Electronic Claims
The 837P
Supporting Code Sets
Grouping of Information for the 837P

HIPAA Standards—A Look at Format 5010
CMS-1500 Form
Possible Problems with Incomplete Claim Forms
Review of CMS-1500
Patient and Insured Information

Items 14-33: Physician or Supplier Information
POS Codes and Definitions
Unit Counts
Billing Multiple Surgeries
Assistance Fees
Bilateral Procedures
Additional Codes

KEY TERMS

Term	Definition
Batching	A deferred or delayed processing method for inputting data for retrieval at a later date.
Beneficiary	In the Medicare program, the person who is eligible to receive a specified payment for either coverage related to illness or injury or for death benefits.
Bundling	Combining lesser services with a major service in order for one charge to include the variety of services.
CCI	Correct Coding Initiative. Bundling edits created by CMS to combine various component items with a major service or procedure.
CMS-1500	A paper claim form submitted to an insurance company to provide billing information regarding patient services.
COB	Coordination of Benefits. A clause that has been written into a health insurance policy stating that the primary insurance will take into account benefits payable by a secondary carrier. Prevents overpayment of the charges billed to the patient.
Component Billing	Billing for each item or service provided to a patient in accordance with insurance carriers' policies.
Covered Entities	Health care providers, health plans, and health care clearinghouses.
DMERC	Durable medical equipment regional carrier.
EDI	Electronic Data Interchange. Computer-to-computer transfer of data between a provider of services and an insurance company or claims-processing clearinghouse.
Encounter Form	Document to record information regarding services provided to a patient; used for billing purposes. Also referred to as a superbill or fee slip.
EPSDT	Early and Periodic Screening, Diagnosis, and Treatment. A Medicaid preventive medical examination.
FECA	Federal Employees' Compensation Act. A program administered by the Office of Workers' Compensation Programs (OWCP), U.S. Department of Labor (DOL). This program decides whether you qualify for medical treatment and compensation under this act.
Fee Slip	Also referred to as a superbill or patient encounter form. A form used to track service information.
Global Period	Specific time frames assigned to a code by an insurance company before additional payment will be made following a surgical procedure.
Global Procedures	Major surgical procedures that typically have a follow-up period of 30, 60, 90, or 120 days, which must elapse before you may begin to bill the patient for services related to the original procedure.
Health Care Clearinghouse	Company that translates electronic transactions between the standard formats and code sets required under HIPAA and nonstandard formats and code sets.
Health Care Provider	Any person who or organization that furnishes, bills, or is paid for health care in the normal course of business.

Health Plans	An individual or group plan that provides or pays for the cost of medical care.
NPI	National Provider Identifier. Number assigned to hospitals, physicians, nursing homes, and other health care providers that contains alphanumeric characters (e.g., E3E30KL74-6).
Ordering Physician	The physician who orders nonphysician services, such as diagnostic laboratory tests, clinical laboratory tests, pharmaceutical services, or DME for the patient.
POS	Place of Service. This term refers to the physical location where services are provided to a patient (e.g., office, inpatient hospital).
Providers	Service providers; for example, physicians, hospitals, pharmacies, nursing homes, DME suppliers, dentists, optometrists, and chiropractors.
Ranking Codes	Listing services in their order of importance by dates of service and values. Codes are usually ranked by value from the highest charge to the lowest charge.
Referring Physician	The physician who requests an item or service for the beneficiary for which payment may be made under the Medicare program.
Relative Value Unit	A method to calculate fees for services. A unit is translated into a dollar value using a conversion factor or dollar multiplier. Assigned value is generally based on three factors: physician work component, overhead practice expense, and malpractice insurance.
Suspended File Report	A listing of claims that have incorrect information such as a posting error or missing information to process the claim.
Timely Filing Clause	The amount of time allowed by an insurance company for a claim to be submitted for payment from the date of the service.
TOS	Type of Service. This refers to the services provided to a patient (e.g., evaluation and management services, surgery, x-rays).
Unbundling Services	Listing services or procedures as separate billable components. Although this practice may generate more revenue, it is often an incorrect reporting technique that could result in an insurance company auditing a practice or asking for refunds of paid monies.
Unit Count	A means to report the number of times a service was provided on the same date of service to the same patient (e.g., removal of 15 lesions).
UPIN	Unique Personal Identification Number. A number assigned to each covered provider in the Medicare program to identify the provider who performed the billed service(s).

OBJECTIVES

After completing this chapter, readers should be able to:

- Read various forms of documentation to obtain coding information.
- Use a patient information sheet.
- Use physician identification numbers.
- Complete CMS-1500 claim forms.
- Define coding and pricing relationships.

INTRODUCTION

All past work, review, and studies bring the reader to the moment of truth! The coder is now ready to translate all the information into the most important step in medical billing: *claim submission*. Before you begin filing claims, you need to understand the basics of claim submission and what information is required to file either electronic or paper claims.

Even though electronic submission is now the standard for most insurance claims, the information on the paper claim form **(CMS-1500)** is still the basis for all insurance claims. Specific information about the CMS-1500 is covered later in this chapter.

HIPAA AND ELECTRONIC CLAIM SUBMISSION

With the implementation of the **Health Insurance Portability and Accountability Act (HIPAA)** of 1996, new standards now exist for claim submission, and almost all physician practices are included under the HIPAA standards. In the past, offices had the option of filing Medicare claims using a paper claim form (CMS-1500) or filing claims electronically. The new HIPAA regulations require the electronic submission of claims to Medicare if the **provider** is a **covered entity** under HIPAA.

A provider is considered a covered entity if the provider submits electronic transactions to any payer or the provider submits paper claims to Medicare and has 10 or more employees. If a practice meets at least one of these criteria, then the provider must be HIPAA-compliant and must submit claims electronically to Medicare.

A practice is not considered a covered entity if the provider has fewer than 10 employees and submits only paper claims to Medicare or if the provider does not send claims to Medicare, but instead only submits paper claims to other insurance carriers. If a practice meets at least one of these criteria, then the provider is not required to submit electronic claims to Medicare.

 ### CODING TIP

> Commercial insurance carriers might not require claims to be submitted electronically. However, if a practice, third-party biller, or **clearinghouse** does submit any electronic claims to any carrier, those claims must be submitted using HIPAA standards.

HIPAA also affects business associates, such as software billing vendors and third-party billing services that do business with a covered entity. Through agreements with these associates, health care providers are responsible for making sure that these companies produce HIPAA-compliant transactions.

STANDARDS FOR CODE SETS

Code sets are the allowable codes that anyone could use when submitting an insurance claim. To be compliant, all health care organizations must use and accept the code set systems required under HIPAA to document different medical conditions, procedures, or supplies. To comply with the HIPAA regulations, billers and coders must use the following standard code sets:

- For disease, injuries, impairments, and other health-related problems: *International Classification of Diseases, Ninth Revision, Clinical Modification* (ICD-9-CM), Volumes 1 and 2
- For procedures or other actions taken to prevent, diagnose, treat, or manage diseases, injuries, and impairments:
  - Inpatient hospital services: ICD-9-CM, Volume 3: Procedures
  - Dental services: *Code on Dental Procedures and Nomenclature* (CDT-4)
  - Physicians' services: *Current Procedural Terminology, Fourth Edition* (CPT)
  - Other hospital-related services: Healthcare Common Procedure Coding System (HCPCS)
- To report retail pharmacy transactions (pharmaceuticals and biologicals): National Drug Codes

Currently, there is no standard for nonretail pharmacy transactions, including medications and biologicals.

These codes have already become a standard in the health care industry, and use of these codes is now simply *mandated* by HIPAA.

STANDARDS FOR ELECTRONIC CLAIMS

HIPAA standard code sets are used in conjunction with the standards for electronic transactions. When a patient comes in for an office visit, his or her confidential information is put into the practice's management system. Codes are assigned to the diagnosis and related procedures, as discussed in Chapters 1 and 2.

When claims are generated for electronic submission, all the collected data are compiled into a HIPAA standard transaction. Providers, clearinghouses, and insurance payers all recognize these standards. To cover the entire life of the insurance claim, there are eight standard transaction functions for electronic submission, as follows:

- Claims or encounters (equivalent to the paper claims [e.g., CMS-1500, UB-92] and American Dental Association claim forms)
- Claim status inquiry and response
- Eligibility inquiry and response
- Enrollment and disenrollment in a **health plan**
- Referral and authorization advice
- Payment and remittance advisory
- First report of injury
- **Coordination of benefits (COB)**
- Health claims attachment

The 837P

A standard transaction is submitted as an electronic file that has medical data compiled in a specific format. For an electronic insurance claim from a physician's office, this format is called the 837P and replaces the paper claim, or CMS-1500. This is an *electronic* data set and *not* a paper form. The provider *cannot* print out the 837P, unlike the CMS-1500. A crosswalk between the 837P and the CMS-1500 is included in this chapter, after the discussion of the paper claim form (Table 7-1).

TABLE 7-1 Comparison of CMS-1500 and 837P

Ref. No. on CMS	CMS-1500 Box No.	CMS-1500 Box Name	837P Data Element No.	837P Data Element Name
1	1	Government program	66	Identification code qualifier
2	1a	Insured ID number	67	Subscriber's primary identifier
3-6	2	Patient's name (last, first, middle initial)	1035 1036 1037 1039	Patient's last name Patient's first name Patient middle name Patient's name suffix
7	3	Patient's date of birth	1251	Patient's date of birth
8	3	Sex	1068	Patient's gender code
9-12	4	Insured's name (L, F, MI)	1035 1037 1039	Patient's last name Patient's first name Patient's middle name
13-14	5	Patient's address	166 166	Patient's address line Patient's address line
15	5	City	19	Patient's city name
16	5	State	156	Patient's state code
17	5	Zip	116	Patient's postal zone or zip code
18	5	Telephone number	—	**Not used in 837P**
19-20	6	Patient's relationship to insured (e.g., self, spouse)	1069	Individual's relationship code

Continued

TABLE 7-1 Comparison of CMS-1500 and 837P—cont'd

Ref. No. on CMS	CMS-1500 Box No.	CMS-1500 Box Name	837P Data Element No.	837P Data Element Name
21-22	7	Insured's address	166 166	Subscriber's address line Subscriber's address line
23	7	City	19	Subscriber's city name
24	7	State	156	State code
25	7	Zip code	116	Subscriber's postal zone or zip code
26	7	Telephone number	—	**Not used in 837P**
27-31	8	Patient's status (e.g., single, married)	1069	Individual's relationship code
	8	Other	1069	Individual's relationship code
	8	Employed	—	**Not used in 837P**
	8	Full-time student	—	**Not used in 837P**
	8	Part-time student	—	**Not used in 837P**
32-35	9	Other insured's name (L, F, MI)	1035 1036 1037 1039	Other insured's last name Other insured's first name Other insured's middle name Other insured's name suffix
36	9a	Other insured's policy or group number	93	Other insured's group name
37	9b	Other insured's date of birth	1251	Other insured's birth date
38	9b	Other insured's sex	1068	Other insured's gender code
39	9c	Employer's name or school name	—	**Not used in 837P**
40	9d	Insurance plan name or program name	93	Other insured's group name
41	10	Is patient's condition related to:		Related causes information:
42	10a	Employment (current or previous)	1362	Related causes code
43	10b	Auto accident	1362	Related causes code
44	10b	Place (state)	156	Auto accident state or province code
45	10c	Other accident	1362	Related causes code
46	11	Insured's policy group or FECA number		
47	11a	Insured's date of birth	1251	Subscriber's birth date
48	11a	Sex	1068	Subscriber's gender code
49	11b	Employer name or school name	—	**Not used in 837P**
50	11c	Insurance plan name or program name	93	Other insured group name
51	11d	Is there another health benefit plan?	98	Entity identifier code
52-53	12	Patient's or authorized person's signature (and date)	1363	Release of information code
54	13	Insured's or authorized person's signature	1351	Patient's signature source code

TABLE 7-1   Comparison of CMS-1500 and 837P—cont'd

Ref. No. on CMS	CMS-1500 Box No.	CMS-1500 Box Name	837P Data Element No.	837P Data Element Name
55-57	14	Date of current: illness, injury, pregnancy (LMP)	1251 1251 1251	Initial treatment date Accident date LMP
58	15	If patient has had same or similar illness, give first date	1251	Similar illness or symptom date
59	16	Dates patient unable to work in current occupation: From MM/DD/YY	1251	Last worked date
60	16	To MM/DD/YY	1251	Work return date
61	17	Name of referring physician or other source		
62	17a	ID number of referring physician		
63	18	Hospitalization dates related to current services: From MM/DD/YY	1251	Related hospitalization
64	18	To MM/DD/YY	1251	Related hospitalization discharge date
65	19	Reserved for local use		
66	20	Outside lab?		
67	20	$ Charges		
68	21	Diagnosis or nature of illness or injury, 1	1271	Diagnosis code
69	21	2	1271	Diagnosis code
70	21	3	1271	Diagnosis code
71	21	4	1271	Diagnosis code
72	22	Medicaid resubmission code	—	**Not used in 837P**
73	22	Original ref. no.	127	Claim's original reference number
74	23	Prior authorization number	127	Prior authorization number
75	24A	Dates of service: From MM/DD/YY	1251	Order date
76	24A	To MM/DD/YY	1251	Order date
77	24B	Place of service	1331	Place of service code
78	24C	Type of service	—	**Not used in 837P**
79	24D	Procedures, services, or supplies CPT/ HCPCS	234	Procedure code
80-81	24D	Modifier	1339 1339 1339	Procedure modifier Procedure modifier Procedure modifier
82-85	24E	Diagnosis code	1328	Diagnosis code pointer
86	24F	$ charges	782	Line-item charge amount
87	24G	Days or units	380	Service unit count
88	24H	EPSDT family plan	1366	Special program indicator
89	24I	EMG	1073	Emergency indicator
90	24J	COB		

Continued

TABLE 7-1 Comparison of CMS-1500 and 837P—cont'd

Ref. No. on CMS	CMS-1500 Box No.	CMS-1500 Box Name	837P Data Element No.	837P Data Element Name
91	24K	Reserved for local use	127	Rendering provider's secondary identifier
92	25	Federal tax ID number	67	Rendering provider's identifier
93	25	SSN, EIN	66	Identification code qualifier
94	26	Patient's account no.	1028	Patient's account number
95	27	Accept assignment	1359	Medicare assignment code
96	28	Total charge	782	Total claim charge amount
97	29	Amount paid	782	Total claim charge amount
98	30	Balance due	782	Patient's amount paid
99-100	31	Signature of physician or supplier (and date)	1073	Provider or supplier signature indicator
101-106; 108-115	32	Name and address of facility where services were rendered	1035	Laboratory or facility name
			166	Laboratory or facility address line
			166	Laboratory or facility address line
			19	Laboratory or facility city
			156	
			116	Laboratory or facility city
			OR	Laboratory or facility state or province code
			1036	
			1035	Laboratory or facility postal zone or zip code
				Submitter's first name
			1036	Billing provider's last name or organizational name
			166	Billing provider's first name
			166	Billing provider's address line
			19	Billing provider's address line
			156	Billing provider's city name
			116	Billing provider's state or province code
				Billing provider's postal zone or zip code
116-122	33	Physicians' suppliers billing name, address, zip code, & telephone number	10351036	Billing provider's last or organizational name Billing provider's first name
			166	Billing provider's address line
			166	Billing provider's address line
			19	Billing provider's city name
			156	Billing provider's state or province code
			116	Billing provider's postal zone or zip code
123	33	PIN#	127	Billing provider's additional identifier
124	33	GRP#	67	Billing provider's identifier

FECA, Federal Employees' Compensation Act; *LMP,* last menstrual period; *CPT,* Current Procedural Terminology; *HCPCS,* Healthcare Common Procedure Coding System; *EPSDT,* early and periodic screening, diagnosis, and treatment; *EMG,* emergency situation; *COB,* coordination of benefits; *SSN,* Social Security Number; *EIN,* employer identification number.

In a HIPAA-compliant medical office, the practice's management software will assemble and submit the required data when the medical billing clerk files an electronic claim with an insurance carrier. However, anyone directly involved in the claims-processing procedures needs to know the specifics of the 837P.

The 837P contains additional information that is not needed for the CMS-1500. Some examples include the following:

- *Taxonomy codes:* Provider specialty codes assigned to each health care provider. Common taxonomy codes include "general practice 203BG0000Y," "family practice 203BF10100Y," and "nurse practitioner 363L00000N."
- *Patient account number:* To be assigned to every claim.
- *Relationship to patient:* Expanded to 25 different relationships, including indicators such as "grandson," "adopted child," "mother," and "life partner."
- *Facility code value:* Identifies the place of service (**POS**), with at least 29 to choose from, including "office," "ambulance, air, or water," and "end-stage renal disease treatment facility."
- *Patient signature source code*: Indicates how a patient or a subscriber signature was obtained for authorization and how it is retained on file.

SUPPORTING CODE SETS

In addition to the major code sets (ICD-9-CM and CPT/HCPCS), several supporting code sets may be needed for both medical and nonmedical data. Because these supporting code sets are identified by HIPAA standard electronic formats, a coder does not need to know all the specific codes to file the claim. However, rejected claims may have to be corrected if they are returned from a clearinghouse or insurance carrier.

These supporting code sets are made up of required and situational data elements, similar to those on the paper claim form. *Required* refers to data elements that must be used in compliance with an HIPAA standard transaction. *Situational* means that the item depends on the data content or context. For example, an infant's birth weight is obviously situational when submitting a claim for the delivery of an infant.

 CODING TIP

Determining the required and situational data elements specifically for the 837P can be quite complex. New HIPAA-compliant software and experience with claims-processing duties will help you to determine this information.

Grouping of Information for the 837P

Because the 837P is an electronic format and not a paper form, data collected to submit a claim are grouped in levels (Table 7-2). Medical coders and billers will likely not need to know exactly how the data are grouped, but it is helpful to be familiar with the groups when following up on claims. For example, if a payer or clearinghouse rejects a claim for an invalid item at the high level, then the person who processed the claim should know to look for information about a provider, subscriber, or payer.

TABLE 7-2 Data Grouping in 837P Standard Transaction Form

Level	Information
High-Level Information: Applies to the entire claim and reflects data pertaining to the billing provider, subscriber, and patient	Billing/Pay-to-Provider Information Subscriber's/Patient's Information Payer's Information
Claim-Level Information: Applies to the entire claim and all service lines and is applicable to most claims	Claim Information
Specialty Claim—Level Information: Applies to specific claim types	Specialty
Service Line—Level Information: Applies to a specific procedure or service that is rendered and is applicable to most claims	Service Line Information
Specialty Service Line—Level Information: Applies to specific claim types. Required data are required only for the specific claim type.	Specialty Service Line Information
Other Information	Coordination of Benefits Repriced Claim/Line Credit/Debit Information/VAN Tracking

HIPAA Standards—a Look at Format 5010

The Centers for Medicare & Medicaid Services (CMS) is underway with implementation activities to convert from HIPAA Accredited Standards Committee (ASC) X12 version 4010A1 to ASC X12 version 5010 and National Council for Prescription Drug Programs (NCPDP) version 5.1 to NCPDP version D.0.

The Secretary of the Department of Health and Human Services (HHS) has adopted ASC X12 version 5010 and NCPDP version D.0 as the next HIPAA standard for HIPAA-covered transactions. The final rule was published on January 16, 2009. Some of the important dates in the implementation process are:

Effective date of the regulation: March 17, 2009
Level I compliance by: December 31, 2010
Level II compliance by: December 31, 2011
All covered entities have to be fully compliant on: January 1, 2012

Level I compliance means that "a covered entity can demonstrably create and receive compliant transactions, resulting from the compliance of all design/build activities and internal testing."

Level II compliance means that "a covered entity has completed end-to-end testing with each of its trading partners and is able to operate in production mode with the new versions of the standards."

HHS permits dual use of existing standards (4010A1 and 5.1) and the new standards (5010 and D.0) from the March 17, 2009 effective date until the January 1, 2012 compliance date to facilitate testing subject to trading partner agreement.

The CMS Medicare Fee-for-Service schedule is:

Level I: April 1, 2010 through December 31, 2010
Level II: January 1, 2011 through December 31, 2011
Fully compliant on January 1, 2012

CMS has prepared a comparison of the current X12 HIPAA EDI standards (Version 4010/4010A1) with Version 5010 and the NCPDP EDI standards Version 5.1 to D.0. The 4010A1 Implementation Guides and the 5010 Technical Report 3 (TR3) documents served as reference materials during the preparation of the comparison excel spreadsheets. The Data Interchange Standards Association (DISA) holds a copyright on the TR3 documents: Copyright © 2009, Data Interchange Standards Association on behalf of ASC X12. Format © 2009, Washington Publishing Company. All Rights Reserved. The TR3 documents can be obtained at http://store.x12.org/.

CMS is making the side-by-side comparison documents available to interested parties without guarantee and without cost. The documents are available for download in both Microsoft Excel and PDF formats. The comparisons were performed for Medicare Fee-for-Service business use and although they may serve other uses, CMS does not offer to maintain for purposes other than Medicare Fee-for-Service. Maintenance will be performed without notification, as needed to support Medicare Fee-for-Service.

To view side-by-side comparisons of the current program 837P versus the proposed guidelines for 5010, go to the following site:

http://www.cms.gov/ElectronicBillingEDITrans/Downloads/ProfessionalClaim4010A1to5010.pdf

Standard Unique Identifiers

The use of standard unique identifiers will improve the efficiency of electronic claim submission across the health care industry by simplifying administrative systems. Currently, only the Standard Unique Employer Identification Number (EIN) has been approved for use. The EIN is used to identify employers rather than the actual company name. Other identifiers, such as the Standard Unique Health Care Provider Identifier, may be approved in the near future.

CMS-1500 FORM

Despite the implementation of HIPAA, it is still important to understand how to properly complete and submit a claim using the CMS-1500 (Fig. 7-1). When a claim form is not fully or correctly completed, several problems can develop to either delay payment or cause the claim to be denied for payment. Be sure to fill out **all** lines on the claim form. The words "Not Applicable" or "N/A" can be used in certain areas.

Possible Problems with Incomplete Claim Forms

- The carrier may reject the claim for payment.
- Because the physician is liable for the information on the form, he or she could be subject to a fine.
- Line completion will prevent tampering with the information on the form.

A key factor for claim submission is determining whether Medicare is the primary insurance or secondary payer. This information affects how the claim form will be completed for reimbursement.

In addition to correctly entering the patient information, coders and billers need to understand the importance of relating the diagnosis to the procedure in order to avoid delays in payment, obtain maximum reimbursement, and avoid a lengthy appeals process.

FIGURE 7-1 CMS-1500 health insurance claim form. *(Source: U.S. Department of Health and Human Services, Centers for Medicare & Medicaid Services.)*

TEST YOUR KNOWLEDGE   Insurance Claims

1.   Match the term to the definition.

   _____ 1. TOS   A. Unique personal identification number

   _____ 2. EPSDT   B. Health Insurance Portability and Accountability Act

   _____ 3. POS   C. Coordination of benefits

   _____ 4. HIPAA   D. Type of service

   _____ 5. UPIN   E. Place of service

   _____ 6. COB   F. Early and periodic screening, diagnosis, and treatment

2.   List the three problems associated with incomplete claims.

   _____

   _____

   _____

3.   A method used to calculate fees for service is called a _____.

4.   An individual or group plan that provides or pays for the cost of health care is called a

   _____.

5.   A _____ is a listing of claims that have incorrect information.

6.   A _____ is a way to report the number of times a service was provided to a patient.

REVIEW OF CMS-1500

Patient and Insured Information

Item 1: Show the type of health insurance coverage applicable to this claim by checking the appropriate box. For example, if a group insurance claim is being filed, check the group plan box.

1. MEDICARE	MEDICAID	TRICARE CHAMPUS	CHAMPVA	GROUP HEALTH PLAN	FECA BLK LUNG	OTHER
☐ (Medicare #)	☐ (Medicaid #)	☐ (Sponsor's SSN)	☐ (Member ID#)	☐ (SSN or ID)	☐ (SSN)	☐ (ID)

Item 1a: Enter the patient's Medicare Health Insurance Claim Number (HICN), whether Medicare is the primary or secondary payer. This is a required field.

1a. INSURED'S I.D. NUMBER	(For Program in Item 1)
X0123456789	

Item 2: Enter the patient's last name, first name, and middle initial, if any, as shown on the patient's Medicare card. This is a required field.

2. PATIENT'S NAME (Last Name, First Name, Middle Initial)
DOE JR, JOHN, J

Item 3: Enter the patient's eight-digit birth date (MM/DD/CCYY) and sex.

3. PATIENT'S BIRTH DATE			SEX	
MM	DD	YY		
01	01	1987	M [X]	F [ ]

Item 4: List the name of the *primary* insured here. When the insured and the patient are the same, enter the word *same.* If Medicare is primary, leave blank.

Item 5: Enter the patient's mailing address and telephone number. On the first line, enter the street address; the second line, the city and state; the third line, the zip code and telephone number.

5. PATIENT'S ADDRESS (No., Street)	
123 MAIN STREET	
CITY	STATE
ANYTOWN	IL
ZIP CODE	TELEPHONE (Include Area Code)
60610	(312) 5551212

Item 6: Check the appropriate box for the patient's relationship to the insured when item 4 is completed (e.g., wife, child).

6. PATIENT RELATIONSHIP TO INSURED
Self [ ]   Spouse [ ]   Child [X]   Other [ ]

Item 7: Enter the insured's address and telephone number. When the address is the same as the patient's, enter the word *same.* Complete this item only when items 4 and 11 are completed.

Item 8: Check the appropriate box for the patient's marital status and whether he or she is employed or a student.

8. PATIENT STATUS
Single [X]   Married [ ]   Other [ ]
[X] Full-Time Student   [ ] Part-Time Student

Item 9: If item 11d is marked, complete fields 9 and 9a-d; otherwise leave blank. When additional group health coverage exists, enter the enrollee's full last name, first name, and middle initial if it is different from that shown in item 2. If the insured uses a surname suffix (e.g., Jr., Sr.), enter it after the last name and before the first name. Titles (e.g., Sister, Capt., and Dr.) and professional suffixes (e.g., Ph.D., M.D., and Esq.) should not be included with the name. Participating physicians and suppliers must enter information required in item 9 and its subdivision if requested by the beneficiary (patient).

9. OTHER INSURED'S NAME (Last Name, First Name, Middle Initial)
DOE, MARY, A

Item 9a: Enter the policy and/or group number of the Medigap insured preceded by Medigap, MG, or MGAP. Item 9d must be completed if the provider enters a policy and/or group number in item 9a.

a. OTHER INSURED'S POLICY OR GROUP NUMBER
X9876543210

Item 9b: Enter the Medigap insured's eight-digit birth date (MM/DD/CCYY) and sex.

```
b. OTHER INSURED'S DATE OF BIRTH          SEX
    MM    DD    YY
    01    01    1960          M☐      F☒
```

Item 9c: Leave blank if a Medigap payer identification number is entered in item 9d. Otherwise, enter the claims-processing address of the Medigap insurer. Use an abbreviated street address, two-letter postal code, and zip code copied from the Medigap insured's Medigap ID card.

```
c. EMPLOYER'S NAME OR SCHOOL NAME
   COMMUNITY HOSPITAL
```

Item 9d: Enter the nine-digit payer ID number of the Medigap insurer. If no payer ID number exists, then enter the Medigap insurance program or plan name.

```
d. INSURANCE PLAN NAME OR PROGRAM NAME
   XYZ INSURANCE COMPANY
```

```
10. IS PATIENT'S CONDITION RELATED TO:            10. IS PATIENT'S CONDITION RELATED TO:

a. EMPLOYMENT? (Current or Previous)              a. EMPLOYMENT? (Current or Previous)
         ☐ YES    ☐ NO                                     ☐ YES    ☒ NO
b. AUTO ACCIDENT?                                 b. AUTO ACCIDENT?
                    PLACE (State)                                    PLACE (State)
         ☐ YES    ☐ NO                                     ☐ YES    ☒ NO
c. OTHER ACCIDENT?                                c. OTHER ACCIDENT?
         ☐ YES    ☐ NO                                     ☐ YES    ☒ NO
```

Items 10a through 10c: Check *yes* or *no* to indicate whether employment, auto liability, or other accident involvement applies to one or more of the services described in item 24. Enter the state postal code. Any item checked *yes* indicates there may be other insurance primary to Medicare. Identify primary insurance information in item 11.

Item 10d: Use this item exclusively for Medicaid (MCD) information. If the patient is entitled to Medicaid, enter the patient's Medicaid number preceded by MCD.

Item 11 (a-d): Provide information requested concerning primary insurance data. Enter the insured's policy or group number as it appears on the insured's health care ID card and then proceed to items 11a through 11c. Items 4, 6, and 7 must also be completed.

The insured's policy, group, or FECA number refers to the alphanumeric identifier for the health, auto, or other insurance plan coverage. For worker's compensation claims the worker's compensation carrier's alphanumeric identifier would be used.

Item 11a: Enter the insured's eight-digit birth date (MM/DD/CCYY) and sex if different from item 3.

Item 11b: Enter employer's name, if applicable. If there is a change in the insured's insurance status (e.g., retired), enter either a six-digit (MM/DD/YY) or eight-digit retirement date (MM/DD/CCYY) preceded by the word *retired.*

Item 11c: Enter the nine-digit payer ID number of the primary insurer. If no payer ID number exists, then enter the *complete* primary payer's program or plan name. If the primary payer's EOB does not contain the claims-processing address, then record the primary payer's claims-processing address directly on the EOB. This is required if there is insurance primary to Medicare that is indicated in item 11.

```
11. INSURED'S POLICY GROUP OR FECA NUMBER
    A1234
```

Item 11d: This field indicates that the patient has insurance coverage other than the plan indicated in item 1.

d. IS THERE ANOTHER HEALTH BENEFIT PLAN?
[X] YES [ ] NO   *If yes*, return to and complete item 9 a-d.

Item 12: Obtain the signature of the **beneficiary** or authorized representative.

READ BACK OF FORM BEFORE COMPLETING & SIGNING THIS FORM.
12. PATIENT'S OR AUTHORIZED PERSON'S SIGNATURE I authorize the release of any medical or other information necessary to process this claim. I also request payment of government benefits either to myself or to the party who accepts assignment below.

SIGNED___SOF___ DATE_____

Item 13: The signature in this item authorizes payment of mandated Medigap benefits to the participating physician or supplier.

13. INSURED'S OR AUTHORIZED PERSON'S SIGNATURE I authorize payment of medical benefits to the undersigned physician or supplier for services described below.

SIGNED ___SOF___

 CODING TIP

To complete items 12 and 13, you can use the phrase "Signature on File," provided you have a signed authorization from the patient.

Items 14-33: Physician or Supplier Information

Item 14: Enter date of any prior, same, or similar illness (not required by Medicare). For chiropractic services, enter the eight-digit date (MM/DD/CCYY) of the initiation of the course of treatment.

14. DATE OF CURRENT: MM 09 DD 30 YY 2005 ◀ ILLNESS (First symptom) OR INJURY (Accident) OR PREGNANCY(LMP)

Item 15: If the patient has had the same or a similar illness, enter the first date the patient had the same or a similar illness. Enter the date in the six-digit format (MM/DD/YY) or eight-digit format (MM/DD/CCYY). Previous pregnancies are not a similar illness. Leave blank if unknown.

15. IF PATIENT HAS HAD SAME OR SIMILAR ILLNESS. GIVE FIRST DATE MM 09 DD 25 YY 2005

Item 16: If the patient is employed and is unable to work in the current occupation, then enter an eight-digit date (MM/DD/CCYY) or six-digit date (MM/DD/YY) during which the patient is unable to work. An entry in this field may indicate employment-related insurance coverage.

16. DATES PATIENT UNABLE TO WORK IN CURRENT OCCUPATION FROM MM 09 DD 25 YY 2005 TO MM 10 DD 28 YY 2005

Item 17: Enter the name of the **referring** or **ordering physician** if the service or item was ordered or referred by a physician.

| 17a. | 1 B ABC1234567890 |
| 17b. NPI | 0123456789 |

Item 17a: Use the other ID number if the number of the referring provider, ordering provider, or other source should be reported in the shaded area. The qualifier indicating what the number represents should be reported in the qualifier field to the immediate right of 17a. The following is a list of qualifiers:

0B	State License Number
1B	Blue Shield Provider Number
1C	Medicare Provider Number
1D	Medicaid Provider Number
1G	Provider UPIN
1H	CHAMPVA Identification Number
EI	EIN
G2	Provider Commercial Number
LU	Location Number
N5	Provider Plan Network Identification Number
SY	Social Security Number (The Social Security number may not be used for Medicare.)
X5	State Industrial Accident Provider Number
ZZ	Provider Taxonomy

Item 17b: Enter the National Provider Identifier (NPI) of the referring or ordering provider or other source. The NPI refers to the HIPAA NPI. This field allows for the entry of a 10-digit NPI.

Item 18: Enter either an eight-digit (MM/DD/CCYY) or six-digit date (MM/DD/YY) when a medical service is furnished as a result of or subsequent to a related hospitalization. Enter the date of hospitalization relating to the patient's condition. When submitting a claim before the discharge date, use the term "Still in hospital" as the discharge date. This box must be completed before the claim can be processed.

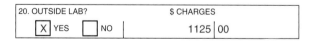

Item 19: Reserved for local use. Please refer to the most current instructions from the applicable public or private payer regarding the use of this field. Some payers ask for certain identifiers in this field. If identifiers are reported in this field, the appropriate qualifiers describing the identifier should be used.

(See item 17a for a list of qualifiers.)

Item 20: Indicate whether an outside laboratory was used and the dollar amount of the charge.

20. OUTSIDE LAB?		$ CHARGES
X YES	☐ NO	1125 00

 Special Note

Item 20 is a required field when billing for diagnostic tests subject to purchase price limitations. A *yes* indicates that another entity provided the service than the one billing for the service. A *no* indicates there were no purchased tests. When *yes* is checked, item 32 must be completed.

Item 21: Enter the patient's diagnosis/condition. With the exception of claims submitted by ambulance suppliers (specialty type 59), all physician and nonphysician specialties (e.g., physician assistant, nurse practitioner, clinical nurse specialist, certified registered nurse anesthetist) must use an ICD-9-CM code number and code to the highest level of specificity. Enter up to four codes in priority order (primary, secondary condition). An independent laboratory must enter a diagnosis only for limited-coverage procedures.

21. DIAGNOSIS OR NATURE OF ILLNESS OR INJURY (Relate Items 1, 2, 3 or 4 to Item 24E by Line)	
1. ⌊ 998 .59	3. ⌊ V18 .0
2. ⌊ 780 .6	4. ⌊ E878 .8

Item 22: Medicaid resubmission codes. These must indicate the original claim reference number assigned by Medicaid. This field is not required by Medicare.

22. MEDICAID RESUBMISSION CODE	ORIGINAL REF. NO.
123	ABC1234567890

Item 23: Enter any of the following: prior authorization number, referral number, mammography precertification number, or Clinical Laboratory Improvement Amendments (CLIA) number, as assigned by the payer for the current service. The prior authorization number refers to the payer-assigned number authorizing the service(s).

23. PRIOR AUTHORIZATION NUMBER
1234567890A

24. A. DATE(S) OF SERVICE						B. PLACE OF SERVICE	C. EMG	D. PROCEDURES, SERVICES, OR SUPPLIES (Explain Unusual Circumstances) CPT/HCPCS | MODIFIER	E. DIAGNOSIS POINTER	F. $ CHARGES	G. DAYS OR UNITS	H. EPSDT Family Plan	I. ID. QUAL.	J. RENDERING PROVIDER ID. #
From			To											
MM	DD	YY	MM	DD	YY									
1													NPI	
2													NPI	
3													NPI	
4													NPI	
5													NPI	
6													NPI	

Item 24A: Enter an eight-digit date (MM/DD/CCYY) for each procedure, service, or supply. When "from" and "to" dates are shown for a series of identical services, enter the number of days or units in column G. This is a required field.

24. A. DATE(S) OF SERVICE					
From			To		
MM	DD	YY	MM	DD	YY
09	30	05	09	30	05

Item 24B: Enter the appropriate POS code(s). Identify the location, using a POS code, for each item used or service performed. This is a required field.

B. PLACE OF SERVICE
11

Item 24C: Originally, this space was used to enter the TOS code. However, because this information is no longer required, the field has been changed to indicate an emergency situation (EMG).

Item 24D: Enter the appropriate CPT or HCPCS codes. When applicable, show modifiers.

Item 24E: Enter the diagnosis code reference number as shown in item 21 to relate the date of service and the procedures performed to the primary diagnosis. Enter only one reference number per line item. When multiple services are performed, enter the primary reference number for each service: 1, 2, 3, or 4. This is a required field.

 CODING TIP

If a situation arises in which two or more diagnoses are required for a procedure code (e.g., Pap smears), the contractor must reference only one of the diagnoses in item 21 1B Blue Shield Provider Number.

Item 24F: Enter the charge amount for each listed service.

Item 24G: Enter the number of days or units. This field is most commonly used for multiple visits, units of supplies, anesthesia minutes, or oxygen volume. If only one service is performed, then the numeral 1 must be entered. For anesthesia, show the elapsed time (minutes) in item 24G. Convert hours into minutes, and enter the total minutes required for this procedure. This field should contain at least one day or unit. Carrier should program their systems to automatically default to a "1" unit when the information in this field is missing to avoid having the form returned as non-processable.

 CODING TIP

Some services require that the actual number or quantity billed be clearly indicated on the claim form (e.g., multiple ostomy or urinary supplies, medication dosages, or allergy testing procedures). When multiple services are provided, enter the actual number provided.

Item 24H: EPSDT. Medicaid-preventive medical examination. This field is not required for Medicare.

Item 24I: This field was originally labeled EMG. However, EMG is now located in 24C. Enter in the shaded area of 24I the qualifier identifying whether the number is a non-NPI. The other ID number of the rendering provider should be reported in 24J, in the shaded area.

Item 24J: Rendering provider ID number. The individual rendering the service should be reported in 24J. The original fields for 24J and 24K have been combined and renumbered as 24J. Enter the non-NPI in the shaded area of the field. Enter the NPI in the unshaded area of the field. This field allows for the entry of 11 characters in the shaded area and the entry of a 10-digit NPI in the unshaded area.

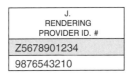

Completing Block 24

Anesthesia Services, when payment is based on 15-minute units:

24. A. DATE(S) OF SERVICE From MM DD YY	To MM DD YY	B. PLACE OF SERVICE	C. EMG	D. PROCEDURES, SERVICES, OR SUPPLIES (Explain Unusual Circumstances) CPT/HCPCS | MODIFIER	E. DIAGNOSIS POINTER	F. $ CHARGES	G. DAYS OR UNITS	H. EPSDT Family Plan	I. ID. QUAL.	J. RENDERING PROVIDER ID. #
				Begin 1245 End 1415 Time 90 minutes					1B	12345678901
10 01 05	10 01 05	22		00770 P2	134	875 00	6	N	NPI	0123456789

Anesthesia Services, when payment is based on actual number of minutes that are used as the unit count:

24. A. DATE(S) OF SERVICE From MM DD YY	To MM DD YY	B. PLACE OF	C. EMG	D. PROCEDURES, SERVICES, OR SUPPLIES (Explain Unusual Circumstances) CPT/HCPCS | MODIFIER	E. DIAGNOSIS POINTER	F. $ CHARGES	G. DAYS OR UNITS	H. EPSDT Family Plan	I. ID. QUAL.	J. RENDERING PROVIDER ID. #
				Begin 1245 End 1415					1B	12345678901
10 01 05	10 01 05	22		00770 P2	134	875 00	90	N	NPI	0123456789

24. A. DATE(S) OF SERVICE From MM DD YY	To MM DD YY	B. PLACE OF SERVICE	C. EMG	D. PROCEDURES, SERVICES, OR SUPPLIES (Explain Unusual Circumstances) CPT/HCPCS | MODIFIER	E. DIAGNOSIS POINTER	F. $ CHARGES	G. DAYS OR UNITS	H. EPSDT Family Plan	I. ID. QUAL.	J. RENDERING PROVIDER ID. #
				N400026064871 Immune Globulin Intravenous			2		1B	12345678901
10 01 05	10 01 05	11		J1563	13	500 00	20	N	NPI	0123456789

Item 25: Enter the provider of service or supplier federal tax employer ID number (EIN) or Social Security number. The participating provider of service or supplier federal tax ID number is required for a mandated Medigap transfer.

25. FEDERAL TAX I.D. NUMBER	SSN EIN
	☐ ☐

Item 26: Enter the patient's account number assigned by the provider's or supplier's accounting system. This field is optional to assist the provider in patient identification. As a service, any account numbers entered here will be returned to the provider.

Item 27: Check the appropriate block to indicate whether the provider of service or supplier accepts assignment of Medicare benefits. If Medigap is indicated in item 9 and Medigap payment authorization is given in item 13, the provider of service or supplier must also be a Medicare-participating provider of service or supplier and must accept assignment of Medicare benefits for all covered charges for all patients.

```
27. ACCEPT ASSIGNMENT?
   For govt. claims, see back
  [ ] YES      [ ] NO
```

 Special Note

The following providers of service/suppliers and claims can only be paid on an assignment basis:
- Clinical diagnostic laboratory services
- Physician services to patients dually entitled to Medicare and Medicaid
- Participating physician/supplier services
- Services of physician assistants, nurse practitioners, clinical nurse specialists, nurse midwives, certified registered nurse anesthetists, clinical psychologists, and clinical social workers
- Ambulatory surgical center (ASC) services for covered ASC procedures
- Home dialysis supplies and equipment paid under method II
- Ambulance services
- Drugs and biologicals
- Simplified billing roster for influenza and pneumococcal vaccines

```
28. TOTAL CHARGE
   $      1125 00
```

Item 28: Enter total charges for the services (i.e., the total of all charges in item 24F).

Item 29: Enter the total amount the patient paid on the covered services only.

Item 30: Enter the difference between item 28 and item 29 (not required by Medicare).

Item 31: Enter the signature of the provider of service or supplier or his/her representative, and either the six-digit date (MM/DD/YY), the eight-digit date (MM/DD/CCYY), or the alphanumeric date (e.g., January 1, 1998) the form was signed.

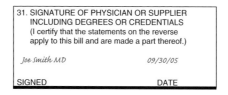

 Special Note

Note: Item 31 is a required field; however, the claim can be processed without it if a physician, supplier, or authorized person's signature is missing, but the signature is on file; if any authorization is attached to the claim; or if the signature field has "Signature on File" or a computer-generated signature.

Item 32: Enter the name, address, city, state, and zip code of the location where the services were rendered. Providers of service (i.e., physicians) must give the supplier's name, address, zip code, and NPI when billing for purchased diagnostic tests. When more than one supplier is used, a separate CMS-1500 claim form should be used to bill for each supplier.

Enter the name and address information in the following format:

First line: Name

Second line: Address

Third line: City, state, and zip code

```
32. SERVICE FACILITY LOCATION INFORMATION
    PHYSICIAN PRACTICE INC
    1234 HEALTHCARE STREET
    ANYTOWN IL 60610-1234
a.  9876543210 (NPI)   b.  1BZ5678901234
```

Item 33: Enter the provider of service or supplier's billing name, address, zip code, and telephone number. This is a required field. Enter the UPIN for the performing provider of service or supplier who is *not* a member of a group practice. This includes the PIN of a billing "absentee" physician in a solo practice. Enter the group PIN for the performing provider of service or supplier who is a member of a group practice. Suppliers billing the **durable medical equipment regional carrier (DMERC)** will use the National Supplier Clearinghouse number in this field.

```
33. BILLING PROVIDER INFO & PH #   ( 314 ) 555-2222
    PHYSICIAN PRACTICE INC
    1234 HEALTHCARE STREET
    ANYTOWN IL 60610-1234
a.  9876543210 (NPI)   b.  1BZ5678901234
```

POS CODES AND DEFINITIONS

Table 7-3 gives the **POS** code set accepted by Medicare and instructions for using it. An asterisk (*) flags new codes. Carriers and DMERCs implement this code set, along with the related system changes required by January 1, 2003. CMS will update this code set on a quarterly basis as needed.

Figures 7-2, 7-3, and 7-4 illustrate the correct completion of claim forms using Medicare as a primary payer or as a secondary payer and as a claim for a typical commercial claim for a hospital visit.

TABLE 7-3   POS Codes and Full Descriptions

POS Code/Name	Payment Rate
01 to 02—Unassigned	—
03—School A facility whose primary purpose is education.	*NF*
04*—Homeless Shelter A facility or location whose primary purpose is to provide temporary housing to homeless individuals (e.g., emergency shelters, individual or family shelters).	*NF*
05*—Indian Health Service Free-Standing Facility A facility or location owned and operated by the Indian Health Service that provides diagnostic, therapeutic (surgical and nonsurgical), and rehabilitation services to American Indians and Alaska Natives who do not require hospitalization.	*Not applicable for adjudication of Medicare claims; systems must recognize for HIPAA*
06*—Indian Health Service Provider-Based Facility A facility or location owned and operated by the Indian Health Service that provides diagnostic, therapeutic (surgical and nonsurgical), and rehabilitation services rendered by or under the supervision of physicians to American Indians and Alaska Natives admitted as inpatients or outpatients.	*Not applicable for adjudication of Medicare claims; systems must recognize for HIPAA*
07*—Tribal 638 Free-Standing Facility A facility or location owned and operated by a federally recognized American Indian or Alaska Native tribe or tribal organization under a 638 agreement that provides diagnostic, therapeutic (surgical and nonsurgical), and rehabilitation services to tribal members who do not require hospitalization.	*Not applicable for adjudication of Medicare claims; systems must recognize for HIPAA*
08*—Tribal 638 Provider-Based Facility A facility or location owned and operated by a federally recognized American Indian or Alaska Native tribe or tribal organization under a 638 agreement that provides diagnostic, therapeutic (surgical and nonsurgical), and rehabilitation services to tribal members admitted as inpatients or outpatients.	*Not applicable for adjudication of Medicare claims; systems must recognize for HIPAA*
09 to 10—Unassigned	—
11—Office Location other than a hospital, SNF, military treatment facility, community health center, state or local public health clinic, or ICF where the health professional routinely provides health examinations, diagnosis, and treatment of illness or injury on an ambulatory basis.	*NF*
12—Home Location other than a hospital or other facility where the patient receives care in a private residence.	*NF*
13*—Assisted Living Facility Congregate residential facility with self-contained living units that provides assessment of each resident's needs and on-site support 24 hours a day, 7 days a week, with the capacity to deliver or arrange for services including some health care and other services.	*NF*
14*—Group Home Congregate residential foster care setting for children and adolescents in state custody that provides some social, health care, and educational support services and that promotes rehabilitation and reintegration of residents into the community.	NF
15*—Mobile Unit A facility or unit that moves from place to place and is equipped to provide preventive, screening, diagnostic, and/or treatment services.	*NF*
16 to 19—Unassigned	—

Continued

TABLE 7-3 POS Codes and Full Descriptions—cont'd

POS Code/Name	Payment Rate
20—Urgent Care Facility Location distinct from a hospital emergency room, an office, or a clinic whose purpose is to diagnose and treat illness or injury for unscheduled, ambulatory patients seeking immediate medical attention.	*NF*
21—Inpatient Hospital A facility other than a psychiatric one that primarily provides diagnostic, therapeutic (surgical and nonsurgical), and rehabilitation services by or under the supervision of physicians to patients admitted for a variety of medical conditions.	*F*
22—Outpatient Hospital A section of a hospital that provides diagnostic, therapeutic (surgical and nonsurgical), and rehabilitation services to sick or injured persons who do not require hospitalization or institutionalization.	*F*
23—Emergency Room, Hospital A section of a hospital where emergency diagnosis and treatment of illness or injury are provided.	*F*
24—ASC A free-standing facility other than a physician's office where surgical and diagnostic services are provided on an ambulatory basis.	*Note: Pay at the NF rate for payable procedures not on the ASC list*
25—Birthing Center A facility other than a hospital's maternity facilities or a physician's office that provides a setting for labor, delivery, and immediate postpartum care as well as immediate care of newborns.	*NF*
26—MTF A medical facility operated by one or more of the Uniformed Services. MTF also refers to certain former U.S. Public Health Service facilities now designated Uniformed Service Treatment Facilities.	*F*
27 to 30—Unassigned	—
31—Skilled Nursing Facility A facility that primarily provides inpatient skilled nursing care and related services to patients who require medical, nursing, or rehabilitative services but does not provide the level of care or treatment available in a hospital.	*F*
32—Nursing Facility A facility that primarily provides to residents skilled nursing care and related services for the rehabilitation of injured, disabled, or sick persons, or, on a regular basis, health-related care services above the level of custodial care to persons who are not developmentally disabled.	*NF*
33—Custodial Care Facility A facility that provides room, board, and other personal assistance services, generally on a long-term basis, and that does not include a medical component.	*NF*
34—Hospice A facility other than a patient's home in which palliative and supportive care for terminally ill patients and their families are provided.	*F*
35 to 40—Unassigned	—
41—Ambulance, Land A land vehicle specifically designed, equipped, and staffed for life-saving and transporting the sick or injured.	*F*

TABLE 7-3   POS Codes and Full Descriptions—cont'd

POS Code/Name	Payment Rate
42—Ambulance, Air or Water An air or water vehicle specifically designed, equipped, and staffed for life-saving and transporting the sick or injured.	*F*
43 to 48—Unassigned	—
49*—Independent Clinic A location not part of a hospital and not described by any other POS code that is organized and operated to provide preventive, diagnostic, therapeutic, rehabilitative, or palliative services to outpatients only.	*NF*
50—Federally Qualified Health Center A facility located in a medically underserved area that provides Medicare beneficiaries preventive primary medical care under the general direction of a physician.	*F*
51—Inpatient Psychiatric Facility A facility that provides inpatient psychiatric services for the diagnosis and treatment of mental illness on a 24-hour basis, by or under the supervision of a physician.	*F*
52—Psychiatric Facility, Partial Hospitalization A facility for the diagnosis and treatment of mental illness that provides a planned therapeutic program for patients who do not require full-time hospitalization, but who need broader programs than are possible from outpatient visits to a hospital-based or hospital-affiliated facility.	*F*
53—CMHC A facility that provides the following services: outpatient services, including specialized outpatient services for children, the elderly, persons who are chronically ill, and residents of the CMHC's service area who have been discharged from inpatient treatment at a mental health facility; 24-hour emergency care services; day treatment, other partial hospitalization services, or psychosocial rehabilitation services; screening for patients being considered for admission to state mental health facilities to determine the appropriateness of such admission; and consultation and education services.	*F*
54—ICF; Developmentally Disabled A facility that primarily provides health-related care and services above the level of custodial care to developmentally disabled individuals but does not provide the level of care or treatment available in a hospital or SNF.	*NF*
55—Residential Substance Abuse Treatment Facility A facility that provides treatment for substance (alcohol and drug) abuse to live-in residents who do not require acute medical care. Services include individual and group therapy and counseling, family counseling, laboratory tests, medications and supplies, psychological testing, and room and board.	*NF*
56—Psychiatric Residential Treatment Center A facility or distinct part of a facility for psychiatric care that provides a total 24-hour therapeutically planned and professionally staffed group environment for living and learning.	*F*
57*—Nonresidential Substance Abuse Treatment Facility A location that provides treatment for substance (alcohol and drug) abuse on an ambulatory basis. Services include individual and group therapy and counseling, family counseling, laboratory tests, drugs and supplies, and psychological testing.	*NF*
58 to 59—Unassigned	—

Continued

TABLE 7-3   POS Codes and Full Descriptions—cont'd

POS Code/Name	Payment Rate
60—Mass Immunization Center A location where providers administer pneumococcal pneumonia and influenza virus vaccinations and submit these services using electronic media claims, paper claims, or the roster billing method. This generally takes place in a mass immunization setting, such as a public health center, pharmacy, or mall but may include a physician office setting.	*NF*
61—Comprehensive Inpatient Rehabilitation Facility A facility that provides comprehensive rehabilitation services under the supervision of a physician to inpatients with physical disabilities. Services include physical therapy, occupational therapy, speech pathology, social or psychological services, and orthotic and prosthetic services.	*F*
62—Comprehensive Outpatient Rehabilitation Facility A facility that provides comprehensive rehabilitation services under the supervision of a physician to outpatients with physical disabilities. Services include physical therapy, occupational therapy, and speech pathology services.	*NF*
63 to 64—Unassigned	—
65—End-Stage Renal Disease Treatment Facility A facility other than a hospital that provides dialysis treatment, maintenance, and/or training to patients or caregivers on an ambulatory or home care basis.	*NF*
66 to 70—Unassigned	—
71—State or Local Public Health Clinic A facility maintained by either state or local health departments that provide ambulatory primary medical care under the general direction of a physician.	*NF*
72—Rural Health Clinic A certified facility that is located in a rural, medically underserved area that provides ambulatory primary medical care under the general direction of a physician.	*NF*
73 to 80—Unassigned	—
81—Independent Laboratory A laboratory certified to perform diagnostic and clinical tests independent of an institution or a physician's office.	*NF*
82 to 98—Unassigned	—
99—Other Place of Service Other place of service not identified previously.	*NF*

POS, Place of service; *NF*, nonfacility; *HIPAA*, Health Insurance Portability and Accountability Act; *SNF*, skilled nursing facility; *ICF*, intermediate care facility; *F*, facility; *ASC*, ambulatory surgical center; *MTF*, military treatment facility; *CMHC*, Community Mental Health Center.
*New code or code not previously implemented by Medicare.

UNIT COUNTS

During the review of the claim form, the phrase **unit count** was mentioned as it relates to line 24G. Unit counts are used to indicate concurrent or consecutive care. This occurs when the patient is seen for the same service for several days in a row. In consecutive care, the coder may only bill treatment for days when there has been no interruption of care and the same type of service was provided each time to the patient. The unit count column will alert the carrier that the charges are a total of units (days) multiplied by the daily rate or charge for the service (e.g., 5 days × $15 = $75) (Fig. 7-5).

CARRIER

1500
HEALTH INSURANCE CLAIM FORM
APPROVED BY NATIONAL UNIFORM CLAIM COMMITTEE 08/05

[ ] [ ] PICA   PICA [ ] [ ]

| 1. MEDICARE [X] (Medicare #) MEDICAID [ ] (Medicaid #) TRICARE CHAMPUS [ ] (Sponsor's SSN) CHAMPVA [ ] (Member ID#) GROUP HEALTH PLAN [ ] (SSN or ID) FECA BLK LUNG [ ] (SSN) OTHER [ ] (ID) | 1a. INSURED'S I.D. NUMBER   (For Program in Item 1) 234-56-7890-A |

2. PATIENT'S NAME (Last Name, First Name, Middle Initial)
SMITH, MARY JANE

3. PATIENT'S BIRTH DATE MM 02 DD 15 YY 30   SEX M [ ] F [X]

4. INSURED'S NAME (Last Name, First Name, Middle Initial)
SAME AS 2

5. PATIENT'S ADDRESS (No., Street)
2221 EVERGREEN ST. APT 2-G

6. PATIENT RELATIONSHIP TO INSURED
Self [X] Spouse [ ] Child [ ] Other [ ]

7. INSURED'S ADDRESS (No., Street)
SAME AS 5

CITY ST. LOUIS   STATE MO

8. PATIENT STATUS
Single [ ] Married [X] Other [ ]

CITY   STATE

ZIP CODE 63131   TELEPHONE (Include Area Code) (314) 222-5566

Employed [ ] Full-Time Student [ ] Part-Time Student [ ]

ZIP CODE   TELEPHONE (Include Area Code) (   )

9. OTHER INSURED'S NAME (Last Name, First Name, Middle Initial)
SMITH, MARY JANE

10. IS PATIENT'S CONDITION RELATED TO:

11. INSURED'S POLICY GROUP OR FECA NUMBER
NONE

a. OTHER INSURED'S POLICY OR GROUP NUMBER
T04-12345678

a. EMPLOYMENT? (Current or Previous)
[ ] YES [X] NO

a. INSURED'S DATE OF BIRTH MM DD YY   SEX M [ ] F [ ]

b. OTHER INSURED'S DATE OF BIRTH MM 02 DD 15 YY 30   SEX M [ ] F [X]

b. AUTO ACCIDENT? PLACE (State)
[ ] YES [X] NO

b. EMPLOYER'S NAME OR SCHOOL NAME

c. EMPLOYER'S NAME OR SCHOOL NAME

c. OTHER ACCIDENT?
[ ] YES [X] NO

c. INSURANCE PLAN NAME OR PROGRAM NAME

d. INSURANCE PLAN NAME OR PROGRAM NAME
BLUE CROSS BLUE SHIELD OF MO

10d. RESERVED FOR LOCAL USE

d. IS THERE ANOTHER HEALTH BENEFIT PLAN?
[ ] YES [ ] NO   If yes, return to and complete item 9 a-d.

READ BACK OF FORM BEFORE COMPLETING & SIGNING THIS FORM.
12. PATIENT'S OR AUTHORIZED PERSON'S SIGNATURE I authorize the release of any medical or other information necessary to process this claim. I also request payment of government benefits either to myself or to the party who accepts assignment below.

SIGNED SIGNATURE ON FILE   DATE

13. INSURED'S OR AUTHORIZED PERSON'S SIGNATURE I authorize payment of medical benefits to the undersigned physician or supplier for services described below.

SIGNED SIGNATURE ON FILE

PATIENT AND INSURED INFORMATION

14. DATE OF CURRENT: MM 01 DD 02 YY 9X   ◄ ILLNESS (First symptom) OR INJURY (Accident) OR PREGNANCY(LMP)

15. IF PATIENT HAS HAD SAME OR SIMILAR ILLNESS. GIVE FIRST DATE MM DD YY

16. DATES PATIENT UNABLE TO WORK IN CURRENT OCCUPATION
FROM MM DD YY   TO MM DD YY

17. NAME OF REFERRING PROVIDER OR OTHER SOURCE

17a.
17b. NPI

18. HOSPITALIZATION DATES RELATED TO CURRENT SERVICES
FROM MM DD YY   TO MM DD YY

19. RESERVED FOR LOCAL USE

20. OUTSIDE LAB? [ ] YES [ ] NO $ CHARGES

21. DIAGNOSIS OR NATURE OF ILLNESS OR INJURY (Relate Items 1, 2, 3 or 4 to Item 24E by Line)
1. [379 . 23]   3. [___ . ___]
2. [___ . ___]   4. [___ . ___]

22. MEDICAID RESUBMISSION CODE   ORIGINAL REF. NO.

23. PRIOR AUTHORIZATION NUMBER

24. A. DATE(S) OF SERVICE From MM DD YY To MM DD YY	B. PLACE OF SERVICE	C. EMG	D. PROCEDURES, SERVICES, OR SUPPLIES (Explain Unusual Circumstances) CPT/HCPCS	MODIFIER	E. DIAGNOSIS POINTER	F. $ CHARGES	G. DAYS OR UNITS	H. EPSDT Family Plan	I. ID. QUAL.	J. RENDERING PROVIDER ID. #
1	01 10 XX	21	1	99221		1	35 00	1		NPI	
2										NPI	
3										NPI	
4										NPI	
5										NPI	
6										NPI	

25. FEDERAL TAX I.D. NUMBER 43-00000   SSN [ ] EIN [X]

26. PATIENT'S ACCOUNT NO. 12345

27. ACCEPT ASSIGNMENT? (For govt. claims, see back) [X] YES [ ] NO

28. TOTAL CHARGE $ 35 00

29. AMOUNT PAID $

30. BALANCE DUE $ 35 00

31. SIGNATURE OF PHYSICIAN OR SUPPLIER INCLUDING DEGREES OR CREDENTIALS (I certify that the statements on the reverse apply to this bill and are made a part thereof.)
A GOOD SURGEON, MD   01-12-XX
SIGNED   DATE

32. SERVICE FACILITY LOCATION INFORMATION

a. NPI   b.

33. BILLING PROVIDER INFO & PH # (   )
A GOOD CLINIC
123 HOPE STREET
ST. LOUIS, MO 63124

a. NPI   b. 00012345

PHYSICIAN OR SUPPLIER INFORMATION

NUCC Instruction Manual available at: www.nucc.org   APPROVED OMB-0938-0999 FORM CMS-1500 (08/05)

FIGURE 7-2 Medicare primary payer claim. *(Source of CMS-1500 form: U.S. Department of Health and Human Services, Centers for Medicare & Medicaid Services.)*

1500

HEALTH INSURANCE CLAIM FORM

APPROVED BY NATIONAL UNIFORM CLAIM COMMITTEE 08/05

PICA PICA

CARRIER

1. MEDICARE [X] (Medicare #) MEDICAID [ ] (Medicaid #) TRICARE CHAMPUS [ ] (Sponsor's SSN) CHAMPVA [ ] (Member ID#) GROUP HEALTH PLAN [ ] (SSN or ID) FECA BLK LUNG [ ] (SSN) OTHER [ ] (ID)

1a. INSURED'S I.D. NUMBER (For Program in Item 1): 234-56-7890-A

2. PATIENT'S NAME (Last Name, First Name, Middle Initial): SMITH, MARY JANE

3. PATIENT'S BIRTH DATE MM DD YY: 02 15 65 SEX M [ ] F [X]

4. INSURED'S NAME (Last Name, First Name, Middle Initial): SMITH, JAMES C

5. PATIENT'S ADDRESS (No., Street): 2221 EVERGREEN ST. APT 2-G

6. PATIENT RELATIONSHIP TO INSURED: Self [ ] Spouse [X] Child [ ] Other [ ]

7. INSURED'S ADDRESS (No., Street): SAME AS 5

CITY: ST. LOUIS STATE: MO

8. PATIENT STATUS: Single [ ] Married [X] Other [ ]; Employed [ ] Full-Time Student [ ] Part-Time Student [ ]

CITY STATE

ZIP CODE: 63131 TELEPHONE (Include Area Code): (314) 222-5566

ZIP CODE TELEPHONE (Include Area Code) ( )

9. OTHER INSURED'S NAME (Last Name, First Name, Middle Initial): PATIENT

10. IS PATIENT'S CONDITION RELATED TO:

11. INSURED'S POLICY GROUP OR FECA NUMBER: ABC-12345678

a. OTHER INSURED'S POLICY OR GROUP NUMBER

a. EMPLOYMENT? (Current or Previous) [ ] YES [X] NO

a. INSURED'S DATE OF BIRTH MM DD YY: 01 05 60 SEX M [X] F [ ]

b. OTHER INSURED'S DATE OF BIRTH MM DD YY SEX M [ ] F [ ]

b. AUTO ACCIDENT? [ ] YES [X] NO PLACE (State)

b. EMPLOYER'S NAME OR SCHOOL NAME: GENERAL MILK COPORATION

c. EMPLOYER'S NAME OR SCHOOL NAME

c. OTHER ACCIDENT? [ ] YES [X] NO

c. INSURANCE PLAN NAME OR PROGRAM NAME: BLUE CROSS BLUE SHIELD OF MO

d. INSURANCE PLAN NAME OR PROGRAM NAME

10d. RESERVED FOR LOCAL USE

d. IS THERE ANOTHER HEALTH BENEFIT PLAN? [ ] YES [ ] NO *If yes*, return to and complete item 9 a-d.

READ BACK OF FORM BEFORE COMPLETING & SIGNING THIS FORM.

12. PATIENT'S OR AUTHORIZED PERSON'S SIGNATURE I authorize the release of any medical or other information necessary to process this claim. I also request payment of government benefits either to myself or to the party who accepts assignment below.

SIGNED SIGNATURE ON FILE DATE

13. INSURED'S OR AUTHORIZED PERSON'S SIGNATURE I authorize payment of medical benefits to the undersigned physician or supplier for services described below.

SIGNED MARY JANE SMITH

PATIENT AND INSURED INFORMATION

14. DATE OF CURRENT: MM DD YY 01 02 9X ◀ ILLNESS (First symptom) OR INJURY (Accident) OR PREGNANCY(LMP)

15. IF PATIENT HAS HAD SAME OR SIMILAR ILLNESS. GIVE FIRST DATE MM DD YY

16. DATES PATIENT UNABLE TO WORK IN CURRENT OCCUPATION MM DD YY FROM TO MM DD YY

17. NAME OF REFERRING PROVIDER OR OTHER SOURCE: JOHN GREEN MD

17a. 000000000

17b. NPI

18. HOSPITALIZATION DATES RELATED TO CURRENT SERVICES MM DD YY FROM TO MM DD YY

19. RESERVED FOR LOCAL USE

20. OUTSIDE LAB? [ ] YES [ ] NO $ CHARGES

21. DIAGNOSIS OR NATURE OF ILLNESS OR INJURY (Relate Items 1, 2, 3 or 4 to Item 24E by Line)

1. 379 . 23
2. ___ . ___
3. ___ . ___
4. ___ . ___

22. MEDICAID RESUBMISSION CODE ORIGINAL REF. NO.

23. PRIOR AUTHORIZATION NUMBER

24.

	A. DATE(S) OF SERVICE From MM DD YY	To MM DD YY	B. PLACE OF SERVICE	C. EMG	D. PROCEDURES, SERVICES, OR SUPPLIES (Explain Unusual Circumstances) CPT/HCPCS	MODIFIER	E. DIAGNOSIS POINTER	F. $ CHARGES	G. DAYS OR UNITS	H. EPSDT Family Plan	I. ID. QUAL.	J. RENDERING PROVIDER ID. #
1	01 10 XX		11	1	99213		1	35 00			NPI	
2											NPI	
3											NPI	
4											NPI	
5											NPI	
6											NPI	

25. FEDERAL TAX I.D. NUMBER: 43-00000 SSN [ ] EIN [X]

26. PATIENT'S ACCOUNT NO.: 12345

27. ACCEPT ASSIGNMENT? (For govt. claims, see back) [X] YES [ ] NO

28. TOTAL CHARGE $ 35 00

29. AMOUNT PAID $

30. BALANCE DUE $ 35 00

31. SIGNATURE OF PHYSICIAN OR SUPPLIER INCLUDING DEGREES OR CREDENTIALS (I certify that the statements on the reverse apply to this bill and are made a part thereof.)

A GOOD SURGEON, MD 01-12-XX

SIGNED DATE

32. SERVICE FACILITY LOCATION INFORMATION

a. NPI b.

33. BILLING PROVIDER INFO & PH # (314) 000-0000

A GOOD CLINIC
123 HOPE STREET
ST. LOUIS, MO 63124

a. NPI b. 00012345

PHYSICIAN OR SUPPLIER INFORMATION

NUCC Instruction Manual available at: www.nucc.org APPROVED OMB-0938-0999 FORM CMS-1500 (08/05)

FIGURE 7-3 Medicare secondary payer claim. *(Source of CMS-1500 form: U.S. Department of Health and Human Services, Centers for Medicare & Medicaid Services.)*

1500

HEALTH INSURANCE CLAIM FORM

APPROVED BY NATIONAL UNIFORM CLAIM COMMITTEE 08/05

PICA   PICA

1. MEDICARE (Medicare #)   MEDICAID (Medicaid #)   TRICARE CHAMPUS (Sponsor's SSN)   CHAMPVA (Member ID#)   GROUP HEALTH PLAN (SSN or ID) [X]   FECA BLK LUNG (SSN)   OTHER (ID)

1a. INSURED'S I.D. NUMBER (For Program in Item 1)
234-56-7890

2. PATIENT'S NAME (Last Name, First Name, Middle Initial)
SMITH, MARY JANE

3. PATIENT'S BIRTH DATE: MM 02 | DD 15 | YY 65   SEX: M [ ] F [X]

4. INSURED'S NAME (Last Name, First Name, Middle Initial)
SMITH, JAMES C

5. PATIENT'S ADDRESS (No., Street)
2221 EVERGREEN ST. APT 2-G

6. PATIENT RELATIONSHIP TO INSURED
Self [ ] Spouse [X] Child [ ] Other [ ]

7. INSURED'S ADDRESS (No., Street)
SAME AS 5

CITY: ST. LOUIS   STATE: MO

8. PATIENT STATUS
Single [ ] Married [X] Other [ ]
Employed [ ] Full-Time Student [ ] Part-Time Student [ ]

CITY   STATE

ZIP CODE: 63131   TELEPHONE (Include Area Code): (314) 222-5566

ZIP CODE   TELEPHONE (Include Area Code): ( )

9. OTHER INSURED'S NAME (Last Name, First Name, Middle Initial)

10. IS PATIENT'S CONDITION RELATED TO:

11. INSURED'S POLICY GROUP OR FECA NUMBER
234-56-7890

a. OTHER INSURED'S POLICY OR GROUP NUMBER

a. EMPLOYMENT? (Current or Previous) YES [ ] NO [X]

a. INSURED'S DATE OF BIRTH: MM 01 | DD 05 | YY 60   SEX: M [X] F [ ]

b. OTHER INSURED'S DATE OF BIRTH: MM DD YY   SEX: M [ ] F [ ]

b. AUTO ACCIDENT? YES [ ] NO [X]   PLACE (State)

b. EMPLOYER'S NAME OR SCHOOL NAME
GENERAL MILK COPORATION

c. EMPLOYER'S NAME OR SCHOOL NAME

c. OTHER ACCIDENT? YES [ ] NO [X]

c. INSURANCE PLAN NAME OR PROGRAM NAME
INSURANCE OF AMERICA CORP

d. INSURANCE PLAN NAME OR PROGRAM NAME

10d. RESERVED FOR LOCAL USE

d. IS THERE ANOTHER HEALTH BENEFIT PLAN?
YES [ ] NO [X]   *If yes,* return to and complete item 9 a-d.

READ BACK OF FORM BEFORE COMPLETING & SIGNING THIS FORM.

12. PATIENT'S OR AUTHORIZED PERSON'S SIGNATURE I authorize the release of any medical or other information necessary to process this claim. I also request payment of government benefits either to myself or to the party who accepts assignment below.
SIGNED MARY JANE SMITH   DATE

13. INSURED'S OR AUTHORIZED PERSON'S SIGNATURE I authorize payment of medical benefits to the undersigned physician or supplier for services described below.
SIGNED MARY JANE SMITH

14. DATE OF CURRENT: MM 01 | DD 02 | YY 9X   ILLNESS (First symptom) OR INJURY (Accident) OR PREGNANCY(LMP)

15. IF PATIENT HAS HAD SAME OR SIMILAR ILLNESS. GIVE FIRST DATE MM | DD | YY

16. DATES PATIENT UNABLE TO WORK IN CURRENT OCCUPATION: FROM MM | DD | YY   TO MM | DD | YY

17. NAME OF REFERRING PROVIDER OR OTHER SOURCE
17a.
17b. NPI

18. HOSPITALIZATION DATES RELATED TO CURRENT SERVICES: FROM MM 01 | DD 10 | YY 9X   TO MM 01 | DD 15 | YY 9X

19. RESERVED FOR LOCAL USE

20. OUTSIDE LAB? YES [ ] NO [ ] $ CHARGES

21. DIAGNOSIS OR NATURE OF ILLNESS OR INJURY (Relate Items 1, 2, 3 or 4 to Item 24E by Line)
1. 250 . 91
2.
3.
4.

22. MEDICAID RESUBMISSION CODE   ORIGINAL REF. NO.

23. PRIOR AUTHORIZATION NUMBER

24. A. DATE(S) OF SERVICE From MM DD YY	To MM DD YY	B. PLACE OF SERVICE	C. EMG	D. PROCEDURES, SERVICES, OR SUPPLIES (Explain Unusual Circumstances) CPT/HCPCS	MODIFIER	E. DIAGNOSIS POINTER	F. $ CHARGES	G. DAYS OR UNITS	H. EPSDT Family Plan	I. ID. QUAL.	J. RENDERING PROVIDER ID. #
1	01 10 XX		21	1	99221		1	100 00	1		NPI	
2	01 11 XX 01 13 XX		21	1	99231		1	60 00	3		NPI	
3	01 14 XX		21	1	99232		1	75 00	1		NPI	
4	01 15 XX		21	1	99238		1	60 00	1		NPI	
5											NPI	
6											NPI	

25. FEDERAL TAX I.D. NUMBER   SSN EIN [X]
43-00000

26. PATIENT'S ACCOUNT NO.
12345

27. ACCEPT ASSIGNMENT? (For govt. claims, see back) YES [X] NO [ ]

28. TOTAL CHARGE $ 245 00

29. AMOUNT PAID $

30. BALANCE DUE $ 245 00

31. SIGNATURE OF PHYSICIAN OR SUPPLIER INCLUDING DEGREES OR CREDENTIALS (I certify that the statements on the reverse apply to this bill and are made a part thereof.)
A GOOD SURGEON, MD   01-20-XX
SIGNED   DATE

32. SERVICE FACILITY LOCATION INFORMATION
WONDERFUL HOSPITAL
2 GET WELL
ST. LOUIS, MO 63111
a. NPI   b.

33. BILLING PROVIDER INFO & PH # (314) 000-0000
A GOOD CLINIC
123 HOPE STREET
ST. LOUIS, MO 63124
a. NPI   b.

NUCC Instruction Manual available at: www.nucc.org   APPROVED OMB-0938-0999 FORM CMS-1500 (08/05)

CARRIER — PATIENT AND INSURED INFORMATION — PHYSICIAN OR SUPPLIER INFORMATION

FIGURE 7-4 Commercial insurance—hospital visit. *(Source of CMS-1500 form: U.S. Department of Health and Human Services, Centers for Medicare & Medicaid Services.)*

Dx Code: 702.1

24.	A						B	C	D		E	F	G
	DATE(S) OF SERVICE						Place of Service	TYPE of Service	PROCEDURES, SERVICES, OR SUPPLIES (Explain Unusual Circumstances)		DIAGNOSIS CODE	$ CHARGES	DAYS OR UNITS
	From			To					CPT/HCPCS	MODIFIER			
	MM	DD	YY	MM	DD	YY							
1	01	01	XX				11	2	17000		1	$50 00	1
2	01	11	XX				11	2	17003		1	$100 00	2
3													
4	01	01	XX	01	04	XX	21	1	99231		1	$400 00	4

FIGURE 7-5 CMS-1500 unit counts. *(Source of CMS-1500 form: U.S. Department of Health and Human Services, Centers for Medicare & Medicaid Services.)*

Unit counts are also used for multiple procedures (e.g., skin lesions). The use of the units will allow the carrier to reimburse the office based on the actual number of lesions removed (e.g., 15 lesions × $10 = $150).

In psychiatry, unit counts are used to show time increments for the time codes. Again, the purpose is to alert the carrier to the multiplier in order to receive correct reimbursement.

BILLING MULTIPLE SURGERIES

Insurance companies have varying payment schedules and guidelines for payments. When billing procedures whereby separate incisions are made to perform the surgery, a general rule of thumb is to bill the services as separate procedures (Fig. 7-6).

Medicare guidelines are to pay 100% of the allowed amount for the primary procedure, 50% for the secondary procedure, and 25% for subsequent procedures. Commercial carriers may reimburse 70% to 100% for separate procedures through separate incisions. It could be to the advantage of the practice to bill these procedures at the full charge and allow the carrier to make any adjustments based on its reimbursement policy.

Assistance Fees

Assistance fees are allowed for many complicated procedures (Fig. 7-7). Use of modifier -80 does not identify a service as being a reduced-for-assistance fee; rather, it is an indication that a surgical assistant was required for a procedure. Carriers typically pay 20% to 35% of the allowed amount for the assistance fee. In the case of Medicare, payment is typically 16% of the allowed amount. For example, if the full fee for code 12007, Simple repair of superficial wound, is $150, then the payable amount for the assistance fee would be $24 by Medicare standards or $30 for a commercial payer.

 CODING TIP

Reducing fees results in lost revenue. Bill the full fee. Modifiers do not show fee reductions, and payment is based on the lower of the billed amount or the carrier's allowed amount.

The information for the claim should indicate the ICD-9-CM code and the CPT code.

EXAMPLE	
881.00	Open wound forearm
12007-80	Simple repair superficial wound with surgical assistant

FIGURE 7-6 Coding bilateral procedures. *(Source of CMS-1500 form: U.S. Department of Health and Human Services, Centers for Medicare & Medicaid Services.)*

FIGURE 7-7 CMS-1500 assistance fee. *(Source of CMS-1500 form: U.S. Department of Health and Human Services, Centers for Medicare & Medicaid Services.)*

727.1   = Bunion
28292   = McBride procedure
28292-50 = McBride procedure with bilateral modifier

FIGURE 7-8 Bilateral procedure.

Bilateral Procedures

Bilateral procedures differ from multiple or separate procedure codes. A bilateral procedure involves similar anatomical sites on both sides of the body (e.g., right arm, left arm) (Fig. 7-8).

Bilateral procedures, as a general rule, are not subject to the reductions applied to multiple-procedure codes. Bilateral procedures should not be reduced when billing a carrier unless the coder has checked with the carrier to determine benefit payments for a specific procedure.

When coding bilateral procedures, the coder should contact the carrier to determine whether the modifier -50 or the code followed by RT (right) and LT (left) to distinguish between the service areas should be used. This will aid reimbursement and help ensure correct payment of the claim. In the case of Medicare, reducing the secondary procedure for a bilateral procedure could result in incorrect profile data.

Additional Codes

In discussing surgical coding, we must include a small, select number of codes that indicate the number count of an item for surgical removal (Fig. 7-9). These codes are found primarily in the integumentary section of the CPT manual.

21. DIAGNOSIS OR NATURE OF ILLNESS OR INJURY. (RELATE ITEMS 1,2,3 OR 4 TO ITEM 24E BY LINE)								22. MEDICAID RESUBMISSION CODE		

1.| __702.1__   3.|____.__

                                     22. MEDICAID RESUBMISSION CODE |

2.|____.__   4.|____.__

23. PRIOR AUTHORIZATION NUMBER

24.	A						B	C	D		E	F	G	H
	DATE(S) OF SERVICE						Place of Service	TYPE of Service	PROCEDURES, SERVICES, OR SUPPLIES (Explain Unusual Circumstances)		DIAGNOSIS CODE	$ CHARGES	DAYS OR UNITS	EPSDT Family Plan
	From			To					CPT/HCPCS	MODIFIER				
	MM	DD	YY	MM	DD	YY								
1	00	00	00				3	2	17000				1	
2	00	00	00				3	2	17003				13	
3	00	00	00				3	2						

702.1: Actinic keratosis
17000: Removal of first lesion
17001: Removal of second and third lesions
17002: Removal of fourth through twentieth lesions

FIGURE 7-9 Addition codes with unit counts. *(Source of CMS-1500 form: U.S. Department of Health and Human Services, Centers for Medicare & Medicaid Services.)*

The 17000 code series will be used to demonstrate additional count codes.

E X A M P L E

A patient presented to the office for the removal of 14 premalignant lesions from the face.

Correct coding: 17000   First lesion (1)

                     17003   Second through 14th lesions (13)

The total equals 14 lesions removed.

To correctly file such a claim, the coder needs to put the number of lesions in the unit section count of the claim form (item 24G). It is also advisable to list the count in the descriptive part of the claim. By doing this, the coder ensures that the person processing the claim will obtain the correct count. In the descriptive area for ICD-9-CM, the coder should list the total number of lesions to help the claims processor correctly adjudicate the claim.

On the basis of the information regarding claims forms and coding techniques, you are now ready to complete insurance claims with the use of charted information. Please refer to Chapter 10: Putting It All Together, which will help you place claim submissions into perspective and promote a better understanding of the location of the codes and applications. (Use the blank CMS-1500 forms at the end of Chapter 10 to complete these exercises.)

Accounts Receivable

CHAPTER OUTLINE

Introduction
> Pegboard Systems
> Computer Systems

Insurance Participation
> Common Claim Errors
> Payment Responsibility
> Collection Policies

Collection Letters
Bad Debt Collection
General Claims Information

Medicare and Reimbursement
> Fee Schedule
> Payments

Allowed Amounts
> Medicare Payment Formulas

Third-Party Payers
> Usual, Customary, and
> Reasonable Payment Plans

Medicaid

KEY TERMS

Term	Definition
Accepting Assignment	The provider of service agrees or is willing to accept as payment the amount allowed/approved by an insurance company as the maximum amount that will be paid for the claim. After the patient has met the annual deductible, the insurance will pay a percentage of the approved/allowed amount and the patient will have a co-payment.
Accounts Payable	Amounts owed by the practice to creditors for property, supplies, equipment, etc.
Accounts Receivable	A/R. The total amount of money owed to the physician for professional services provided to a patient.
Adjustment	The amount corrected on a patient ledger due to an error or the difference in the amount billed by a practice and the amount allowed by the insurance company for payment of a claim.
Aging Accounts	Analysis of accounts receivable that indicate delinquency of 60, 90, to 120 days.
Appeal	A request sent to an insurance company or other payer asking that a submitted claim be reconsidered for payment or processing.
Assignment	Authorization by a policy holder to allow a third-party payer to pay benefits to a heath care provider.
Collection Ratio	The relationship between the amount of money owed and the amount of money collected.
Conversion Factor	The dollar amount determined by dividing the actual charge of a service or procedure by a relative value.
Co-payment	The amount the insured has to pay toward the amount allowed by the insurance company for services.
Cycle Billing	Breaking the account receivable amounts into portions for billing at a specific date of the month.
Deductible	The amount the insured must pay before the insurance company will begin benefit payments.
Dun/Dunning	A request or message to remind a patient that the account is over due or delinquent.
EOB	Explanation of Benefits. Form accompanying an insurance remittance with a breakdown and explanation of payments for a claim. Also referred to as a remittance advisory (RA).
EOMB	Explanation of Medicare Benefits. Form accompanying an insurance remittance with a breakdown and explanation of payments for a claim.
Fee Schedule	An established price set by a medical practice for professional services.
Inquiry	Checking or tracing a claim sent to an insurance company to determine payment or processing status.

229

Ledger Card	A record to track patient charges, payments, adjustments, and balances due.
Limiting Charge	Typically applies to Medicare reimbursement. This is the absolute maximum fee a physician may charge a Medicare patient when not accepting assignment on the claim. This fee is set by the Centers for Medicare & Medicaid Services (CMS).
Open Account	Accounts that are subject to charges from time to time.
Posting	A process of transferring account information from a journal to a ledger.
Professional Courtesy	A discount or fee exception given to a patient at the discretion of the physician.
Profile	A list of CPT codes used by a physician with a corresponding fee that is usually calculated and maintained by a third-party payer.
RBRVS	Resource-Based Relative Value Scale. A system of assigning values to CPT codes developed for Medicare to determine reimbursement amounts for services.
Relative Value Unit (RVU)	A method to calculate fees for services. A unit is translated into a dollar value using a conversion factor or dollar multiplier. The assigned value is generally based on three factors: physician work component, overhead practice expense, and malpractice insurance.
Review	Process of looking over a claim to assess payment amounts.
Skip	A patient who owes a balance on the account who has moved without a forwarding address.
Specificity	Using ICD-9-CM codes to the highest degree of certainty. Using fourth and fifth digits, as appropriate, while avoiding over use of the unspecified codes.
Statement	An itemized bill sent to the patient describing professional services provided. A request for payment.
Superbill	A multipurpose billing form to track procedure and diagnosis codes during a patient encounter or visit.
Truth in Lending	An agreement between the patient and the physician regarding monthly installments to pay a bill. A truth in lending statement must be signed when payments exceed a 4-month period.
TWIP	Take What Insurance Pays.
UCR	Usual, Customary, and Reasonable. The reimbursement method that establishes a maximum fee an insurance company will pay for services.
Utilization Review	A process of assessing medical services to assure medical necessity and the appropriateness of treatment.
Withhold Incentive	The percentage of payment held back for a risk account in the HMO program. Withhold arrangements are used to share potential losses or profits with providers of service.

OBJECTIVES

After completing this chapter, readers should be able to:

- Read an explanation of benefits (EOB) form.
- Read and retrieve information from a Medicare profile.
- Evaluate reimbursement amounts.
- Explain the impact of deductibles.
- Explain how to calculate co-payment amounts.

INTRODUCTION

Because the reader has achieved a better understanding of insurance carriers, our focus will shift to **accounts receivable.**

Whether coders have a manual system or a computer, without a basic knowledge of insurance programs, one will not be able to properly credit accounts or collect money from patients.

In this segment, insurance profiles, explanations of benefits **(EOB)** (remittance advisory), and **adjustments** or write-offs will be examined.

The following is a quick review of the two types of accounting systems used in medical practices. Regardless of the system used by the practice, the system must accomplish a few basic functions to be effective in ensuring reimbursement.

Pegboard Systems

Although this is an outdated system for most practices, there are a few smaller practices that use this system to tract patient financials. This information is presented for several reasons: (1) it is still a viable system; and (2) this format is used in a later chapter to allow the student to manually tract billing and payment transactions. This type of system incorporates basic bookkeeping skills and requires manual labor to function properly. With this system, copies of the ledger serve as **statements.**

A pegboard system, also referred to as a "one-write system," is a manual accounting system to track accounts receivable activity. This type of system requires **superbills** (Fig. 8-1), **ledger cards** or statements (Fig. 8-2), a day transaction sheet, a monthly journal form, and a special board to ensure the information is correctly entered on the forms.

Although this is a labor-intensive system, it may be less expensive than the investment of a computer system for a small practice or a practice just starting up. This system allows for account accuracy, centralized information, and quick review of charges.

Pegboard Elements

Ledger: Tracks patient billing activity, including charges, payments, and account activity.

Day Sheet/Journal: Tracks practice billing and collection activity, including patient charges, insurance payments, and cash transactions.

Statements/Ledger Card: A method to remind patients that their account has an open balance; this is usually sent on a 30-day rotation.

Computer Systems

A computer system can record patient data, charges, and payments from patients and insurance companies and relate those payments to a specific date of service. The system can balance and control all transactions on a daily basis, make necessary payment adjustments, maintain accounts receivable information and ledger transactions, and record all bank deposits.

Systems complete claim forms, track claims for reimbursement, and generate second insurance claims, as well as maintain records of all outstanding insurance claims.

2 Hope Street
Any Town, Missouri 60600
(314) 123-4444

MIRACLE CLINIC

A. Good Surgeon, M.D.

BILLING INFORMATION

DATE:_____ ACCT. #_____ DR. #_____ PREV. BAL._____

NAME:_____ DOB:_____
           LAST   FIRST   M

ADDRESS:_____
           STREET   CITY   STATE   ZIP

TYPE OF INSURANCE:_____

DIAGNOSIS: (1)_____   (3)_____

(2)_____   (4)_____

OFFICE CODES					CONSULTATIONS					HOSPITAL SERVICES			
X	CPT	DESCRIPTION	DX	AMT	X	CPT	DESCRIPTION	DX	AMT	X	CPT	DESCRIPTION	DX	AMT
	90000	N.P. BRIEF				90600	LIMITED CONSULT				90200	ADMIT, BRIEF		
	90010	N.P. LIMILTED				90605	INTERMEDIATE				90215	INTERMEDIATE		
	90015	N.P. INTERMEDIATE				90610	EXTENDED				90220	COMPREHENSIVE		
	90017	N.P. EXTENDED				90620	COMPREHENSIVE				90240	DAILY CARE, BRIEF		
	90020	N.P. COMPREHENSIVE				90630	COMPLEX				90250	DAILY CARE, LIMITED		
	90030	EST. PT. MINIMUM				90640	FOLLOW UP BRIEF				90260	INTERMEDIATE		
	90040	EST. PT. BRIEF				90641	FOLLOW UP LIMITED				90270	DAILY, EXTENDED		
	90050	EST. PT. LIMITED				90642	INTERMEDIATE				90280	COMPREHENSIVE		
	90060	INTERMEDIATE				90643	COMPLEX				90292	DISCHARGE MGMT.		
	90070	EXTENDED				90652	CONFIRMATORY EXTENDED							
	90080	COMPREHENSIVE									ADMIT:		DISCHARGE:	

X	CPT	DESCRIPTION	DX	AMT	X	CPT	DESCRIPTION	DX	AMT	X	CPT	DESCRIPTION	DX	AMT
		PROCEDURE CODES				43264	For Removal Stones				45910	Dilate Rectum		
	43200	Esoph.-Diag.				43265	For Des. Litho. Stone				46600	Anoscopy-Diagnostic		
	43202	For Biopsy				43267	For Insert. Drain Tube				4700	Liver Biop.-Needle		
	43204	For Inj. Sclerosis				43269	For Remov/Chg. Tube					**LABORATORY**		
	43219	For Inser. Stent				43271	For Balloon Dilation				86038	ANA		
	43226	For Inser. Guide Wire				43268	For Insert. Stents				82948	Blood Sugar		
	43235	**Upper G.I.-Diag.**				44380	**Ileoscopy through Stoma**				85031	CBC		
	43239	For Blopsy/Brush.				44382	With Blopsy/Brush.				80019	Chemistry Profile		
	43243	For Inj. Sclerosis				45300	Protosigmoidoscopy				90004	Electrolytes		
	43245	Dil. Gas. out. Obst.				45330	**Sigmoid.-Flexible**				82728	Ferritin		
	43246	For Placement PEG				45331	For Biopsy				82941	Gastrin Lev.		
	43453	Esoph. Dil.-Guide Wire				45333	For Polyp Removal				82951	Glucose Tol. Test (3)		
	43455	Esoph. Dil. Pneu.				45334	For Control Hemor.				82952	Glucose Tol. Test +		
	43760	Change of G-Tube				45336	For Electro./Laser				85014	Hematocrit		
	44372	Placement J-Tube				45337	For Decompre. of Volv.				80059	Hepatitis Panel		
	43247	For Remov. For. Body				45378	**Colonoscopy-Diag.**				80061	Lipid Profile		
	43255	For Control Hemor.				45382	For Control Hemor.				86300	Mono Test		
	43258	For Electro.g/Laser				45383	For Electro./Laser				87177	Ova Parasite		
	43260	**ERPC-Diag.**				45385	For Removal Polyp				88150	Pap Smear		
	43262	For Sphincterotomy				4538522	Additional Polyp				85610	Prothrombin		

	CPT	DESCRIPTION (cont.)									CPT	DESCRIPTION		
											86430	RA Latex		
											36415	Rout. Venipuncture		
											85650	Sediment Rate		
											82270	Stool for Occult Blood		
											87045	Stool Culture		
											86585	TB/Tine		
											87060	Throat Culture		
											81000	Urinalysis w/Micro		
											81002	Urine without Micro		
											87086	Urine Culture		
												MISCELLANEOUS		
											95125	Allergy Injection		
											71020	Chest X-ray		
											93000	Electrocardiogram		
											90724	Influenza Injection		
											90732	Pneumo. Injection		

ICD-9-CM DIAGNOSIS CODES

789.0	Abdominal pain	562.11	Diverticulitis	577.0	Pancreatitis	780.7	Fatigue, Malaise
794.8	Abn Liver Funct	562.10	Diverticulosis	211.3	Polyp of Colon	784.0	Headaches
280	Anemia	532	Duodenal Ulcer	564.8	Pseudo Obstruction	272.0	Hypercholesterolemia
448.9	Angiodysplasia	787.2	Dysphagia	448.9	Radiation Proctitis	401	Hypertension
154.0	CA of Colon	530.3	Esoph. Stricture	569.3	Rectal Bleeding	729.9	Musculoskeletal Pain
150.9	CA of Esophagus	530.2	Esophageal Ulcer	751.1	Small Bowel Obstruction	V70.0	Physical/No Comp.
235.3	CA of Liver	530.1	Esophagitis			486	Pneumonia
157.9	CA of Pancreas	531	Gastric Ulcer	477	Allergic Rhinitis	782.1	Rash
151.9	CA of Stomach	535	Gastritis/Duodenitis	715	Arthritis	461	Sinusitis
558	Colitis	578.9	Gastro. Bleeding	493	Asthma	785.0	Tachycardia
V76.41	Colon Cancer Screening	536.8	Gastroparesis	490	Bronchitis	465.9	Upper Respiratory
574.5	Common Duct Stone	455	Hemorrhoids	786.50	Chest pain	599.0	UTI
564.0	Constipation	553.3	Hiatal Hernia	250	Diabetes	790.8	Viremia
555	Crohn's Disease	564.1	Irritable Colon	786.09	Dyspnea		
558.9	Diarrhea	782.4	Jaundice				

TO FILE INSURANCE: Complete the personal information on your claim form.
Attach this copy and mail to your insurance company. This copy contains all
the information the doctor is required to furnish.

☐ CASH ☐ CHECK ☐ CHARGE

TOTAL CHARGES	
AMT PAID	
BAL. DUE	

Physician Signature_____ Date_____

FIGURE 8-1 Superbill/encounter form.

STATEMENT

DATE	FAMILY MEMBER	DESCRIPTION	CHARGE	CREDITS		CURRENT BALANCE
				Payments	Adj.	

PLEASE PAY LAST AMOUNT IN THIS COLUMN

THIS IS A COPY OF YOUR ACCOUNT AS IT APPEARS ON YOUR LEDGER CARD

FIGURE 8-2 Ledger card/statement.

INSURANCE PARTICIPATION

The fundamental aspects of reimbursement consist of learning to read EOB forms and understanding participatory agreements. Perhaps the first issue to be examined is: What does it mean to participate in an insurance program?

The primary element related to this question is that the physician must accept as payment the amount allowed by the insurance company. In other words, the physician must write off the difference of the actual, submitted charge and the insurance carrier's allowed amount.

E X A M P L E
A doctor bills $40 for a service; however, the carrier only allows $30 for the service. Therefore, the doctor forfeits $10 every time he performs this service for this particular insurance carrier.

The physician's office must file all insurance claims to the carrier for any services rendered to the patient.

The physician must wait until the carrier makes payment before collecting monies from the patient. The one exception to this rule involves health maintenance organizations (HMOs) and preferred provider organizations (PPOs). With these programs, the patient will have a **co-payment** based on the individual insurance program. The co-payment amount is usually listed on the back of the insurance card. These co-payments must be collected at the time of the service.

The office is responsible for the timely filing of insurance claims based on carrier determination. Each carrier has a preset time limit during which a claim may be submitted to qualify for payment (e.g., 90 days, 12 months).

The office must write off any incentive pools or withhold amounts per contract agreements. An incentive withhold pool is usually a percentage of the allowed amount that is retained by the carrier to offset operational expenses. Physicians are prohibited from collecting this amount from the patient. However, if the carrier makes a profit during a given time, the carrier will reimburse a portion of the incentive withhold back to the physician.

The physician also agrees to abide by the rules for participation as determined by the insurance carriers. Some of these rules include:

- Precertification when necessary
- Utilization reviews
- Obtaining authorization for service when necessary
- Utilizing other physicians who participate with the insurance program
- Utilizing hospital and outpatient facilities that participate with the insurance program

☑ Claims Processing Timetable by Carrier

Blue Shield:	6-8 weeks
TRICARE:	3-6 weeks
Commercial:	6-10 weeks
Medicaid:	8-10 weeks
Medicare:	
Participating:	19 days
Nonparticipating:	27 days
Electronic:	14 days
Workers' Compensation:	3-8 weeks

Common Claim Errors

Errors in completing a claim form affect reimbursement because the claim may be denied for payment or payment may be reduced. Claims are denied for a variety of reasons. The following is a list of the more common reasons a claim may be denied for payment.

Diagnosis

- ICD-9-CM codes missing or not carried to the highest level of **specificity**
- Diagnosis does not correspond to treatment or procedure
- Reporting suspected conditions as confirmed conditions
- Diagnosis does not relate to the gender of the patient

Dates of Service

- Incomplete or incorrect
- More than one calendar year on same claim form

Charges

- Missing or incomplete
- Charges not itemized

Identification Numbers

- Number is missing
- Number is incomplete
- Number is incorrect

Procedure Coding

- Code is incorrect
- Number and description do not match
- Code is missing or incomplete
- Current Procedure Terminology (CPT) code does not relate to diagnosis

Payment Responsibility

How does one determine who is responsible for payment and when the patient is responsible for payment? In most cases it is ultimately the patient who is responsible for payment. The following are a few guidelines.

- A husband is responsible for his wife. However, a wife is not always responsible for claims incurred by the husband.
- A father is usually responsible for bills incurred on behalf of his children.
- An insurance company is responsible for claims under the Workers' Compensation Act.
- In special circumstances a third-party guarantor may be responsible for the bill in the following cases:
  - Court-ordered examinations
  - An attorney for third-party liability suits
  - An employer for pre-employment examinations or drug screens

Collection Policies

The best policy is to collect from the patient at the time of service. However, based on participation agreements, this may not always be possible. In that event, there are a few basic rules or guidelines to follow.

- Advise patients of office payment policies before beginning treatment. When using this policy, the patient will know, before entering the office, whether payment is due at time of service or if the office will file the insurance before collecting from the patient.
- Establish and enforce a well-defined collection policy. Develop a specific method to monitor and handle accounts before they become a problem. Use a collection follow-up system for all patients in the practice.

One of the best result-oriented methods used by most practices is the policy of follow-up letters for delinquent accounts. Some general rules for sending letters are as follows:

- Send patients a statement every 30 days.
- Send a second letter for accounts over 60 days.
- Send a notice informing the patient when the account will be turned over to a collection agency, usually after 90 days.

If the office has time, incorporating phone calls into the collection process beginning with the 60th day of a delinquent account is sometimes effective. When using phone calls, one should follow up the call with a letter. Whatever course of action one tells the patient one plans to take regarding the account, make sure that action is taken. Otherwise, the office could be sued by the patient for harassment.

Collection Letters

Writing a collection letter is not always an easy task. However, there are some important points that should be part of every letter created. The letter should inform the patient of the following items:

- How much is owed on the account
- What the services are or the reason for the charges
- What the patient needs to do regarding the account
- When, where, and why patient should pay the account
- How the patient can make a payment

An effective collection letter does not have to be harsh in nature. The intent is to advise the patient that payment is needed. The consequences of not paying the account should be explained.

The following pages illustrate some examples of collection letters. Each person or office has to develop the style most suited to the office and the personality of the physician for the letter to be effective.

> ## EXAMPLE
>
> **Initial Letter**
> Dear Patient:
> Our records indicate you have an outstanding balance in the amount of $_____ for your _____ visit.
> Please send payment today so we can keep your account current. If you have a question concerning your account, please give me a call so that I may discuss it with you.
>
> _____
>
> **Alternate Wording**
> Dear Patient:
> We have not heard from you regarding your account in the amount of $_____.
> Please send your payment today. If there is a problem with the account, please give us a call.

EXAMPLE

Second Letter

Dear Patient:

We have not heard from you regarding your account in the amount of $_____. Because this account is now 60 days past due, please call me today so that we may discuss arrangements for payment.

_____

Alternate Wording

Dear Patient:

We wrote you 3 weeks ago requesting that you contact our office concerning your overdue account in the amount of $_____.

Please make arrangements to pay this account today.

If you are unable to pay the account in full at this time, please call our office manager, (name), so that (he or she) may assist you in establishing a payment plan for your account.

EXAMPLE

Third Letter

Dear Patient:

Our previous attempts to contact you regarding your unpaid account in the amount of $_____ have been ignored. Please contact our office immediately to discuss this account.

If we have not heard from you by (specify a date), we will be forced to turn this account over to a collection agency.

_____

Alternate Wording

Dear Patient:

Please be advised this is our final attempt to contact you regarding your overdue account in the amount of $_____.

Your failure to work with us concerning payment of this account leaves us no recourse but to turn your account over to our collection agency on (specify a date).

This action can be avoided if you send your payment in full within 10 days of the date of this letter. If you are unable to pay the account in full, please contact our office manager, _____, within 7 days so that she may arrange a payment program.

Reimbursement Tip

The best collection policy is to ask the patient for payment at the time of service.

Bad Debt Collection

Statute of Limitation

Open Book Accounts

An open book account is an account where charges are made from time to time. This is also the most common type of collection account. Open book accounts generally have a 5-year limitation for collection from the date the charge incurred.

Written Contracts

Written contract accounts are an agreement signed by a patient in which specific payment amounts are made on the account on a monthly basis. These accounts usually have high amounts that will take over 4 months to repay.

Written contracts generally have a 6-year limitation for collection. Because collection limitations may vary from state to state, one should contact the local bar association or Insurance Commissioner to determine any time limits that have been set for your specific state.

General Claims Information

Remittance Advisory or Explanation of Benefits

The remittance advisory or explanation of benefits must include the following information:
- Patient information
  - Name
  - Address
  - Identification number
- Provider of service
  - Name
  - Address
  - Identification numbers when appropriate
- Date(s) of service
- Type of service
- Allowed amounts
- Carrier payments
- Adjustments or write-offs based on special programs or participation agreements
- Patient responsibility
- Reason for nonpayment of a claim
  The following pages contain excerpts of various types of explanation of benefits (Figs. 8-3 to 8-6).

	PHYSICIAN OR SUPPLIED NUMBER	DATE OF STATEMENT MO. DAY YR.	Item 1

Item 2

B.A. Doctor, M.D.
1 Getwell
Anytown, MO 63111

Physician or Supplied Number: 0000
Check No 0099480771
Date of Statement: 04 29 92

Item: 3 4 5 6 7 8 9 10 11 12 13 14 15

NAME OF PATIENT	HEALTH INSURANCE CLAIM NUMBER	PHYSICIAN OR SUPPLIER NAME	SERVICE DATES FROM TO MO DAY MO DAY YR	Type	Place	PROCEDURE CODE	TOTAL CHARGES	REMARKS CODES A B	NON-ALLOWED CHARGES	DEDUCTIBLE	CO-INSURANCE	PAYMENT TO PATIENT	PAYMENT TO PHYSICIAN OR SUPPLIER
		Account PT 2637; ENB. 3441											
	497167009A	00000	022792	1	IH		8383 43		1397	00	1397	00	5589
	497167009A	00000	022892	1	IH		4134 43		690	00	689	00	2755
	497167009A	00000	022992	1	IH		4134 43		690	00	689	00	2755
	497167009A	00000	031692	1	IH		4134 43		690	00	689	00	2755
	497167009A	00000	031792	1	IH		4134 43		690	00	689	00	2755
	497167009A	00000	031892	1	IH		6552 43		1092	00	1092	00	4368
	9210790016119		CLAIM TOTALS				31471		5249	00	5245	00	20977
		ACCOUNT - PT 2670;INV 3442											
	486661953A	00000	032492	1	IH		6552 43 03		1092	00	1092	00	4368
	9210790016120		CLAIM TOTALS				6552		1092	00	1092	00	4368
		ACCOUNT - PT 2670;INV 3442											
	486661953A	00000	032592	1	IH		6552 43 03		1092	00	1092	00	4368
	9210790016121		CLAIM TOTALS				6552		1092	00	1092	00	4368
		ACCOUNT - PT 2670;INV 3443											
	486661953A	00000	032692	1	IH		6552 43 03		1092	00	1092	00	4368
	9210790016122		CLAIM TOTALS				6552		1092	00	1092	00	4368
		ACCOUNT - PT 2670;INV 3443											
	486661953A	00000	032792	1	IH		6552 43 03		1092	00	1092	00	4368
	9210790016123		CLAIM TOTALS				6552		1092	00	1092	00	4368
		ACCOUNT - PT 2670;INV 3450											
	486661953A	00000	033092	1	IH		4134 43 03		690	00	689	00	2755
	9210790016125		CLAIM TOTALS				4134		690	00	689	00	2755
		ACCOUNT - PT 2670;INV 3450											
	486661953A	00000	040192	1	IH		4134 43 03		690	00	689	00	2755
	9210790016126		CLAIM TOTALS				4134		690	00	689	00	2755
		ACCOUNT - PT 2670;INV 3450											
	486661953A	00000	040292	1	IH		4134 43 03		690	00	689	00	2755
	9210790016127		CLAIM TOTALS				4134		690	00	689	00	2755
		ACCOUNT - PT 2670;INV 3450											
	486661953A	00000	040392	1	IH		4134 43 03		690	00	689	00	2755
	9210790016128		CLAIM TOTALS				4134		690	00	689	00	2755
		ACCOUNT - PT 2670;INV 3440											
	489075488A	00000	040192	T	OF		4134 32 U		690	00	1722	00	1722
	9210790016118		CLAIM TOTALS				4134		690	00	1722	00	1722

THE 1991 VISIT CODES ARE NO LONGER VALID AFTER DECEMBER 31, 1991

GRAND TOTALS	10	783.49	130.67	.00	140.91	.00	.00	511.91
	TOTAL NO. OF CLAIMS	TOTAL CHARGES	TOTAL NON-ALLOWED CHARGES	TOTAL DEDUCTIBLE	TOTAL CO-INSURANCE	TOTAL INTEREST	TOTAL PAID TO PATIENTS	TOTAL PHYSICIAN OR SUPPLIER PAYMENT

Medicare Explanation of Benefits

Item 1: Contains information regarding date of statement, Medicare carrier address and phone number, and supplier/provider I.D. number and check number
Item 2: Address of physician or supplier
Item 3: Name of the patient
Item 4: Patient's Medicare number and control number (Refer to the control number when making claim inquiries.)
Item 5: Physician patient account information (patient account number or invoice number)
Item 6: Dates when service was rendered to patient
Item 7: Type of service (medical/surgical) Place of service (office/hospital)
Item 8: CPT or procedure code
Item 9: Total submitted charge for the service
Item 10: Remarks codes supply information regarding why payment was or was not made. Some carriers list the coded definitions on the bottom of the EOB. Other carriers supply providers with a master key list so the office may verify the reason for nonpayment or discounted fees.

Item 11: Total amount of charges not allowed by Medicare for a particular procedure code (Always refer to the remarks codes to determine if this is a write-off for the office or patient responsibility.)
Item 12: Information concerning the amount of the yearly deductible remaining on the patient's account. Amounts in this column should be collected from the patient.
Item 13: Amount patient owes based on copayments.
Item 14: If the office overcharged a patient, Medicare will send the overpayment back to the patient.
Item 15: Amount Medicare will pay the provider of the service

Remarks Codes: Columns A & B
143: Approved amount limited by fee schedule
32: Charge reflects 62.5% psychiatric outpatient limit
U: Claim was forwarded to Blue Cross Blue Shield
03: Claim has been forwarded to Medicaid

FIGURE 8-3 Medicare remittance advisory/explanation of benefits. (*Source: U.S. Department of Health and Human Services, Centers for Medicare & Medicaid Services.*)

Medicare Patient Explanation of Benefits

Oct 21, 1991

Your Health Insurance Claim Number:
000-00-0000-A

Patient Name
Patient Address
City, State, Zip

For more information call or write
General American Life Ins. Co
P.O. Box 505
St. Louis MO 63166
Local Telephone 843-8880
Toll Free 1-800-392-3070
Walk-in: 13045 Tesson Ferry Rd

Page 1 of 2
Check No. 0019845503

Item 1: Patient information

Item 2: Address and phone numbers of the carrier. Check number for reference.

Item 3: Explanation of type of service, date, and payment information

Participating doctors and suppliers always accept assignment of Medicare claims. See back of this notice for an explanation of assignment. Write or call us for the name of a participating doctor or supplier or for a free list of participating doctors and suppliers.

Item 4: Total approved amount. Medicare payment based on applicable formulas.

Your doctor or supplier did not accept assignment on your claim (Control No. 91280-0003086500) for ($610.00). See item 4 on back.

Item 5: Advising patient of balance due to physician

B.A. Doctor, MD		Billed	Approved
1 Inpatient Service	Aug 01, 1991	$125.00	$61.84
Approved amount limited by item 5c on back.			
4 Inpatient Services	Aug 02-Aug 08, 1991	$360.00	$197.60
Approved amount limited by item 5c on back.			
Charges were reduced for the same reason and by the same amount.			
1 Inpatient Service	Aug 07, 1991	$125.00	$64.00
A special method was used to set the approved amount because not enough charge data was available.			
Total approved amount			$323.44
Medicare payment (80% of the approved amount)			$258.75

You are responsible for a total of $351.25, the difference between the billed amount and the Medicare payment. You could have avoided paying $286.56, the difference between the billed and approved amounts, if the claim(s) had been assigned.

We are paying a total of $258.75 to you on the enclosed check. Please cash it as soon as possible. If you have other insurance, it may help with the part Medicare did not pay.

A copy of this claim has been forwarded to Blue Cross Blue Shield of Missouri for supplemental claims processing. You do not need to file a supplemental claim; you will receive an explanation of benefits from Blue Cross Blue Shield.

FIGURE 8-4 Medicare patient explanation of benefits. *(Source: U.S. Department of Health and Human Services, Centers for Medicare & Medicaid Services.)*

EXAMPLE: HMO PRODUCT

	Item 1	Item 2	Item 3
HMO of St. Louis	P.O. Box 1234 St. Louis, MO 63333 (314) 000-0000	B.A. Doctor, M.D. 1 Get Well St. Louis, MO 63333	Check Date: 05-06-9x

Item: 4	5	6	7	8		9		10	11
CLAIM NUMBER	PROVIDER ACCT NO	SERVICE DATE	BILLING CODE/CPT	ALLOWABLE		DEDUCTIONS		INCENTIVE WITHHOLD	TOTAL PAID / NET AMTS
				AMOUNT	CODE	CO-PAY OTHER	EXP CODE		

PATIENT NAME: Dough, Jane   SUBSCRIBER NAME: Dough, John
ID Number: 48760408641

CLAIM NUMBER	PROVIDER ACCT NO	SERVICE DATE	BILLING CODE/CPT	AMOUNT	CODE	CO-PAY OTHER	EXP CODE	INCENTIVE WITHHOLD	TOTAL PAID	NET AMTS
0220221	12345	12-04-9x	99231	30.00	30.00	15.00		3.75	11.25	
0220221	12345	12-23-9x	99233	60.00	55.00 02	25.00		7.50	22.50	
0220221	12345	04-06-9x	14011	100.00	74.00 02	25.00		12.25	36.75	
				$190.00	$159.00			$23.50	$70.50	$70.50

Check Number 489204 Check Date: 05-06-9x   PAYEE: B. A. Doctor, MD   AMOUNT $70.50

02   FEE EXCEEDS ALLOWABLE

Item 1: Address of carrier
Item 2: Name and address of provider
Item 3: Date check was issued
Item 4: Use this number when referring to claim
Item 5: Patient account number at office
Item 6: Actual date of service
Item 7: CPT code or procedure
Item 8: Actual charge versus allowed amount and explanation code
Item 9: Amount of copayment due from patient
Item 10: Incentive withholds must be written off by the office.
         These may be refunded at end of year if carrier makes a profit.
Item 11: Actual amount paid to the provider

FIGURE 8-5 HMO product update.

EXPLANATION OF PROVIDER PAYMENT

ENCLOSED IS A DRAFT (50-52343505) IN THE AMOUNT OF $90.00 IN PAYMENT OF THE
FOLLOWING ASSIGNED BENEFITS. IF YOU HAVE ANY QUESTIONS ABOUT THE INDIVIDUAL
PAYMENTS LISTED BELOW, PLEASE CONTACT THE APPROPRIATE ISSUING OFFICE.

NOTE: ALL INQUIRIES AND CLAIMS SHOULD REFERENCE THE INSURED ID NUMBER FOR PROMPT RESPONSE.

Item: 2	3	4	5	6	7		8		9	10
SERVICE DATES PL	SERVICE CODE NO.	SUBMITTED EXPENSES	NEGOTIATED ADJUSTMENT	COPAY AMOUNT	PENDING OR NONPAYABLE	SEE RMRKS	DEDUCT-IBLE	CO-INSURANCE	PATIENT RESP	PAYABLE AMOUNT

Item 1

NETWORK   PARTNERS-ST. LOUIS
ISSUING CLAIM OFFICE – P.O. BOX 2520, TYLER, TX 75710 – (214) 534-6180
PAYOR ID   SUB-ID   GROUP NO -

INSURED: INSURED ID:
PATIENT: RELATION: PATIENT NO: NA   DIAG: 3090   DRG: TCN:

SERVICE DATES PL	SERVICE CODE NO.	SUBMITTED EXPENSES	NEGOTIATED ADJUSTMENT	COPAY AMOUNT	PENDING OR NONPAYABLE	SEE RMRKS	DEDUCT-IBLE	CO-INSURANCE	PATIENT RESP	PAYABLE AMOUNT
OF 90020 1	125.00	30.00	5.00						5.00	90.00
CLAIM TOTALS:	125.00	30.00	5.00						5.00	90.00
								ISSUED AMOUNT		$90.00

NETWORK   PARTNERS-ST. LOUIS
ISSUING CLAIM OFFICE – P.O. BOX 937 FOUR SEAGATE, TOLEDO, OH 43695 – TEL. (419) 321-2400
PAYOR ID   SUB-ID   GROUP NO -

INSURED: INSURED ID:
PATIENT: RELATION: PATIENT NO: DIAG: 3129   DRG: TCN:

SERVICE DATES PL	SERVICE CODE NO.	SUBMITTED EXPENSES	NEGOTIATED ADJUSTMENT	COPAY AMOUNT	PENDING OR NONPAYABLE	SEE RMRKS	DEDUCT-IBLE	CO-INSURANCE	PATIENT RESP	PAYABLE AMOUNT
OF 90020 1	125.00				125.00				125.00	0.00
OF 90844 1	100.00				100.00				100.00	0.00
OF 90844 1	60.00				60.00				60.00	0.00
CLAIM TOTALS:	285.00				285.00				285.00	0.00
								ISSUED AMOUNT		NO PAY

                                                            ** TOTAL ** $90.00
                                                      ** DRAFT AMOUNT ** $90.00

Commercial Carrier (PPO)

Item 1:	Name and location of insurance program	Item 6:	Patient copay amounts
Item 2:	Date of service	Item 7:	Amount not being paid / Reason(s) for nonpayment
Item 3:	CPT or procedure code	Item 8:	Any outstanding deductible amounts
Item 4:	Actual submitted charge / Type of service	Item 9:	Amount that is patient responsibility
Item 5:	Amount to be written off by office	Item 10:	Amount carrier paid to physician

FIGURE 8-6 Explanation of provider payment.

TEST YOUR KNOWLEDGE

1. Match the term to the definition.

    _____1. Skip

    _____2. Appeal

    _____3. Dunning

    _____4. Adjustment

    _____5. Profile

    _____6. Assignment

    A. Request or message to remind patient an account is overdue

    B. A fee schedule with CPT codes to advise a practice how much an insurance company will pay

    C. Transfer right to collect revenue

    D. Patient owing a balance who moves without leaving a forwarding address

    E. A correction amount or write-off

    F. Request for additional payment consideration

2. _____ is an agreement to pay a balance in monthly installments.

3. List the five items to be included in a collection letter.

    A. _____

    B. _____

    C. _____

    D. _____

    E. _____

4. A _____ is an itemized bill sent to the patient describing professional services.

5. A _____ is the relationship between the amount of money owed and the amount of money collected.

Claim Follow-Up Guidelines
- Establish a claim-tracking system for the office.
- Send a copy of the claim with a cover letter or insurance inquiry card to the carrier.
- Call the carrier to inquire about the claim.

Reimbursement Tip

Send a copy of the claim with an inquiry letter. If the claim has been lost or not processed, the carrier will have a copy available to begin processing the claim.

MEDICARE AND REIMBURSEMENT

Fee Schedule

A **fee schedule** (or **profile**) is the means developed by Medicare to advise physicians as to the amount Medicare will pay for a given procedure or service. Profiles are generally sent to physicians by the first of December. Because physicians must make changes in participation status before December 31, it is important that this comparison data be available to the physician before that deadline.

Following is an excerpt of a Medicare fee schedule.

CPT Code	Fee Schedule		Limiting Charge
	Participating	Nonparticipating	
11404	$119.98	$113.98	$136.78
	$98.16*	$93.25*	$111.90†
11424	$113.64	$126.96	$152.35
	$111.68*	$106.10*	$126.32*
99204	$72.64	$69.01	$82.81
	$61.32*	$58.25*	$69.90*

*Denotes limiting charge is less than 120% of non par fee schedule
†Fee amount and limiting charge apply when the place of service is hospital outpatient department.

As discussed in detail in Chapter 6, there are two types of providers in the Medicare system, participating providers and nonparticipating providers. Because of the two types of providers, Medicare had to develop two allowed amount columns for the profile based on the physician's contract status with Medicare.

Payments

In 1992, Medicare adopted a relative value system. The unit value of a procedure is composed of a work value, overhead value, and malpractice insurance value. This system was designed to make uniform the Medicare reimbursement system by basing payment on units instead of geographic regions. The idea behind the system is that a physician in New York will receive the same reimbursement for the work as a physician in Alaska when performing the same service.

Payment is based on a **relative value unit (RVU)** multiplied by a **conversion factor** (CF). In 1992, Medicare had only one conversion factor. In 1993, Medicare began using a two–conversion factor system. In the new system, you have a separate conversion factor or multiplier for all surgical procedures, and another conversion factor for all nonsurgical procedures and services.

In addition to the relative value component, Medicare also bases allowed amounts for the physician on the location or where the service was provided (e.g., office versus hospital outpatient department). (Please refer to the profile excerpt.)

ALLOWED AMOUNTS

Allowed amounts are divided into three separate categories.

- **Participating Providers:** Fees are based on the Medicare fee schedule.
- **Nonparticipating Providers:** Fees are based on the fee schedule minus 5% differential from the participating physician's column and apply for payment when the nonparticipating provider accepts assignment on a claim.

- **Limiting Charge:** Fees set by Medicare when a nonparticipating provider does not accept assignment on a Medicare claim. The limiting charge is typically 115% of the nonparticipating allowed amount column.

Allowed amounts for some CPT codes are also based on location of service. If a service that could have been performed in the office was performed in another location, Medicare reduces the physician's allowed amount and the limiting charge amount.

Medicare Payment Formulas

Deductible

A **deductible** is the amount that must be paid by the patient before a carrier will begin making payment on a claim. With Medicare, even though the patient has not met the yearly deductible ($140), the physician may not bill a Medicare patient more than the amount allowed by Medicare.

 Reimbursement Tip

When accepting assignment, fees are based on the allowed amount.

When not accepting assignment, fees are based on the limiting charge amount.

Medicare Payment Formula

Typical Medicare payment

Allowed amount × 80% = Medicare payment

Example: $100 × 80% = $80 Medicare payment

Typical Patient Payment Formula

Allowed amount × 20% = Patient co-payment

Example: $100 × 20% = $20 Patient co-payment

Psychiatric Payment Formula

The psychiatric payment formula pertains to outpatient services only. Inpatient services follow the payment guidelines listed previously.

Medicare Payment: Outpatient

Allowed amount × 62.5% × 80% = Medicare payment

Example: $100 × 62.5% = $62.50

$62.50 × 80% = $50

Patient Payment

Allowed amount × 62.5% × 20% = Patient co-payment

Example: $100 × 62.5% = $62.50

$62.50 × 20% = $12.50

Allowed amount × 37.5% = Additional patient obligation

Example: $100 × 37.5% = $37.50

Reimbursement Tip

On outpatient psychiatric charges, one may collect up to the allowed amount. In this example, the allowed amount was $100. Medicare paid $50.

Patient obligation: Co-payment ($12.50) + Psychiatric limit ($37.50) = $50

Multiple Surgery

First Procedure

Allowed amount × 80% = Medicare payment
Example: $100 × 80% = $80

Second Procedure

Allowed amount × 50% × 80% = Medicare payment
Example: $100 × 50% = $50
$50 × 80% = $40

Third Procedure

Allowed amount × 25% × 80% = Medicare payment
Example: $100 × 25% = $25
$25 × 80% = $20
(Fourth and fifth procedures follow the guideline for a third procedure.)

Assistant Surgery Formula

Assigned Claim

Allowed amount × 16% × 80% = Medicare payment
Example: $100 × 16% = $16
$16 × 80% = $12.80
Allowed amount × 16% × 20% = Patient co-payment
Example: $100 × 16% = $16
$16 × 20% = $3.20

Nonassigned Claim

Allowed amount × 16% × 120% = Limiting charge
Example: $100 × 16% = $16
$16 × 125% = $19.20
Allowed amount × 16% × 115% = Limiting charge
Example: $100 × 16% = $16
$16 × 115% = $18.40

Laboratory Fees

Medicare pays 100% of the allowed amount for all approved laboratory services. Fees are currently based on a fee schedule. One should contact the local Medicare carrier to determine if the area will be affected by these changes.

Radiology

Radiology is paid based on a fee schedule. Medicare pays 80% of the allowed amount with the patient having a 20% co-payment after the yearly deductible has been met. Currently, the deductible is $140 per calendar year.

☑ *Understanding Medicare Reimbursement*

When Office Accepts Assignment	
Actual fee	$150.00
Medicare allowed amount	$125.00
Medicare payment	$100.00
Patient co-payment	$ 25.00
Total reimbursement	$125.00
Adjustment/write-off	$ 25.00*
When Office Does not Accept Assignment	
Actual fee	$150.00
Limiting charge amount	$135.00
Patient receives Medicare payment	$100.00
Patient owes practice	$135.00†

*Difference between the allowed amount and the actual charge.
†When an office does not accept assignment, Medicare determines the amount the office can bill the patient—*the limiting charge*. Medicare payment is based on the actual allowed charge amount from the profile.

THIRD-PARTY PAYERS

Most insurance companies pay at a difference rate based on the patient's coverage package. In some cases for outpatient surgery, a carrier may pay 100% of the allowed amount but all other services are paid at 70% to 90% of the allowed amount with deductibles varying based on individual policy stipulations.

In the HMO and PPO products, the patient may have a co-payment per visit that is to be collected at the time of service. The carrier will then pay a percentage of the allowed amount or the fee schedule.

Regardless of the carrier, one fact is constant. When the patient has a deductible, the deductible must be met before a carrier will pay the claim.

Usual, Customary, and Reasonable Payment Plans

Usual, customary, and reasonable **(UCR)** plans have become one of the least used methods for payment determination because it is a complex system that compares three sets of fees per each provider. However, a few carriers such as indemnity providers may use this method to calculate reimbursement for a given population or geographic region.

When a carrier uses UCR as a basis for payment, three payment factors are taken into consideration in order for the carrier to establish a payment base for the allowed or covered amount of a service.

Essentially, UCR means payment is determined by: (1) ascertaining the usual fee a doctor charges to the majority of his patients for a particular service; (2) reviewing the geographic location of the practice and the specialty of the physician; and (3) reviewing complications or unusual circumstances or services. In the UCR method, reimbursement is based on the lowest of the usual, customary, or reasonable fees charged by a physician.

Defining UCR

Usual Fee: The fee most often charged by a physician for a service or procedure.
Customary Fee: The fee most often charged by other physicians of similar training and experience within a geographic region for the same service or procedure.
Reasonable Fee: The fee the insurance company considers appropriate reimbursement based on the criteria of usual or customary fees.

MEDICAID

With Medicaid, the patient does not have a co-payment for the doctor's office. Medicaid pays 100% of the Medicaid allowed amount. Offices are required to write off the difference between the allowed amount and the actual charge. Medicaid patients may not be billed for any services covered by Medicaid provided Medicaid coverage was in effect at the time of the visit.

When a patient has both Medicare and Medicaid, Medicare is the primary insurance. Regardless of the physician's contract with Medicare (par vs. non par), the physician must accept assignment on the claim in order to receive the Medicaid benefits payment. The following pages are exercises in calculating reimbursement and adjustments. Based on the Medicare profile and information given for reimbursement, process the following claims for payment.

When working these exercises, give the following information for each problem:
- Allowed amounts
- Write-offs or adjustments
- Expected payments from insurance carrier
- Expected payment from patient

As you review Table 8-1, please note this table is for example only to be used for exercises for problems stated in this book. This table is not intended to reflect any official allowed amounts nor current CPT codes as published by the American Medical Association. Its only purpose is for examples and is to be used to complete certain exercised included in this book.

Table 8-1 Sample Medicare Profile Data

CPT Codes	Medicare Allowed Amount Participating Provider ($)	Limit Charge Non Participating Provider ($)	Amount ($)
99201	21.56	20.48	24.58
99202	6.99	6.64	7.97
99203	29.82	28.33	34.00
	27.11	25.75	30.90*
99204	32.36	30.74	35.35†
	28.02	26.62	31.94*
99205	102.78	97.64	117.17
	92.62	98.99	105.59*
99212	30.88	29.34	35.21
	27.35	25.98	31.18*
99213	118.86	112.92	135.50
99214	23.16	22.00	26.40
	20.10	19.10	22.92
99215	121.86	115.77	138.92
	106.17	100.86	121.03*
10021	30.73	29.19	33.57†
	26.92	25.57	30.68*
11022	102.70	97.57	117.08
	90.30	85.79	102.95*

Table 8-1   Sample Medicare Profile Data—cont'd

CPT Codes	Medicare Allowed Amount Participating Provider ($)	Limit Charge Non Participating Provider ($)	Amount ($)
10040	30.33	28.81	33.13
	26.85	25.51	30.61*
10061	111.59	106.01	127.21
10080	27.54	26.16	30.08†
	23.58	22.40	26.88*
11010	23.61	22.43	26.92
20520	19.57	18.59	22.31
	33.83	32.14	38.57
20550	27.55	26.17	31.40*
	49.85	47.36	56.83
20551	40.88	38.84	46.61*
20552	62.87	59.73	71.68
	52.56	49.93	59.92*
20553	136.38	129.56	155.47
46600	190.49	180.97	217.16
46900	18.86	17.92	21.15†
	14.80	14.06	16.87*
46910	10.83	10.29	12.35
46916	22.58	21.45	25.74
46917	13.26	12.60	15.12
46922	22.14	21.03	25.24
46924	15.90	15.11	18.13
46934	26.70	25.37	30.44
46935	11.94	11.34	13.61
46937	24.99	23.74	28.49
46940	10.26	9.75	11.70
46942	25.60	24.33	29.20
46945	13.87	13.18	15.82
46946	33.35	31.68	38.02
55000	5.92	5.62	6.74
55040	27.44	26.07	31.28
55041	46.03	43.73	52.48
55060	66.60	63.27	75.92
55100	52.19	49.58	59.50
55870	21.10	20.05	24.06
57410	76.97	73.12	87.74
57415	105.14	99.88	119.86
57420	62.58	59.45	71.34

Continued

Table 8-1   Sample Medicare Profile Data—cont'd

CPT Codes	Medicare Allowed Amount Participating Provider ($)	Limit Charge Non Participating Provider ($)	Amount ($)
57452	46.62	44.29	53.15
57455	17.82	16.93	19.47[†]
57456	25.58	24.30	29.16
	19.76	18.77	22.52*
57460	40.32	38.30	45.96
	33.00	31.35	37.62*
57461	48.64	46.21	55.45
	41.03	38.98	46.78*
57500	72.64	69.01	82.81
	62.31	58.25	69.90*
57505	82.05	77.95	93.54
	70.78	67.24	80.69*
57510	11.62	11.04	13.25
	9.00	8.55	10.26*
57511	22.06	20.96	25.15
	17.57	16.69	20.03*
57513	28.00	26.60	31.92
	22.68	21.55	25.86*
58300	41.30	39.24	47.09
	34.02	32.32	38.78*
58301	68.50	65.08	78.10
	56.96	54.11	64.93*
58321	58.64	55.71	66.85
58322	91.93	87.33	104.80
58323	102.80	97.66	117.19
58340	30.98	29.43	35.32
59000	36.82	34.98	41.98
59001	49.43	46.96	56.35
59012	53.33	50.66	60.79
59030	40.81	38.77	46.52
59050	62.20	59.09	70.91
59051	80.24	76.23	91.48
59200	112.32	106.70	128.04
59300	125.82	119.53	143.44
59320	42.95	40.80	48.96
60001	63.82	60.63	72.76
60100	82.16	78.05	93.66
61001	112.46	106.84	128.21

Table 8-1   Sample Medicare Profile Data—cont'd

CPT Codes	Medicare Allowed Amount Participating Provider ($)	Limit Charge Non Participating Provider ($)	Amount ($)
61020	125.72	119.43	143.32
61070	24.43	23.21	27.85
62310	41.31	39.24	47.09
62311	56.28	53.47	64.16
62318	46.44	44.12	52.94
62319	48.14	45.73	54.88
64400	71.61	68.03	81.64
64402	82.08	77.98	93.58
64405	126.76	120.42	144.50
64408	25.21	23.95	28.74
64410	43.46	30.84	37.01
64412	45.09	43.41	52.09
64416	79.38	75.41	90.49
69100	102.99	97.84	117.41
69105	125.04	118.79	142.55
69205	59.24	56.28	67.54
69210	35.83	34.04	40.85
69220	42.59	40.46	48.55
69222	53.66	50.98	61.18
69400	23.26	22.10	26.52
69410	32.77	31.13	37.36
69433	37.02	35.17	42.20
70030	35.59	33.81	40.57
70100	42.64	40.51	48.61
92002	61.26	58.20	69.84
92012	23.73	22.54	27.05
92014	26.53	25.20	30.24
92100	33.20	31.54	37.85
92130	46.00	43.70	52.44
92584	51.85	49.26	59.11
92601	65.78	62.49	74.99
92602	31.02	29.47	35.36
96400	44.78	42.54	51.05
96405	53.40	50.73	56.46

*Fee amount and limiting charge apply when the place of service is a hospital.
†Denotes limiting charges for less than 120% of the nonparticipant fee schedule.

REIMBURSEMENT EXERCISES

Directions: Based on the information provided, complete the following exercises to show payments, co-payments, and adjustments.

1. Patient has Blue Cross Blue Shield. Actual charge was $125. Blue Shield allowed $97.50 for the service payable at 80% of the allowed amount.

   Actual Charge _____

   Allowed Amount _____

   Payment Amount _____

   Co-Payment _____

   Adjustment _____

2. Patient is a Medicaid recipient. Your actual charge for the service is $45. Medicaid allowed $22.

   Actual Charge _____

   Allowed Amount _____

   Payment Amount _____

   Co-Payment _____

   Adjustment _____

   The following problems are based on a Medicare fee schedule (see Table 8-1). Use the schedule to determine correct billing information, allowed amounts, payment, co-payments, and adjustments.

3. Code: 58323   Nonparticipating   Accepting Assignment

   Actual Charge _____

   Allowed Amount _____

   Payment Amount _____

   Co-Payment _____

   Adjustment _____

4. Code: 55041   Nonparticipating   Not Accepting Assignment

Actual Charge _____

Allowed Amount _____

Payment Amount _____

Co-Payment _____

Adjustment _____

5. Code: 60100   Nonparticipating   Not Accepting Assignment

Actual Charge _____

Allowed Amount _____

Payment Amount _____

Co-Payment _____

Adjustment _____

6. Code: 96405   Participating Physician

Actual Charge $65.00

Allowed Amount $53.40

Payment Amount _____

Co-Payment _____

Adjustment _____

7. Code: 57505   Participating Physician

(Patient seen in hospital outpatient department.)

Actual Charge $125

Allowed Amount _____

Payment Amount _____

Co-Payment _____

Adjustment _____

8. Code: 58300   Participating

(Patient seen in office.)

Actual Charge $50

Allowed Amount _____

Payment Amount _____

Co-Payment _____

Adjustment _____

9. Code: 20553   Participating Physician

$45 Remaining on Deductible

(Patient seen in office.)

Actual Charge $165

Allowed Amount _____

Payment Amount _____

Co-Payment _____

Adjustment _____

10. Patient has commercial insurance that pays 60% UCR after $100 deductible. The patient has not met the deductible for this visit.

Actual Charge $225

Allowed Amount $225

Insurance Payment _____

Patient Payment _____

11. Patient has a commercial insurance that will pay 80% UCR after a deductible of $250. To date, the patient has not met any portion of his deductible. Your bill is $195. List all payments and adjustments.

    Actual Charge $195

    Allowed Amount $195

    Insurance Payment _____

    Patient Payment _____

12. Code 55041   Participating Provider

    Remaining Deductible: $50

    Actual Charge: $60

    Allowed Amount _____

    Mm Payment _____

    Co-Payment _____

    Adjustment _____

9 Legal Issues

CHAPTER OUTLINE

KEY TERMS

Term	Definition
Abuse	Unknowingly defrauding the Medicare program by obtaining payment for items or services when there is not legal entitlement to the payment.
Arbitration	Legal method where the patient and physician may agree to resolve any controversy that may occur before an impartial panel.
Civil Law	Law that enforces private rights and liabilities, as distinguished from criminal law.
Defamation	Slander or libel or injury to reputation.
Defendant	Person defending a case. In a malpractice case this is usually the physician.
Deposition	Taking of testimony from a witness made under oath although not in an open court. Information is written down or taped to be used in the case of a trial.
Embezzlement	Willful act of illegally taking an employer's money by an employee.
Ethics	Moral principles and standards in the ideal relationship between a physician and patient or between physicians.
Fraud	An intentional misrepresentation of facts to deceive or mislead another.
Judgment	The official decision of the court in regard to an action or suit.
Litigation	A lawsuit.
Locum Tenens	A physician who substitutes for another physician who is out of the office for an extended period of time.
Malfeasance	Wrongful treatment of a patient.
Misfeasance	Lawful treatment performed or provided in the wrong way.
Negligence	Omission to do something that should be done under ordinary circumstances. Negligence can involve a wrongful action or an omission of care.
Nonfeasance	Failure by a physician to anything in regard to a patient's medical condition when the physician has an obligation to act.
Open Contract	An account where charges are made from time to time with a 5-year limitation for collection from the date the charge incurred.
PHI	Protected Health Information. Data that could be used to learn a person's health information.
Qui Tam	Recovery of a penalty brought by an informer in a situation. Generally, a percentage of the recovery is given to the informer for payment.
Statute of Limitations	The time limit in which a lawsuit may be filed.
Written Contract	An agreement signed by a patient in which specific payment amounts are made on the account on a monthly basis. These accounts usually have high amounts that will take over 4 months to repay and generally have a 6-year limitation for collection.

OBJECTIVES

After completing this chapter, readers should be able to:

- Describe legal issues concerning medical records.
- Discuss ways to comply with privacy regulations.
- Define fraud and fraudulent billing.
- Explain the importance of record keeping.
- Describe subpoena and the consequence in receiving a subpoena.
- Understand the statute of limitation on accounts for collection.

INTRODUCTION

The purpose of this chapter is to describe some of the problems encountered in the performance of practice duties and to provide guidance on ways to avoid legal issues in medical records, billing, and collection activities.

The best policy for any practice is to practice within the guidelines of the law and to have an attorney who is skilled in laws concerning medical practices and policies. When in doubt concerning practice policy or guidelines, one should contact an attorney to determine the various rules and regulations for the particular state and circumstances.

It is not the author's intent to replace legal counsel or to offer advice on legal matters. The intent is to direct the reader in identifying problems and situations that may require assistance from those who are versed in the rules and regulations governing your state policies and laws.

MEDICAL ETHICS

According to *Mosby's Medical, Nursing, & Allied Health Dictionary*, **ethics** is defined as the science or study of moral values or principles, including ideals of autonomy, beneficence, and justice. Ethics are standards in which a medical practice determines the propriety of conduct in relationship to patients, physicians, and coworkers. Our modern code of medical ethics was adopted by the American Medical Association and is known as the "Principles of Medical Ethics." Often in medicine, medical ethics and medical professional liability sometimes overlap.

Medical ethics and patient privacy have several factors in common. In forming the privacy rules discussed later in this chapter, you can see the parallel between ethics and HIPAA rulings. The following represent some of the standard guidelines of medical ethics used by medical practices.

- Everything you see, hear, or read about a patient remains confidential and does not leave the office.
- Never make critical remarks about the physician to a patient.
- Do not discuss a patient's condition within hearing distance of other patients.
- Do not discuss patient information with acquaintances (yours or the patient's).
- Do not leave patient records or appointment books exposed on your desk.
- Do not make critical statements about treatment given to a patient by another physician.

To obtain an in-depth understanding of the Code of Ethics for professional associations, visit the following web sites:

American Association of Medical Assistants   http://www.aama-ntl.org
American Health Information Management Association   http://www.ahima.org

MEDICAL RECORDS

A medical record is a written account of the reason a patient sought medical care and the treatment rendered by the physician. Records include:

- Notes written in an office chart (progress notes)
- Operative reports
- Hospital summaries
- Consultation notes
- Laboratory/diagnostic studies
- Radiology reports

Patients' medical records and financial records contain health information. Health information includes any facts that relate to the past, present, or future physical or mental health or condition of an individual, the health care they received, or the payment for that health care.

The data that could be used to learn a person's health information is called **protected health information, or PHI.** Under federal regulations, medical offices, insurance carriers, and any other company that processes patients' health information electronically must protect the privacy and security of this PHI.

PROTECTED HEALTH INFORMATION: THE HIPAA PRIVACY RULE

Congress passed the **Health Insurance Portability and Accountability Act (HIPAA)** in 1996 because of concerns regarding fraud (e.g., coding irregularities, medical necessity issues, and waiving co-pays and deductibles). Although the authority granted under the Federal False Claims Act provided CMS with regulatory authority to enforce fraud and abuse statutes, HIPAA extends that authority to all federal and state health care programs.

HIPAA provisions were designed to improve the portability and continuity of heath care coverage by:

- Limiting exclusions for preexisting medical conditions.
- Providing credit for prior health coverage and a process for transmitting certificates and other information concerning prior coverage to a new group health plan.
- Providing new rights that allow individuals to enroll for health coverage when they lose other coverage, change from a group to individual plan, or have a new dependent.
- Prohibiting discrimination in enrollment and premiums against employees and their dependents based on health status.
- Guaranteeing availability of insurance coverage for small employers and renewability of coverage in both the small and large group markets.
- Preserving the states' traditional role through narrow preemption provisions in regulating health insurance.

Privacy Rule

The final HIPAA Privacy Rule was published by the Department of Health and Human Services (HHS) on December 28, 2000. The final rule took effect on April 14, 2003. The Privacy Rule creates national standards to protect individuals' medical records and other PHI. The rule also gives patients greater access to their own medical records and more control over how their personal health information is used. The rule addresses the obligations of health care providers and health plans to protect health information.

The Privacy Rule requires the implementation of activities that include:

- Providing information to patients about their privacy rights and how their information can be used.
- Adopting clear privacy procedures for the practice, hospital, or plan.
- Training employees so they understand the privacy procedures.

- Designating an individual to be responsible for seeing that the privacy procedures are adopted and followed.
- Securing patient records containing individually identifiable health information so they are not readily accessible to those who do not need them.

The **HIPAA Privacy Rule** covers patients' protected health information. Under the Privacy Rule, medical practices may not use or disclose protected health information, except as the individual who is the subject of the information (or the individual's personal representative) authorizes in writing or as needed for treatment, payment, and health care operations.

These terms refer to:

Treatment	Providing, coordinating, and managing health care for the patient, such as asking the patient's insurance carrier for an authorization, a consultation between doctors on the patient's case, or the referral of a patient from one physician to another.
Payment	All the activities the medical office does to be reimbursed by insurance companies and government health plans, including billing and collection activities.
Health Care Operations	Administrative, financial, and legal activities necessary to run the business of the medical office.

If a practice thinks it best, it may obtain patient consent for uses and disclosures of protected health information for treatment, payment, and health care operations. This consent is not required by the Privacy Rule, however. An **authorization** from the patient is required by the Privacy rule for the practice, hospital, or plan to use and disclose protected health information not otherwise allowed by the rule. Where the Privacy Rule requires patient authorization, voluntary consent is not sufficient to permit use or disclosure of protected health information unless it also satisfies the requirements of a valid authorization. A valid authorization is a detailed document that gives covered entities permission to use protected health information for specified purposes, which are generally other than treatment, payment, or health care operations.

An authorization must have:

- A description of the protected health information to be used and disclosed.
- The person authorized to make the use or disclosure.
- The person to whom the covered entity may make the disclosure.
- An expiration date.
- Usually, the purpose for which the information may be used or disclosed.

How Practices Comply

To comply with the HIPAA Privacy Rule, practices must:

- Tell patients about their privacy rights and how their information can be used.
- Have privacy procedures and train employees so that they understand how to follow them.
- Have a staff member who is appointed to be responsible for seeing that the privacy procedures are adopted and followed.
- Make patient records that have PHI secure, so that they cannot be accessed by those who do not need the information.

Offices usually create written privacy policies called a Notice of Privacy Practices. The main points of this document are summarized on a form called the **Acknowledgment of Receipt of Notice of Privacy Practices**. Patients of the practice are asked to sign this form and can take a copy of the privacy practices if they wish. If a particular patient refuses to sign, a note of this is made in the medical record to show that the practice attempted in good faith to get a signature.

The Privacy Rule also must be followed by vendors outside the practice that work with or provide services to the practice if the work involves the use of protected health information. Such **business associates** of the practice must sign agreements that they will follow the regulations and keep the data secure. Examples are outside billing service companies, attorneys, and accounting firms.

When using or disclosing protected health information, medical office staff must try to limit the use or disclosure to the minimum amount of PHI necessary—just what is needed to accomplish the intended purpose. This **minimum standard** does not apply to disclosures, including oral disclosures, among physicians who are treating the patient. For example, a physician is not required to apply the minimum necessary standard when discussing a patient's medical chart with another doctor also handling the case.

Physician's offices may use patient sign-in sheets or call out patient names in waiting rooms, as long as the information disclosed is appropriately limited. The HIPAA Privacy Rule explicitly permits the incidental disclosures that may result from this practice—for example, when other patients in a waiting room hear the identity of the person whose name is called, or see other patients' names on a sign-in sheet. Reasonable safeguards need to be in place. For example, the sign-in sheet may not display medical information that is not necessary for the purpose of signing in (e.g., the medical problem for which the patient is seeing the physician).

The Privacy Rule also addresses records that have been written or dictated by the physician while rendering the service in that particular office. Records from hospitals, laboratories, x-ray departments, or other physicians are not part of the physician's records. Information of this type should be requested from the agency or party that actually performed the service. When a physician has dictated notes or operative reports at a hospital, this information should be requested from and sent by the hospital even though the physician has a copy of the information in the office chart.

Patient Rights

Patients also have rights under the HIPAA Privacy Rule, such as the right to:

- Access, copy, and inspect their health information.
- Request an amendment to their health care information.
- Obtain an accounting of certain disclosures of their health information.
- Another means of receiving communications from providers.
- Complain about alleged violations of the regulations and the provider's own information policies.

If patients ask for copies of their records, the medical practice is permitted to charge for this service. The amount charged should be reasonable and stated in the Notice of Privacy Policies. Fees should be established based on the type of information requested and comply with the state limitations on copy fees. Items subject to fees are as follows:

- Copy of records only
- Office **depositions**
- Court appearance
- Written narrative reports
- Written narrative report with copy of record

Patients who feel their privacy rights have been violated can complain to the Office of Civil Rights, a federal agency, which will investigate the charges and take the necessary legal actions if physicians or other health care providers are guilty of a violation.

E X A M P L E

Authorization for Release of Medical Information

To Dr Hope T. Getwell:

I authorize you to furnish a copy of the medical records for Wanda L. Adams for service dates January 2, 20XX to February 5, 20XX. Records are to be sent to Dr. John L. Smith, Villa, New Mexico, for review of my case. I release you from all legal responsibility or liability that may arise from this authorization.

Witnessed By: _____   Authorized Signature _____

Date _____

HIPAA Security Rule

The **HIPAA Security Rule** requires medical offices to have safeguards to protect the confidentiality, integrity, and availability of health information covered by HIPAA. The security rule specifies how the practice must secure such PHI on computer networks, the Internet, and storage devices such as disks.

FEDERAL LAW AND STATE LAWS

The HIPAA Privacy and Security Rules are federal law. Most states also have laws and regulations about the privacy of patients' medical information. The general rule is that if the state law is more restrictive than the federal law, then the state law applies. If there is no state law, then medical practices follow the federal law. The office should consult with an attorney, state medical association, or the liability carrier to determine which laws apply and include these in the privacy policies and procedures. For example, most states require disclosure of public health information relating to births, deaths, and certain communicable diseases such as AIDS.

Because of these differences in state laws, the medical office may have procedures requiring patients to sign a release of information form, even if the information falls under HIPAA Privacy Rule guidelines.

State Insurance Commissions

Each state has a department or division to watch over and regulate the activities of insurance companies. These commissions monitor carriers to ensure that they are financially sound, the interests of the policy holders are protected, and agents, brokers, or organizations who transact insurance business are in compliance with the laws of the state.

When an office is experiencing problems with an insurance carrier, the office should notify the state insurance commission. Written notification to the commission should include:
- Nature of the problem
- Frequency of the situation
- Any other problems experienced with the carrier

The commission may hold a hearing or investigation to determine if the carrier is acting in accordance with contract agreements or help settle disputes.

Some problems that may need involvement by the commission include but are not limited to the following situations:
- Delay in payments for claims
- Payment denials based on contract agreements
- Lowering payment amounts when documentation supports a higher fee
- Unlawful termination or cancellation of an insurance policy
- Problems with charges for premiums
- Misrepresentation by an insurance agent or broker concerning policy benefits and payments

SUBPOENAS

A subpoena is a written legal order directing a physician to either give testimony or provide copies of the medical record. Subpoenas are usually issued in the case of child abuse or Workers' Compensation cases.

When issued a subpoena, the office may bill the requesting party for copies of records or special reports with one exception—the insurance carrier for a Workers' Compensation case when that carrier requests a copy of the records.

Before accepting a subpoena, staff should determine, when possible, the content of the subpoena (e.g., court appearance, deposition, copying the records). The office should have a written policy for staff members to following concerning the acceptance of a subpoena. This policy will help avoid crisis or problems for the physician.

 Legal Tip

Once a subpoena is accepted by a staff member, the physician is obligated to comply with the contents of the summons.

WORKERS' COMPENSATION CLAIMS

Workers' Compensation cases are exempt from HIPAA regulations. An office usually bills the Workers' Compensation carrier provided the patient has been declared eligible for Workers' Compensation by either the carrier or the attorney for that carrier. If the Workers' Compensation carrier requests regular medical records, the office should not bill for this service. However, if the carrier has requested a special report or requires special testimony from the physician, it is generally a safe rule to charge the carrier for these special conditions as long as the reports or testimony are not part of the original record. However, because rules governing Workers' Compensation vary from state to state, you should check with your state agency for exact information.

RECORD RETENTION

A question often asked by medical offices concerns how long medical and business records should be kept for legal purposes. It is generally a good rule to keep pertinent records for the life of the practice. However, when space is limited and this is not feasible, the following rules listed in Table 9-1 should help you maintain good records to support physician billing and service. Because regulations vary from state to state, you should contact local agencies such as the state's medical association or bar association for more accurate information.

TABLE 9-1   General Guidelines for Retaining Medical Records

Type of Record	Length of Retention
Medical records	10 years from the date of most recent encounter
X-ray film	5 years
Cases involving radiological injury	Indefinitely
Cases involving minors	3 to 4 years after the patient reaches legal age
Laboratory reports; pathology reports	Indefinitely
Calendars; appointment books; phone logs	Indefinitely
Assigned Medicare and Medicaid	7 years
Records of HIPAA compliance	6 years

COLLECTIONS

Collecting overdue payments from patients is regulated by federal and state law. The Fair Debt Collection Practices Act of 1977 and the Telephone Consumer Protection Act of 1991 regulate debt collections, forbidding unfair practices. General guidelines include:

- Do not call a patient before 8 AM or after 9 PM.
- Do not make threats or use profane language.
- Do not discuss the patient's debt with anyone except the person who is responsible for payment.
- If the patient has a lawyer, then problems may be discussed with the lawyer based on patient authorization.
- Do not use any form of deception or violence to collect a debt. As an example, do not impersonate a law officer to try to force a patient to pay.
- If the practice's printed or displayed payment policy covers adding finance charges on late accounts, it is acceptable to do so. The amount of the finance charge must comply with federal and state law.

 R E M I N D E R

Always check with the medical or bar association of your state to determine if specific retention guidelines have been established.

Statute Of Limitations

In Chapter 8, readers were introduced to the terms **open account** and **written contract accounts**. Table 9-2 provides information for each state regarding the time limits for collection of these accounts.

Small Claims Court

An office may take a patient to court for an unpaid bill. This type of court action is generally transacted through small claims courts. Each state sets a specific dollar amount limit on the accounts that can be handled by small claims courts. Using this collection method is often an inexpensive way to handle a collection problem. An office needs to show proof of the account to the judge and verify that the account is delinquent in payment.

 Special Note

Once an account has been turned over to a collection agency, the account cannot be processed by a small claims court. Legal action must be obtained through a municipal court hearing.

In a court action, the following information is required in order to begin the proceedings:

- Name, address, and phone number of the physician
- Patient's name and address
- The amount of the claim
- A brief description or summary of the account (include date the bill was due when a treatment series is in dispute)
- Date of last visit or payment
- Balance due amount

In small claims court, the court only rules if the debt is valid or not. It does not guarantee a payment. It is still the responsibility of the practice to collect the debt.

TABLE 9-2   State Timelines for Account Collections

ACCOUNT CONTRACT LIMITATION GUIDELINES (YEARS)					
State	Open	Written	State	Open	Written
Alabama	3	6	Montana	5	8
Alaska	6	6	Nebraska	4	5
Arizona	3	6	Nevada	4	6
Arkansas	3	5	New Hampshire	6	6
California	4	4	New Jersey	6	6
Colorado	6	6	New Mexico	4	6
Connecticut	6	6	New York	6	6
Delaware	3	6	North Carolina	3	3
District of Columbia	3	3	North Dakota	6	6
Florida	4	5	Ohio	6	15
Georgia	4	6	Oklahoma	3	5
Hawaii	6	6	Oregon	6	6
Idaho	4	5	Pennsylvania	6	6
Illinois	5	10	Rhode Island	6	6
Indiana	6	10	South Carolina	6	6
Iowa	5	10	South Dakota	6	6
Kansas	3	5	Tennessee	6	6
Kentucky	5	15	Texas	4	4
Maine	6	6	Utah	4	6
Maryland	3	3	Vermont	6	6
Massachusetts	6	6	Virginia	3	5
Michigan	6	6	Washington	3	6
Minnesota	6	6	West Virginia	5	10
Mississippi	3	6	Wisconsin	6	6
Missouri	5	10	Wyoming	8	10

Estate Claims

Estate claims are made against the estate of a deceased patient (Fig. 9-1). Many states have established time limits governing the filing of a claim against the patient's estate. Once the office receives notification of the patient's death, the office must submit a claim for the unpaid balance to the administrator for the estate.

If one has been unable to locate the name of the administrator for an estate, one should contact the probate department of the Superior Court, County Recorder's Office. After obtaining the name of the administrator:

- Send an itemized statement of the account by certified mail with a request for a return receipt.
- If there is no reply after 10 days, contact the executor or county clerk where the estate is being settled and obtain correct forms for filing a claim against the estate.
- If the administrator rejects the claim for payment, the physician should file a claim against the administrator of the estate.

Department of Health and Human Services
Centers for Medicare and Medicaid Services

Form Approved
OMB No. 0938-0020

REQUEST FOR INFORMATION — MEDICARE PAYMENT FOR
SERVICES TO A PATIENT NOW DECEASED

No further monies or other benefits may be paid out under this program unless this report is completed and filed as required by existing law and regulations (20 C.F.R. 405 1683).

When completed, send this form to:	Deceased patient
	Health insurance claim number of deceased patient

For services provided by:

PART I — PAID BILL (If the bill is not paid go to part II)

If bills for medical or other health services were paid by or for the deceased person, Medicare benefits may be due. We hope you will be able to help us determine who should receive payment. The person who paid the deceased's bill(s) has first right to any payment due. If the deceased or his estate paid the bill(s), benefits will be paid to the legal representative of the estate. If there is no legal representative, payment will be made to the person who stands highest in the list of relatives below. If the person who paid the bill(s) dies before being reimbursed, payment is also made to the person standing highest in the list of relatives. If there are no living relatives or legal representatives, no payment will be made. Please answer the questions, sign on the reverse side, and return this form in the enclosed envelope.

ALWAYS INCLUDE EVIDENCE OF PAYMENT SUCH AS A RECEIPTED BILL OR OTHER RECEIPT

1. Who paid the deceased bills for medical or other health services?
   - ☐ The deceased or his estate (Answer (2) below)
   - ☐ Yourself (Sign on reverse side and return form)
   - ☐ Other person or organization (Enter the person's or organization's name and address in item 4 below. If there is more than one person or organization, attach a listing of names and addresses of these persons or organizations to this form.)

2. Is there a legal representative of the estate?
   - ☐ Yes (If "Yes," print his name and address below, sign on reverse side, and return form.) If you are the legal representative, submit a copy of your appointment papers with this form.
   - ☐ No (If "No," answer item 3 below.)

3. This item is answered only if item 2 above is checked "No." Put a check in the box next to the living relative that stands highest on the following list, and then write that relative's name and address in item 4 below. (If you check the box for child or children and there is more than one child, attach a listing of the names and address of all the children to this form.)
   - ☐ Widow or widower living in the same household as the deceased at the time of death, or entitled to a monthly Social Security or Railroad Retirement benefit on the same earnings record as the deceased in the month of death.
   - ☐ A child or children of the deceased entitled to monthly Social Security or Railroad Retirement benefits or the same earnings record as the deceased in the month of death. (List the names and addresses of all entitled children of the deceased.)
   - ☐ A parent or parents of the deceased entitled to monthly Social Security or Railroad Retirement benefits on the same earnings record as the deceased in the month of death.
   - ☐ A widow or widower who was neither living with the deceased at the time of death nor at that time entitled on the same earnings record to a Social Security or Railroad Retirement benefit.
   - ☐ A child or children of the deceased who were not entitled in the month of death to monthly Social Security or Railroad Retirement benefits on the same earnings record as the deceased. (List the names and addresses of all such children.)
   - ☐ A parent or parents not entitled in the month of death to monthly Social Security or Railroad Retirement benefits on the same earnings record as the deceased.

4. Name | Address

FIGURE 9-1 Request for information: Medicare Payment for Services to a Patient Now Deceased. *(Source: U.S. Department of Health and Human Services, Centers for Medicare & Medicaid Services.)*

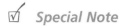 *Special Note*

Claims must be filed in the county where the estate is being settled, not where the debt occurred.

Each state has different rules and regulations concerning the filing of an estate claim. In some states the physician must file a claim against the estate within a specific time period based on:

- The date the court of probate recognizes an administrator
- The date the first notice of creditors was published
- The date of the second notice of publication
- The date of the death of the patient

States also differ regarding with whom the claim must be filed. In some states the physician must file the claim with a court-appointed official, the court of probate, or the administrator or representative of the estate. To ensure the office is correctly filing your claims, check with the individual state probate court or the attorney for the practice to determine the rules and regulations concerning time limits and where the claim has to be filed.

FRAUD AND ABUSE

Fraud is knowingly and willfully executing, or attempting to execute, a scheme or artifice against the Medicare program to obtain payment. Fraud may be committed either for the person's own benefit or the benefit of some other party. **Abuse** is unknowingly defrauding the Medicare program by obtaining payment for items or services when there is not legal entitlement to the payment.

A frequently asked question in the medical community is: How is fraud uncovered?

- Carriers audit physicians who routinely have excessive charges or vague diagnosis codes.
- If an office is suspected of wrongful doing, undercover agents may go to the office as patients.
- Questionnaires are sent to patients asking patients to verify types or dates of services.

The following are examples of the most common types of fraud and **embezzlement:**

- Billing for services not rendered to a patient
- Altering fees on a claim form
- Omitting relevant information on a claim (e.g., spouse's insurance information)
- Changing a date of service to an incorrect date
- Changing a diagnosis to ensure insurance coverage

The following are examples of the most common types of abuse:

- Billing for services or items in excess of those needed by the patient
- Routinely filing duplicate claims, even if it does not result in duplicate payments
- Inappropriate or incorrect information filed on cost reports

Although inappropriate billing or reporting may initially appear abusive, it could evolve into fraud, such as:

- Collecting in excess of the deductible or coinsurance amounts due from the patient
- Requiring a deposit or other payment from a patient as a condition of admission, continued care, or other provision of services

When a provider commits fraud, an investigation is conducted by the Office of the Inspector General (OIG). The OIG Office of Investigations prepares the case for referral to the Department of Justice for criminal and/or civil prosecution. A person(s) found guilty of Medicare fraud could face criminal, civil, and/or administrative sanctions. Penalties for Medicare fraud include:

- Civil penalties of $5,000 to $10,000 per false claim plus triple damages under the False Claims Act. (If found guilty, the provider pays an amount equal to three times the amount submitted on the claim plus the civil penalty fine.)

- Criminal fines and/or imprisonment of up to 10 years if convicted of health care fraud.
- For violations of the Medicare/Medicaid anti-kickback statute, imprisonment of up to 5 years and/or a criminal fine of up to $25,000.
- Administrative sanctions include up to a $10,000 civil monetary penalty claim form, assessment of up to triple the amount falsely claimed, and/or exclusion from participating in Medicare and state health care programs.

 Legal Tip

In addition to the previous penalties, offices who commit health care fraud can also be tried for mail and wire fraud.

TIPS FOR A CLEAN PRACTICE

As a first step, a practice should establish a policy or plan of action to identify erroneous and fraudulent claims by reviewing claims for accuracy to minimize billing mistakes and avoid conflicts with self-referrals and anti-kickback statutes.

Practices can work to identify risk areas based on the practice's specific history with billing problems and other compliance issues.

- Keep accurate, legible records.
- Perform periodic reviews to internally monitor billing practices. Although there is not a set rule for frequency, it is recommended that an office review these practices at least twice a year.
- Conduct appropriate training and education sessions to keep staff knowledgeable of practice standards and procedures.
- Enforce disciplinary standards through well-publicized guidelines.

When correcting an entry, cross out incorrect data, enter correct data, initial the correction, and give an explanation for the reason for the error. Never use correction fluid or erase information already in the patient's record. Review insurance forms before mailing them. An insurance company can sue the physician for incomplete records. Be sure to complete all blank lines on the form because this will prevent tampering with your submitted claim. Record missed or cancelled appointments. This can assist the office in showing patient compliance in case of a malpractice suit. Do not release confidential information without a signed permission form from patient. Avoid having office staff give patients test or laboratory results. The physician is the only one qualified to interpret data. Ensure services are reasonable and necessary. Avoid improper inducements, kickbacks, and self-referrals.

REVIEW QUESTIONS   Legal Issues

1. What are the two types of accounts that have a statute of limitation for collection?

_____

_____

2. Before a physician may release records to another physician, what must the physician obtain from the patient?

_____

_____

3. Can a staff member accept a subpoena on behalf of the physician?

_____

_____

4. A new patient came into the office. After the visit, she stated she did not like the doctor and would not be coming back to the office. Would you keep this patient's records in your files? Why or why not?

_____

_____

5. List the different levels of appeal in the Medicare system.

_____

_____

6. When a patient asks for a copy of his or her records, what portion of the record may the office release?

_____

_____

7. What is a subpoena?

_____

_____

8. In the case of a deceased patient, where would you find information regarding the administrator of the estate?

_____

_____

9. In the event of a Workers' Compensation case, who may be billed for copies of medical records?

_____

_____

10. List three ways fraud is discovered in a medical practice.

_____

_____

KEY TERMS

Term	Definition
Actual Charge	The amount charged by a practice when providing services.
Adjudicate	A term for processing payment of a claim.
Adjudicator	Person who reviews a claim to determine payments.
Adjustment	The amount corrected on a patient ledger due to an error or the difference in the amount billed by a practice and the amount allowed by the insurance company for payment of a claim.
Adjustment Codes	Codes used by insurance companies to explain actions taken on a remittance notice.
Aging Report	A report to track claim status of patient accounts and to identify individual accounts requiring additional workup for payments and collections.
Allowed Charge	The amount set by the carrier for the reimbursement of services.
Assignment	Authorization by a policyholder to allow a third-party payer to pay benefits to a health care provider.
Assignment of Benefits	A request that money be paid directly to the physician for services rendered on a given claim. In some instances, accepting assignment may result in adjustments or write-offs.
Beneficiary	In the Medicare program, one who is eligible to receive Medicare benefits for medical coverage.
Commercial Payer	Private health insurance company or employer-based group insurance plan that pays claims for eligible participants.
Co-payment	The amount the insured has to pay toward the amount allowed by the insurance company for services.
Customary Charge	The amount representing the charge most frequently used by a physician in a given period of time.
Deductible	The dollar amount that must be paid by the patient before insurance will pay a claim based on coverage plans and benefits.
Demographic Information	Patient identification information. Contains complete patient name, date of birth, Social Security number, and insurance information.
DOS	Date of Service.
EIN	National standard Employer Identification Number. An IRS federal tax identification number adopted as the national employer identifier (e.g., 42-1212123).
Encounter Form	Document to record information regarding services provided to a patient; used for billing purposes.
EOB	Explanation of Benefits. A form accompanying an insurance remittance with a breakdown and explanation of payments for a claim. Also referred to as a remittance advisory.
Fee Schedule	An established price set by a medical practice for professional services.
Insurance Adjustment or Write-Off	Amount required by an insurance company that must be taken off of a patient's account based on contract agreement and participation.
Ledger Card	A record to track patient charges, payments, adjustments, and balances due.
NPI	National Provider Identifier. A number assigned to hospitals, physicians, nursing homes, and other health care providers containing alphanumeric characters plus a check digit (e.g., E3E30KL74-6).
POS Codes	Place-of-Service Codes. Codes used on insurance claim forms to specify the location where services were provided. A complete list is found in the introduction section of the professional version of the CPT manual.
Remittance Advisory	Statement sent by an insurance company detailing how submitted claims were processed for payment along with payment amounts.
Superbill	A multipurpose billing form to track procedure and diagnosis codes during a patient encounter or visit.

OBJECTIVES

After completing this chapter, readers should be able to:

- Organize and process claims appropriately.
- Complete insurance claims based on patient demographic information.
- Code ICD-9-CM and CPT codes as applicable for correct placement on a CMS-1500 claim form.
- Assign fees based on a fee schedule.
- Read a remittance advisory and correctly apply payments and adjustments.

INTRODUCTION

This chapter will allow you to apply all the information learned from this text by providing an opportunity to work up a patient from the time of service, through the billing cycle, and ending with applying payments and adjustments.

This chapter will enhance your learning experience by providing insight into the complete billing and reimbursement cycle.

INSURANCE CLAIM FORMS EXERCISES

For the purpose of these exercises, use the following provided physician information for all the claims:

Physician:	A. Good Surgeon, MD
Phone:	(314) 123-4444
Address:	Miracle Clinic
	12 Hope and Get Well
	Any Town, Missouri 63010
Social Security Number:	222-22-2222
Tax ID #:	43-00110000
Insurance ID Numbers:	Medicare Numbers
TRICARE: 002000134567	Clinic: 00001115
Blue Shield: 0101010101010	NPI: 1115222222222
Hospital Address:	Mercy General
	1 Get Well
	Anytown, MO 60600

Please refer to Chapter 7 for additional information on these exercises.

Practice Fee Schedule

Medical Services					
New Patient		**Injections**		**Surgery Cont'd**	
99201	$45.00	90471	$5.00	27506	$1,450.00
99202	$60.00	90742	$5.00	36415	$12.00
99203	$90.00	90701	$15.00	45331	$135.00
99204	$115.00	90702	$12.00	45333	$150.00
99205	$135.00	90703	$15.00	45378	$375.00
		90707	$15.00	45385	$50.00
				49520	$650.00
Est. Patient		**Psychiatric Service**		49525	$825.00
99211	$15.00	90801	$125.00	50075	$2,000.00
99212	$30.00	90804	$55.00	51030	$300.00
99213	$45.00	90805	$65.00	64719	$600.00
99214	$60.00	90806	$125.00	64721	$600.00
99215	$85.00				
Hospital Services		**Special Services**		**X-Ray Services**	
Admissions		99000	$10.00	71010	$40.00
99221	$80.00	99204	-0-	71020	$60.00
99222	$100.00	99058	$10.00	73090	$40.00
99223	$125.00			73110	$60.00
Daily Care		**Surgery**		**Lab/Pathology**	
99231	$40.00	11400	$75.00	81000	$10.00
99232	$45.00	11401	$95.00	82947	$15.00
99233	$60.00	11402	$115.00	82948	$10.00
				82951	$25.00
Discharge		12031	$85.00	85025	$20.00
99238	$75.00	12032	$135.00		
Consult–Office		12034	$160.00	**Misc Services**	
99241	$60.00	21088	$75.00	93000	$35.00
99242	$70.00	25600	$160.00	36415	$7.00
99243	$90.00	25605	$290.00		
99244	$125.00	27500	$850.00		
99245	$150.00	27511	$1350.00		

CPT codes, descriptions, and two-digit numeric modifiers only are copyright 2004 American Medical Association. All rights reserved.

Above fees are for the purpose of practice only and are not intended as a basis to set fees.

Note: The physician information cited first pertains to the first set of patients (ending with Worthington) who do not have ledger cards. The fees on the superbill (pages 287-288) apply to all patients in this chapter.

PATIENT: PAMELA JEAN BROWN (Fig. 10-1)

DATE: February 27, 20XX

COMPLAINT/SYMPTOMS
This 44-year-old married, white woman presented for an initial evaluation on February 27, 20XX, with complaints of severe headaches, chest pain, and difficulty breathing.

HISTORY
No known allergies. The patient is currently taking no prescribed medication. She is active, walking 30 minutes a day. Has history of two live births by cesarean section late in life, ages 27 and 33. She has been obese most of her life, with periodic attempts to lose weight that were unsuccessful. She has a history of underactive thyroid but is not currently undergoing treatment for this problem. Her history is remarkable for urinary infection with kidney stone removal at age 37. She has a history of ovarian infections with severe complication. Patient complains of migraine headaches on average of three to four times a month, with nausea and vomiting and light sensitivity.

PRACTICE ACCOUNT NUMBER	**PATIENT REGISTRATION FORM**	DATE

<table>
<tr><td>PATIENT ACCOUNT NUMBER
54678</td><td>PRACTICE NAME
MIRACLE CLINIC</td><td>02-27-xx

☒NEW ☐ CHANGE</td></tr>
</table>

PATIENT INFORMATION *(Please write information about the patient here.)*

PATIENT'S NAME BROWN, Pamela Jean	SEX ☐ Male ☒ Female	REFERRING DOCTOR N/A		
PATIENT'S ADDRESS 3796 Rose Lane		REFERRING DOCTOR ADDRESS	CITY	STATE
CITY Anytown	STATE ZIP MO 60600	EMPLOYER'S NAME N/A		TELEPHONE
TELEPHONE 314-555-2168	MARITAL STATUS ☒ Single ☐ Separated ☐ Married ☐ Divorced ☐ Widowed DATE OF BIRTH 02/10/46	EMPLOYER'S ADDRESS	CITY	STATE
AGE SOCIAL SECURITY NUMBER 271-18-3640	DRIVERS LICENSE NUMBER	EMPLOYMENT STATUS ☐ Full-Time ☐ Retired ☐ Part-Time ☒ Not Employed STUDENT STATUS: If 19 Years of Older: ☐ Full Time ☐ Part Time ☐ Not a Student		

INSURANCE INFORMATION *(Please write information about the patient's insurance here.)*

PRIMARY INSURANCE COMPANY May Day Insurance Co.	☒ Medical ☐ Dental ☐ Worker's Comp.	SECONDARY INSURANCE COMPANY MEDICARE	☒ Medical ☐ Dental ☐ Worker's Comp.
INSURANCE COMPANY'S ADDRESS 22 May Street		INSURANCE COMPANY'S ADDRESS P.O. Box 505	
CITY Mayville	STATE ZIP Ohio 22441	CITY St. Louis	STATE ZIP MO 63166
GROUP PLAN NUMBER POLICY OR SUBSCRIBER'S NUMBER 288-71-1664		GROUP PLAN NUMBER POLICY OR SUBSCRIBER'S NUMBER 271-18-3640-A	

POLICYHOLDER INFORMATION *Is the secondary policyholder the:* ☐ *Patient*   ☐ *Primary Policyholder*   ☐ *Other*
(Complete the information below if the PATIENT is not the POLICYHOLDER)   *(Complete the information below if you checked "Other")*

PRIMARY POLICYHOLDER'S NAME BROWN, Sideny	DATE OF BIRTH 20 08 42	SECONDARY POLICYHOLDER'S NAME PATIENT	DATE OF BIRTH ___/___/___
PRIMARY POLICYHOLDER'S ADDRESS Same as patient	TELEPHONE	SECONDARY POLICYHOLDER'S ADDRESS	TELEPHONE
CITY	STATE ZIP	CITY	STATE ZIP
EMPLOYER'S NAME Wonderful Department Store	TELEPHONE 314-525-0001	EMPLOYER'S NAME	TELEPHONE
EMPLOYER'S ADDRESS 12 Sell Avenue		EMPLOYER'S ADDRESS	
CITY Anytown	STATE ZIP MO 60600	CITY	STATE ZIP
SOCIAL SECURITY NUMBER RELATIONSHIP TO PATIENT 288-71-1664 ☒ SPOUSE ☐ DEPENDENT ☐ OTHER___		SOCIAL SECURITY NUMBER RELATIONSHIP TO PATIENT ☐ SPOUSE ☐ DEPENDENT ☐ OTHER___	
EMPLOYER PLAN COVERAGE IF CHAMPUS: ☐ Active ☐ Retired ☐ Deceased ☐ YES ☐ No Branch of Service: _____		EMPLOYER PLAN COVERAGE IF CHAMPUS: ☐ Active ☐ Retired ☐ Deceased ☐ YES ☐ No Branch of Service: _____	

RESPONSIBLE PARTY INFORMATION *Responsible party is:* ☐ *Patient* ☐ *Primary Policyholder* ☐ *Secondary Policyholder*
(Please complete the information below if the person responsible for paying the fill is not the PATIENT or the POLICYHOLDER.)

RESPONSIBLE PARTY'S NAME	SEX ☐ Male ☐ Female	SOCIAL SECURITY NO. DRIVERS LICENSE NO. LEGAL REPRESENTATIVE ☐ Yes ☐ No
RESPONSIBLE PARTY'S ADDRESS STATE ZIP		EMPLOYER'S NAME TELEPHONE
TELEPHONE RELATIONSHIP TO PATIENT ☐ SPOUSE ☐ DEPENDENT ☐ OTHER___		EMPLOYER'S ADDRESS STATE ZIP

I AGREE TO THE ASSIGNMENTS AND FINANCIAL RESPONSIBILITIES SHOWN ON THE BACK OF THIS FORM.
<u>YOU SHOULD READ THOSE TERMS CAREFULLY.</u>

X _____ Date _____
   SIGNED (Patient, or parent if under 18 years of age.)

FIGURE 10-1 Patient registration form for Pamela Jean Brown.

FAMILY HISTORY

Paternal grandfather had history of high blood pressure. Maternal grandmother had cervical cancer and died of coronary occlusion on 64th birthday. Mother and sister had total hysterectomies before age 40, with histories of migraine headaches. Father died of heart attack at age 57.

EXAMINATION

Patient received a complete, detailed physical examination, and a routine electrocardiogram was performed. Results were within normal limits. Blood count, hematocrit, automated CBC, and routine urinalysis with microscopy and tablet reagent yielded negative results. Blood pressure was taken at intervals; levels were elevated in all situations.

DECISION-MAKING

Low complexity

RECOMMENDATION

Patient to be placed on 25 mg Tenormin for blood pressure. Patient instructed to return in 4 weeks for reevaluation of blood pressure.

DIAGNOSIS

Hypertension unspecified
Migraine headache, classic
Hiatal hernia

PATIENT: **PAMELA JEAN BROWN**

DATE: February 27, 20XX

HISTORY	EXAMINATION	DECISION MAKING
HPI: Extended	1995:	Diagnosis:
ROS: Extended		Data:
PFSH: Complete	1997:	Risk:
TYPE: Comprehensive	TYPE: Detailed	TYPE: Low
Category/subcategory:		
CPT Code(s):		
ICD-9 Code(s):		

HPI, History of present illness; *ROS*, review of systems; *PFSH*, past family social history.

	PF	Exp. PF	Detail	Complete
HPI: Severity, timing, location, and associated signs	Brief 1-3 elements	Brief 1-3 elements	Extended 4 or more elements	Extended 4 or more elements
ROS Allergy endo GI & GU	None	Pertinent 1 system	Extended 2-9 systems	Complete 10 or more
PFSH: Past, family and social	None	None	Pertinent 1 area	Complete 2-3 areas
	No PFSH required: 99231-33, 99261-63, 99311-33			
	Circle entry farthest to the right for each history area. To determine history level, draw a line down the column with the circle farthest to the left.			
	Problem Focus	E. P. Focus	Detail	Compre-hensive

OFFICE VISIT
PATIENT: **MARY SUE GANNON (Fig. 10-2)**

COMPLAINT
Bicycle accident occurring near home
Date of accident: March 12, 20XX

HISTORY
The patient was involved in a bicycle accident near her home 2 hours before appearance in the office. She fell on her left leg and sustained a laceration to the pretibial area. There was no head trauma or loss of consciousness during the incident. This was the patient's first time on a bicycle, so she was unsure of herself with respect to the mobility of the bike.

PHYSICAL EXAMINATION
Neck: No adenopathy; supple
Lungs: Clear
Abdomen: Soft
Cardio: Normal sinus rhythm

An examination of the extremities revealed a well-demarcated pinpoint 5-cm laceration over the mid-pretibial area. The wound margins are well marginated and discrete, with small amounts of grassy debris. The depth is penetrating down to the periosteum of the tibia. No arterial bleeding is indicated. However, there is some small venous capillary bleeding.
Vascular examination: Bilateral venous pulses in the posterior tibia and dorsalis pedis.
Capillary refill time: Normal
Neurologic examination: Normal
Motor and sensory examination: Normal, without any numbness or paresthesias to the left leg

Irrigated wound copiously with normal saline solution. Wound infiltrated with 1% Xylocaine. Prepped and draped in sterile fashion. Skin and deeper tissues closed in layers. Skin edges reapproximated with 12 3-0 Prolene sutures and alternating vertical mattress interrupted sutures. Skin reapproximated with slight difficulty. Bacitracin ointment and sterile dressing applied. Compression dressing.

DECISION MAKING: Low complexity

PLAN OF TREATMENT
The patient and her parent are instructed in wound-skin precautions. Patient to return tomorrow for recheck of wound. Patient given prescription for Tylenol #3, 1 tablet every 4-6 hours for pain. Keflex, 250 mg, 1 by mouth four times daily.

DIAGNOSIS
Acute laceration to the left pretibia, with extension down to the periosteum

TIME FACTOR
Total time: 40 minutes
Counseling: 25 minutes spent counseling patient and parent about wound care

OFFICE VISIT

DATE: March 14, 20xx
Patient returned for examination of laceration. Patient appears to be recovering from mishap. Wound is clear. Sterile dressing applied with bacitracin ointment. Patient instructed to change bandage daily and to call office if she has a change in condition. Patient to return in 1 week for examination and possible removal of sutures.

DECISION MAKING: Straightforward

DATE: March 20, 20XX
Patient returned for examination of wound. Area appears to be healing without difficulty. Sutures are removed. Patient is instructed in continuing care of wound. Bandage to be applied for next couple of days. Patient is released with instructions to be more careful on her new bicycle.

DECISION MAKING: Straightforward

TIME
Total visit: 20 minutes
Counseling: 10 minutes for wound care

PATIENT REGISTRATION FORM

PRACTICE ACCOUNT NUMBER		DATE
		03-12-xx

PATIENT ACCOUNT NUMBER	PRACTICE NAME	
17261	MIRACLE CLINIC	☐ NEW ☐ CHANGE

PATIENT INFORMATION *(Please write information about the patient here.)*

PATIENT'S NAME	SEX	REFERRING DOCTOR
GANNON, Mary Sue	☐ Male ☒ Female	N/A

PATIENT'S ADDRESS	REFERRING DOCTOR ADDRESS	CITY	STATE
123 My Street			

CITY	STATE	ZIP	EMPLOYER'S NAME	TELEPHONE
Anytown	MO	60600	N/A	

TELEPHONE	MARITAL STATUS		DATE OF BIRTH	EMPLOYER'S ADDRESS	CITY	STATE
314-555-2168	☐ Single ☒ Married	☐ Separated ☐ Divorced ☐ Widowed	03/05/80			

AGE	SOCIAL SECURITY NUMBER	DRIVERS LICENSE NUMBER	EMPLOYMENT STATUS	STUDENT STATUS: If 19 Years of Older:
	123-45-6677		☐ Full-Time ☐ Retired ☐ Part-Time ☒ Not Employed	☐ Full Time ☐ Part Time ☐ Not a Student

INSURANCE INFORMATION *(Please write information about the patient's insurance here.)*

PRIMARY INSURANCE COMPANY		SECONDARY INSURANCE COMPANY	
Great Way Insurance Co.	☒ Medical ☐ Dental ☐ Worker's Comp.	General Insurance Company	☒ Medical ☐ Dental ☐ Worker's Comp.

INSURANCE COMPANY'S ADDRESS	INSURANCE COMPANY'S ADDRESS
121 Insurance Lane	2121 Pay Well Avenue

CITY	STATE	ZIP	CITY	STATE	ZIP
Claimsville	MN	01011	Vicksburg	MS	39111

GROUP PLAN NUMBER	POLICY OR SUBSCRIBER'S NUMBER	GROUP PLAN NUMBER	POLICY OR SUBSCRIBER'S NUMBER
1010	333-43-4433		434-56-1234

POLICYHOLDER INFORMATION *Is the secondary policyholder the:* ☐ Patient ☐ Primary Policyholder ☐ Other
(Complete the information below if the PATIENT is not the POLICYHOLDER)   *(Complete the information below if you checked "Other")*

PRIMARY POLICYHOLDER'S NAME	DATE OF BIRTH	SECONDARY POLICYHOLDER'S NAME	DATE OF BIRTH
GANNON, Raymond B.	02/13/69	GANNON, Mavis J.	08/16/72

PRIMARY POLICYHOLDER'S ADDRESS	TELEPHONE	SECONDARY POLICYHOLDER'S ADDRESS	TELEPHONE
Same as patient		Same as patient	

CITY	STATE	ZIP	CITY	STATE	ZIP

EMPLOYER'S NAME	TELEPHONE	EMPLOYER'S NAME	TELEPHONE
B. F. Goodwill	314-555-2222	Secretaries R Us	314-525-1212

EMPLOYER'S ADDRESS	EMPLOYER'S ADDRESS
222 Work Avenue	1 Type Street

CITY	STATE	ZIP	CITY	STATE	ZIP
Anytown	MO	60600	Cool Ville	MO	60610

SOCIAL SECURITY NUMBER	RELATIONSHIP TO PATIENT	SOCIAL SECURITY NUMBER	RELATIONSHIP TO PATIENT
333-43-4433	☐ SPOUSE ☐ DEPENDENT ☒ OTHER father	434-56-1234	☐ SPOUSE ☐ DEPENDENT ☒ OTHER mother

EMPLOYER PLAN COVERAGE	IF CHAMPUS: ☐ Active ☐ Retired ☐ Deceased	EMPLOYER PLAN COVERAGE	IF CHAMPUS: ☐ Active ☐ Retired ☐ Deceased
☐ YES ☐ No Branch of Service: _____		☐ YES ☐ No Branch of Service: _____	

RESPONSIBLE PARTY INFORMATION *Responsible party is:* ☐ Patient ☐ Primary Policyholder ☐ Secondary Policyholder
(Please complete the information below if the person responsible for paying the fill is not the PATIENT or the POLICYHOLDER.)

RESPONSIBLE PARTY'S NAME	SEX	SOCIAL SECURITY NO.	DRIVERS LICENSE NO.	LEGAL REPRESENTATIVE
GANNON, RAYMOND B	☐ Male ☐ Female			☐ Yes ☐ No

RESPONSIBLE PARTY'S ADDRESS	STATE	ZIP	EMPLOYER'S NAME	TELEPHONE

TELEPHONE	RELATIONSHIP TO PATIENT	EMPLOYER'S ADDRESS	STATE	ZIP
	☐ SPOUSE ☐ DEPENDENT ☐ OTHER_____			

I AGREE TO THE ASSIGNMENTS AND FINANCIAL RESPONSIBILITIES SHOWN ON THE BACK OF THIS FORM.
<u>YOU SHOULD READ THOSE TERMS CAREFULLY.</u>

X _____Date _____
SIGNED (Patient, or parent if under 18 years of age.)

FIGURE 10-2 Patient registration form for Mary Sue Gannon.

PATIENT: **MARY SUE GANNON**

DOS: March 23, 20xx

HISTORY	EXAMINATION	DECISION MAKING
HPI: Timing, Context, Location	# of body systems or areas: 7 systems	Diagnosis:
ROS:		Data:
PFSH:		Risk:
TYPE: Problem-Focused	TYPE: Detailed	TYPE: Low
Category/subcategory:	Established patient (code based on time/counseling aspect)	

Note: Coding is based on AMA guidelines.
According to AMA guidelines, wound repairs do not have follow-up days.

<table>
<tr><th rowspan="2">History</th><th></th><th>PF</th><th>Exp. PF</th><th>Detail</th><th>Complete</th></tr>
<tr><td>**HPI:**
# of elements</td><td>Brief
1-3</td><td>Brief
1-3</td><td>Extended
4 or more</td><td>Extended
4 or more</td></tr>
<tr><td></td><td>**ROS**
# of systems</td><td>None</td><td>Pertinent
1 system</td><td>Extended
2-9 systems</td><td>Complete
10 or more</td></tr>
<tr><td></td><td>**PFSH:**</td><td>None</td><td>None</td><td>Pertinent
1 area</td><td>Complete
2-3 areas</td></tr>
<tr><td></td><td colspan="5">No PFSH required: 99231-33, 99261-63, 99311-33</td></tr>
<tr><td></td><td colspan="5">**Circle entry farthest to the right for each history area. To determine history level, draw a line down the column with the circle farthest to the left.**</td></tr>
<tr><td></td><td></td><td>**Problem Focus**</td><td>**E. P. Focus**</td><td>**Detail**</td><td>**Comprehensive**</td></tr>
</table>

Mary Sue Gannon DOS: March 13, 20xx		
History	Examination	Decision making
HPI	1995:	Dx:
ROS:		Data:
PFSH:	1997:	Risk:
TYPE: Problem focus	TYPE: Problem focus	TYPE: Straightforward
Mary Sue Gannon DOS: March 20, 20xx		
History	Examination	Decision making
HPI	1995:	Dx:
ROS:		Data:
PFSH:	1997:	Risk:
TYPE: Problem focus	TYPE: Problem focus	TYPE: Straightforward
Category/subcategory: Established patient (Code based on time/counseling aspect)		

 CODING TIP

Most insurance carriers allow a 10-day follow-up period on laceration repairs.

OFFICE VISIT
PATIENT: **JOHN J. JOHNSON** (Fig. 10-3)

DATE: January 13, 20XX

PATIENT HISTORY
The patient is 66-year-old white man with a 5-year history of diabetes. Patient has been insulin-dependent for the past 2 years, 25 units bid NPH. No reported allergies. No other reported medications.

FAMILY HISTORY
Family history unremarkable other than mother died 2 years ago of colon cancer and was insulin-dependent for the last year of her life. Father's history unknown. Two sisters and one brother without mention of diabetes.

EXAMINATION
The patient seeks a new physician because previous physician recently retired. Patient's record of blood sugar checks revealed elevation of levels exceeding 300 units. Physical findings reveal patient is slightly overweight.
Neck: Supple, soft with good mobility.
Abdomen: Supple, good interaction of digestive juices.
Lungs: Clear.
Respiration and pulse: Within normal levels of tolerance
   Blood glucose test with reagent strip revealed levels exceeding 275 mg/dL. Routine urinalysis dip test with microscopy reveals trace of sugar, which is not remarkable based on current condition.

DECISION MAKING: Low complexity

PLAN OF TREATMENT
Patient advised to set up appointment with diabetes dietitian at local hospital to begin 2000-calorie diet for weight loss. Patient to return in 4 days for monitoring of glucose levels. Patient to self-check blood levels twice a day: morning and night before meals. Medication increased to 30 units bid NPH.

DIAGNOSIS
Diabetes mellitus, uncontrolled

TIME
Total visit: 40 minutes
Counseling: 20 minutes spent explaining injections and importance of diet and daily checks of blood sugar levels.

OFFICE VISIT
PATIENT: **JOHN J. JOHNSON**

DATE: January 17, 20XX
Patient returns for evaluation of glucose levels he has taken over the past week and conference on laboratory results. Patient's glucose tests showed readings of 225, 225, 250, and 200 mg/dL. Patient is scheduled for glucose tolerance test with fasting, then repeat 2 hours after eating for January 18, in the office. Dosage to remain at 30 units bid NPH at this time. Patient to begin exercise program of walking 30 minutes a day. At this time, the patient has not made an appointment with dietitian to begin diet program. Patient is urged to begin weight loss program immediately. Patient to return in 5 days.

DECISION MAKING: Low complexity

TIME
Total visit: 20 minutes
Counseling: 15 minutes

PRACTICE ACCOUNT NUMBER	**PATIENT REGISTRATION FORM**	DATE
PATIENT ACCOUNT NUMBER 23456	PRACTICE NAME MIRACLE CLINIC	01-13-xx ☒ NEW ☐ CHANGE

PATIENT INFORMATION *(Please write information about the patient here.)*

PATIENT'S NAME JOHNSON, John J	SEX ☒ Male ☐ Female	REFERRING DOCTOR N/A		
PATIENT'S ADDRESS 2122 Greenlawn Lane		REFERRING DOCTOR ADDRESS	CITY	STATE
CITY Anytown	STATE ZIP MO 60600	EMPLOYER'S NAME Retired		TELEPHONE
TELEPHONE 314-555-7771	MARITAL STATUS ☐ Separated DATE OF BIRTH ☐ Single ☒ Divorced ☐ Married ☐ Widowed 11/27/22	EMPLOYER'S ADDRESS	CITY	STATE
AGE SOCIAL SECURITY NUMBER DRIVERS LICENSE NUMBER 321-20-0054		EMPLOYMENT STATUS ☐ Full-Time ☐ Retired ☐ Part-Time ☒ Not Employed	STUDENT STATUS: If 19 Years of Older: ☐ Full Time ☐ Part Time ☐ Not a Student	

INSURANCE INFORMATION *(Please write information about the patient's insurance here.)*

PRIMARY INSURANCE COMPANY MEDICARE	☒ Medical ☐ Dental ☐ Worker's Comp.	SECONDARY INSURANCE COMPANY A.A.R.P	☒ Medical ☐ Dental ☐ Worker's Comp.
INSURANCE COMPANY'S ADDRESS P. O. Box 505		INSURANCE COMPANY'S ADDRESS	
CITY St. Louis	STATE ZIP MO 64161	CITY	STATE ZIP
GROUP PLAN NUMBER POLICY OR SUBSCRIBER'S NUMBER 1010 321-20-0054-A		GROUP PLAN NUMBER POLICY OR SUBSCRIBER'S NUMBER	

POLICYHOLDER INFORMATION *Is the secondary policyholder the:* ☐ Patient ☐ Primary Policyholder ☐ Other
(Complete the information below if the PATIENT is not the POLICYHOLDER)   *(Complete the information below if you checked "Other")*

PRIMARY POLICYHOLDER'S NAME PATIENT	DATE OF BIRTH ___/___/___	SECONDARY POLICYHOLDER'S NAME	DATE OF BIRTH ___/___/___
PRIMARY POLICYHOLDER'S ADDRESS	TELEPHONE	SECONDARY POLICYHOLDER'S ADDRESS	TELEPHONE
CITY	STATE ZIP	CITY	STATE ZIP
EMPLOYER'S NAME	TELEPHONE	EMPLOYER'S NAME	TELEPHONE
EMPLOYER'S ADDRESS		EMPLOYER'S ADDRESS	
CITY	STATE ZIP	CITY	STATE ZIP
SOCIAL SECURITY NUMBER RELATIONSHIP TO PATIENT ☐ SPOUSE ☐ DEPENDENT ☐ OTHER_____		SOCIAL SECURITY NUMBER RELATIONSHIP TO PATIENT ☐ SPOUSE ☐ DEPENDENT ☐ OTHER_____	
EMPLOYER PLAN COVERAGE IF CHAMPUS: ☐ Active ☐ Retired ☐ Deceased ☐ YES ☐ No Branch of Service: _____		EMPLOYER PLAN COVERAGE IF CHAMPUS: ☐ Active ☐ Retired ☐ Deceased ☐ YES ☐ No Branch of Service: _____	

RESPONSIBLE PARTY INFORMATION *Responsible party is:* ☐ Patient ☐ Primary Policyholder ☐ Secondary Policyholder
(Please complete the information below if the person responsible for paying the fill is not the PATIENT or the POLICYHOLDER.)

RESPONSIBLE PARTY'S NAME	SEX ☐ Male ☐ Female	SOCIAL SECURITY NO. DRIVERS LICENSE NO. LEGAL REPRESENTATIVE ☐ Yes ☐ No
RESPONSIBLE PARTY'S ADDRESS	STATE ZIP	EMPLOYER'S NAME TELEPHONE
TELEPHONE	RELATIONSHIP TO PATIENT ☐ SPOUSE ☐ DEPENDENT ☐ OTHER_____	EMPLOYER'S ADDRESS STATE ZIP

I AGREE TO THE ASSIGNMENTS AND FINANCIAL RESPONSIBILITIES SHOWN ON THE BACK OF THIS FORM.
<u>YOU SHOULD READ THOSE TERMS CAREFULLY.</u>

X _____ Date _____
   SIGNED (Patient, or parent if under 18 years of age.)

FIGURE 10-3 Patient registration form for John J. Johnson.

OFFICE VISIT
PATIENT: JOHN J. JOHNSON

DATE: January 22, 20XX

Patient returns for evaluation of blood sugar and results of glucose tolerance test. While in the office, patient is given a blood reagent strip test using an ACCU-CHEK 2. Results show levels at 180. Patient's record of self-checks reveals levels to be at 170, 175, and 170 mg/dL. Patient has begun diet program and continues to walk 30 minutes a day. Patient is counseled to continue diet and exercise program and to remain on 30 units bid NPH. Patient advised of importance of continuing self-checks of blood glucose levels. Patient to return in 1 month and to notify office if levels exceed 250 mg/dL.

DECISION MAKING: Low complexity

TIME
Total visit: 20 minutes
Counseling: 15 minutes

MERCY GENERAL HOSPITAL
PATIENT: TOMMY Q. PUBLIC (Fig. 10-4)

DATE OF OPERATION: May 05, 20XX

SURGEON: A. Good Surgeon, MD

PREOPERATIVE DIAGNOSIS: Inguinal hernia, right and left

POSTOPERATIVE DIAGNOSIS: Left hernia, inguinal simple, recurrent right hernia, sliding type

OPERATION: Repair, hernia, inguinal, recurrent repair, hernia, inguinal, sliding

ANESTHESIA: General

OPERATION

Patient was taken to the operating room and placed supine on the operating table. General anesthesia with endotracheal intubation was performed. The left and right lower areas were then prepped and draped free in the usual sterile manner. A longitudinal incision was made on the lateral aspect of the abdomen. Care was taken to pick up and electrocauterize the bleeding blood vessels and other blood vessels before they bled to maintain hemostasis. The dissection was then continued. Repair was accomplished to the left hernia. Wound was irrigated with a copious amount of bacteriostatic-containing sterile saline solution. Wound was closed with interrupted-tissue 3-0 Vicryl sutures. The subcutaneous tissue was then closed with interrupted buried simple 2-0 Vicryl sutures. The skin was then closed in routine fashion, with excellent apposition of the skin without tension. There were no complications.

The right side was prepped and draped with an incision to the lower right abdominal section. Procedure was completed for right hernia repair. Wound was then irrigated with a copious amount of bacteriostatic-containing sterile saline solution. The wound was then closed with interrupted 0 Vicryl sutures. The subcutaneous tissue was then closed with interrupted buried simple 2-0 Vicryl sutures. The skin was then closed in routine fashion with excellent apposition of the skin without tension. There were no complications. The patient was awakened from general anesthesia and extubated. Patient was then taken to the recovery room in good condition.

PRACTICE ACCOUNT NUMBER	**PATIENT REGISTRATION FORM**	DATE
		05-05-xx
PATIENT ACCOUNT NUMBER	PRACTICE NAME	
24689	MIRACLE CLINIC	☐ NEW ☐ CHANGE

PATIENT INFORMATION *(Please write information about the patient here.)*

PATIENT'S NAME PUBLIC, Tommy Q.	SEX X Male ☐ Female	REFERRING DOCTOR N/A		
PATIENT'S ADDRESS 2 Lonely Avenue		REFERRING DOCTOR ADDRESS	CITY	STATE
CITY Anytown	STATE MO ZIP 60600	EMPLOYER'S NAME Fancy Meat Company		TELEPHONE 314-555-6000
TELEPHONE 314-555-1280	MARITAL STATUS X Single ☐ Separated ☐ Married ☐ Divorced ☐ Widowed DATE OF BIRTH 01 / 15 / 75	EMPLOYER'S ADDRESS 1 Cattle Drive	CITY Anytown	STATE MO
AGE SOCIAL SECURITY NUMBER 123-33-7788 DRIVERS LICENSE NUMBER		EMPLOYMENT STATUS ☐ Full-Time ☐ Retired ☐ Part-Time ☐ Not Employed	STUDENT STATUS: If 19 Years of Older: ☐ Full Time ☐ Part Time ☐ Not a Student	

INSURANCE INFORMATION *(Please write information about the patient's insurance here.)*

PRIMARY INSURANCE COMPANY Cattleman Association of America	X Medical ☐ Dental ☐ Worker's Comp.	SECONDARY INSURANCE COMPANY N/A	☐ Medical ☐ Dental ☐ Worker's Comp.
INSURANCE COMPANY'S ADDRESS 1 Railroad Drive		INSURANCE COMPANY'S ADDRESS	
CITY Dallas	STATE TX ZIP 76765	CITY	STATE ZIP
GROUP PLAN NUMBER POLICY OR SUBSCRIBER'S NUMBER Cattle 101 123-22-7788		GROUP PLAN NUMBER POLICY OR SUBSCRIBER'S NUMBER	

POLICYHOLDER INFORMATION *Is the secondary policyholder the:* ☐ *Patient* ☐ *Primary Policyholder* ☐ *Other*
(Complete the information below if the PATIENT is not the POLICYHOLDER)   *(Complete the information below if you checked "Other")*

PRIMARY POLICYHOLDER'S NAME PATIENT	DATE OF BIRTH ___/___/___	SECONDARY POLICYHOLDER'S NAME	DATE OF BIRTH ___/___/___
PRIMARY POLICYHOLDER'S ADDRESS	TELEPHONE	SECONDARY POLICYHOLDER'S ADDRESS	TELEPHONE
CITY	STATE ZIP	CITY	STATE ZIP
EMPLOYER'S NAME	TELEPHONE	EMPLOYER'S NAME	TELEPHONE
EMPLOYER'S ADDRESS		EMPLOYER'S ADDRESS	
CITY	STATE ZIP	CITY	STATE ZIP

SOCIAL SECURITY NUMBER   RELATIONSHIP TO PATIENT
            ☐ SPOUSE ☐ DEPENDENT ☐ OTHER_____
		SOCIAL SECURITY NUMBER RELATIONSHIP TO PATIENT
		            ☐ SPOUSE ☐ DEPENDENT ☐ OTHER_____	

EMPLOYER PLAN COVERAGE IF CHAMPUS: ☐ Active ☐ Retired ☐ Deceased ☐ YES ☐ No Branch of Service: _____		EMPLOYER PLAN COVERAGE IF CHAMPUS: ☐ Active ☐ Retired ☐ Deceased ☐ YES ☐ No Branch of Service: _____	

RESPONSIBLE PARTY INFORMATION *Responsible party is:* ☐ *Patient* ☐ *Primary Policyholder* ☐ *Secondary Policyholder*
(Please complete the information below if the person responsible for paying the fill is not the PATIENT or the POLICYHOLDER.)

RESPONSIBLE PARTY'S NAME	SEX ☐ Male ☐ Female	SOCIAL SECURITY NO. DRIVERS LICENSE NO. LEGAL REPRESENTATIVE ☐ Yes ☐ No	
RESPONSIBLE PARTY'S ADDRESS	STATE ZIP	EMPLOYER'S NAME	TELEPHONE
TELEPHONE RELATIONSHIP TO PATIENT ☐ SPOUSE ☐ DEPENDENT ☐ OTHER_____		EMPLOYER'S ADDRESS	STATE ZIP

I AGREE TO THE ASSIGNMENTS AND FINANCIAL RESPONSIBILITIES SHOWN ON THE BACK OF THIS FORM.
<u>YOU SHOULD READ THOSE TERMS CAREFULLY.</u>

X _____Date _____
    SIGNED (Patient, or parent if under 18 years of age.)

FIGURE 10-4 Patient registration form for Tommy Q. Public.

MERCY GENERAL HOSPITAL OUTPATIENT SERVICES

PATIENT: **MARY J. PULLINS (Fig. 10-5)**

DATE: September 30, 20XX

PROCEDURE: Release right carpal tunnel

ANESTHESIA: Regional

PREOPERATIVE DIAGNOSIS: Right carpal tunnel syndrome

POSTOPERATIVE DIAGNOSIS: Same

PROCEDURE

This 38-year-old woman presented with complaints of numbness and tingling in her right hand. The patient was evaluated in the office and thought to have carpal tunnel syndrome in the right arm. The patient was sent for EMG and NCB studies, whose results were compatible with bilateral carpal tunnel disease. For this reason, the patient was prepared electively for the operation room for release procedures.

Patient was brought to the operating room, where an intravenous access was established. Patient was then placed in the supine position, and regional anesthesia from a scalene approach was achieved. Adequate anesthesia analgesia was achieved. Patient was prepped and draped in the usual manner. A 4-cm incision was performed over the palm on the ulnar side of the patient's right palm over the third metacarpal. Extension was made onto the flexor creases of the palm. This was performed in a transverse fashion to prevent any scarring contracture from occurring postoperatively. Dissection was carried sharply through the skin and past the dermis. Then, using hemostat and blunt dissection, the palm tissues were separated to identify the transverse carpal ligament at its most proximal extent. A small hemostat was placed underneath the transverse carpal ligament and, using sharp dissection with a #5 blade, a complete transverse carpal ligament was released. Upon performing this, the median nerve was found at the base of the wound; this median nerve was not encountered during the dissection because of the patient's lack of symptoms in this area. The wound was copiously irrigated using normal saline solution. The skin was closed using a horizontal mattress #5-0 nylon suture. Xeroform gauze was placed, then a Kerlix was wrapped around the patient's hand. The patient was placed in a volar splint, which was held in place with an Ace wrap. The patient was returned to the recovery room in stable condition.

PRACTICE ACCOUNT NUMBER	**PATIENT REGISTRATION FORM**	DATE
		09-30-xx
PATIENT ACCOUNT NUMBER	PRACTICE NAME	☐ NEW ☐ CHANGE
13373	MIRACLE CLINIC	

PATIENT INFORMATION *(Please write information about the patient here.)*

PATIENT'S NAME	SEX	REFERRING DOCTOR		
PULLINS, Mary Jane	☐ Male ☒ Female	Samuel Medicine, M.D.		
PATIENT'S ADDRESS		REFERRING DOCTOR ADDRESS	CITY	STATE
34 North Corner		1 Office Plaza	Anytown	MO
CITY	STATE	ZIP	EMPLOYER'S NAME	TELEPHONE
Anytown	MO	60600	Office Cleaners, Inc.	314-555-5000
TELEPHONE	MARITAL STATUS	DATE OF BIRTH	EMPLOYER'S ADDRESS	CITY	STATE
314-555-7980	☐ Single ☒ Married ☐ Separated ☐ Divorced ☐ Widowed	09/16/72	5 Dusty Villa	Anytown	MO
AGE	SOCIAL SECURITY NUMBER 406-06-7652	DRIVERS LICENSE NUMBER	EMPLOYMENT STATUS ☐ Full-Time ☐ Retired ☐ Part-Time ☐ Not Employed	STUDENT STATUS: If 19 Years of Older: ☐ Full Time ☐ Part Time ☐ Not a Student

INSURANCE INFORMATION *(Please write information about the patient's insurance here.)*

PRIMARY INSURANCE COMPANY		SECONDARY INSURANCE COMPANY	
Better Insurance Corp.	☒ Medical ☐ Dental ☐ Worker's Comp.	Insurance World	☒ Medical ☐ Dental ☐ Worker's Comp.
INSURANCE COMPANY'S ADDRESS		INSURANCE COMPANY'S ADDRESS	
5 Insurance Drive		1 Collision Drive	
CITY	STATE ZIP	CITY	STATE ZIP
Gladtown	IA 54543	Wayward	ME 01116
GROUP PLAN NUMBER POLICY OR SUBSCRIBER'S NUMBER		GROUP PLAN NUMBER POLICY OR SUBSCRIBER'S NUMBER	
W562 406-06-7652		Salesmen of the World 406-28-8690	

POLICYHOLDER INFORMATION   Is the secondary policyholder the: ☐ Patient   ☐ Primary Policyholder   ☐ Other

(Complete the information below if the PATIENT is not the POLICYHOLDER)   *(Complete the information below if you checked "Other")*

PRIMARY POLICYHOLDER'S NAME	DATE OF BIRTH	SECONDARY POLICYHOLDER'S NAME	DATE OF BIRTH
PATIENT	___/___/___		11/11/70
PRIMARY POLICYHOLDER'S ADDRESS	TELEPHONE	SECONDARY POLICYHOLDER'S ADDRESS	TELEPHONE
		Same as patient	
CITY	STATE ZIP	CITY	STATE ZIP
EMPLOYER'S NAME	TELEPHONE	EMPLOYER'S NAME	TELEPHONE
		Salesmen of the World Inc.	
EMPLOYER'S ADDRESS		EMPLOYER'S ADDRESS	
		123 High Street	
CITY	STATE ZIP	CITY	STATE ZIP
		Gold Key	MO 60606
SOCIAL SECURITY NUMBER	RELATIONSHIP TO PATIENT ☐ SPOUSE ☐ DEPENDENT ☐ OTHER___	SOCIAL SECURITY NUMBER 406-28-8690	RELATIONSHIP TO PATIENT ☒ SPOUSE ☐ DEPENDENT ☐ OTHER___
EMPLOYER PLAN COVERAGE IF CHAMPUS: ☐ Active ☐ Retired ☐ Deceased ☐ YES ☐ No Branch of Service: ___		EMPLOYER PLAN COVERAGE IF CHAMPUS: ☐ Active ☐ Retired ☐ Deceased ☐ YES ☐ No Branch of Service: ___	

RESPONSIBLE PARTY INFORMATION   Responsible party is: ☐ Patient ☐ Primary Policyholder ☐ Secondary Policyholder

(Please complete the information below if the person responsible for paying the fill is not the PATIENT or the POLICYHOLDER.)

RESPONSIBLE PARTY'S NAME	SEX ☐ Male ☐ Female	SOCIAL SECURITY NO. DRIVERS LICENSE NO. LEGAL REPRESENTATIVE ☐ Yes ☐ No
RESPONSIBLE PARTY'S ADDRESS	STATE ZIP	EMPLOYER'S NAME TELEPHONE
TELEPHONE	RELATIONSHIP TO PATIENT ☐ SPOUSE ☐ DEPENDENT ☐ OTHER___	EMPLOYER'S ADDRESS STATE ZIP

I AGREE TO THE ASSIGNMENTS AND FINANCIAL RESPONSIBILITIES SHOWN ON THE BACK OF THIS FORM.
<u>YOU SHOULD READ THOSE TERMS CAREFULLY.</u>

X _____ Date _____
  SIGNED (Patient, or parent if under 18 years of age.)

FIGURE 10-5 Patient registration form for Mary J. Pullins.

PATIENT: **JOSEPHINE M. SMITH (Fig. 10-6)**

DATE: March 03, 20XX

OPERATION: Excision of two nevi with diameters of 0.5 cm and 1.1 cm

ANESTHESIA: Xylocaine 0.5% with epinephrine

PREOPERATIVE DIAGNOSIS: Dysplastic nevus and probably junctional nevus of the back

POSTOPERATIVE DIAGNOSIS: Intradermal nevus with lymphocytic infiltration: compound nevus with active junctional component

FINDINGS: Patient has two lesions of the back, a 1.1-cm oval lesion and a dark 0.5-cm lesion.

PROCEDURE

In the office, after adequate prepping and draping, Xylocaine 0.5% with epinephrine was infiltrated in a field block pattern for both lesions. The smaller lesion was excised elliptically and closed with 4-0 Vicryl in the subcutaneous tissue and 5-0 nylon on the skin. A towel was placed on top of this, and the upper lesion was elliptically excised down to the subcutaneous tissue. Bleeding points were tied with 3-0 Vicryl and the skin was closed with running 5-0 nylon. Estimated blood loss for both procedures was less than 5 mL. No drains were placed. Specimens were sent for pathological testing, with ellipse of skin on the lower back and upper midback. Dressings were applied, and the procedure was completed.

Patient to return to the office in 5 days for examination of the wounds.

PRACTICE ACCOUNT NUMBER	**PATIENT REGISTRATION FORM**	DATE

03-03-xx

PATIENT ACCOUNT NUMBER	PRACTICE NAME

11146   MIRACLE CLINIC   ☐ NEW ☐ CHANGE

PATIENT INFORMATION *(Please write information about the patient here.)*

PATIENT'S NAME	SEX	REFERRING DOCTOR
SMITH, Josephine	☐ Male ☒ Female	Samuel Medicine, M.D.

PATIENT'S ADDRESS	REFERRING DOCTOR ADDRESS		CITY	STATE
2660 Tree Lane Drive	1 Office Plaza		Anytown	MO

CITY	STATE	ZIP	EMPLOYER'S NAME		TELEPHONE
Anytown	MO	60600	N/A		

TELEPHONE	MARITAL STATUS	☐ Separated	DATE OF BIRTH	EMPLOYER'S ADDRESS	CITY	STATE
314-555-8181	☐ Single ☒ Married	☐ Divorced ☐ Widowed	07 /05 /55			

AGE	SOCIAL SECURITY NUMBER	DRIVERS LICENSE NUMBER	EMPLOYMENT STATUS	STUDENT STATUS: If 19 Years of Older:
	516-64-7237		☐ Full-Time ☐ Retired ☐ Part-Time ☒ Not Employed	☐ Full Time ☐ Part Time ☐ Not a Student

INSURANCE INFORMATION *(Please write information about the patient's insurance here.)*

PRIMARY INSURANCE COMPANY		SECONDARY INSURANCE COMPANY	
Blue Cross Blue Shield of MO	☒ Medical ☐ Dental ☐ Worker's Comp.	N/A	☐ Medical ☐ Dental ☐ Worker's Comp.

INSURANCE COMPANY'S ADDRESS	INSURANCE COMPANY'S ADDRESS
444 Forest Park	

CITY	STATE	ZIP	CITY	STATE	ZIP
St. Louis	MO	63144			

GROUP PLAN NUMBER	POLICY OR SUBSCRIBER'S NUMBER	GROUP PLAN NUMBER	POLICY OR SUBSCRIBER'S NUMBER
1015	VBS 534342066		

POLICYHOLDER INFORMATION *Is the secondary policyholder the:* ☐ *Patient* ☐ *Primary Policyholder* ☐ *Other*

(Complete the information below if the PATIENT is not the POLICYHOLDER)   *(Complete the information below if you checked "Other")*

PRIMARY POLICYHOLDER'S NAME	DATE OF BIRTH	SECONDARY POLICYHOLDER'S NAME	DATE OF BIRTH
SMITH, John B.	12 04 40		___/___/___

PRIMARY POLICYHOLDER'S ADDRESS	TELEPHONE	SECONDARY POLICYHOLDER'S ADDRESS	TELEPHONE
2660 Tree Lane Drive	314-555-8181		

CITY	STATE	ZIP	CITY	STATE	ZIP
Anytown	MO	60606			

EMPLOYER'S NAME	TELEPHONE	EMPLOYER'S NAME	TELEPHONE
Maxwell Powers Inc	314-525-0123		

EMPLOYER'S ADDRESS	EMPLOYER'S ADDRESS
2 Coffee Lane	

CITY	STATE	ZIP	CITY	STATE	ZIP
Anytown	MO	60601			

SOCIAL SECURITY NUMBER	RELATIONSHIP TO PATIENT	SOCIAL SECURITY NUMBER	RELATIONSHIP TO PATIENT
534-34-2066	☒ SPOUSE ☐ DEPENDENT ☐ OTHER_____		☐ SPOUSE ☐ DEPENDENT ☐ OTHER_____

EMPLOYER PLAN COVERAGE	IF CHAMPUS: ☐ Active ☐ Retired ☐ Deceased	EMPLOYER PLAN COVERAGE	IF CHAMPUS: ☐ Active ☐ Retired ☐ Deceased
☐ YES ☐ No Branch of Service: _____		☐ YES ☐ No Branch of Service: _____	

RESPONSIBLE PARTY INFORMATION *Responsible party is:* ☐ *Patient* ☐ *Primary Policyholder* ☐ *Secondary Policyholder*

(Please complete the information below if the person responsible for paying the fill is not the PATIENT or the POLICYHOLDER.)

RESPONSIBLE PARTY'S NAME	SEX	SOCIAL SECURITY NO.	DRIVERS LICENSE NO.	LEGAL REPRESENTATIVE
	☐ Male ☐ Female			☐ Yes ☐ No

RESPONSIBLE PARTY'S ADDRESS	STATE	ZIP	EMPLOYER'S NAME		TELEPHONE

TELEPHONE	RELATIONSHIP TO PATIENT	EMPLOYER'S ADDRESS	STATE	ZIP
	☐ SPOUSE ☐ DEPENDENT ☐ OTHER_____			

I AGREE TO THE ASSIGNMENTS AND FINANCIAL RESPONSIBILITIES SHOWN ON THE BACK OF THIS FORM.
<u>YOU SHOULD READ THOSE TERMS CAREFULLY.</u>

X _____ Date _____

SIGNED (Patient, or parent if under 18 years of age.)

FIGURE 10-6 Patient registration form for Josephine M. Smith.

MERCY GENERAL HOSPITAL
PATIENT: **MARY WORTHINGTON (Fig. 10-7)**

DATE: August 23, 20XX

SURGEON: A. Good Surgeon, MD

ANESTHESIA: General

PREOPERATIVE DIAGNOSIS: Left supracondylar femur fracture

POSTOPERATIVE DIAGNOSIS: Comminuted left supracondylar femur fracture

OPERATIVE PROCEDURE: Open reduction, internal fixation, left supracondylar femur fracture

PROCEDURE

Patient was taken to the operating room and placed in supine position on the operating table. General anesthesia with endotracheal intubation was performed. The left lower extremity was then prepped and draped free in the usual sterile manner. A longitudinal incision was made on the lateral aspect over the left distal thigh, and this was taken down and lateral to the skin incision through the subcutaneous incision down to the fascia. The posterolateral approach was then made to the left distal femur by separating the vastus lateralis off the intramuscular septum with care being taken to pick up and electrocauterize the bleeding blood vessels and other blood vessels before they bled to maintain hemostasis. This dissection was then continued to the periosteum and continued in the subperiosteal plane, exposing the bone at the left distal half of the femur and using large bone clamps, an open reduction was then performed and maintained in anatomical position. Multiple lag screws were then placed with 10-hole, 90-degree barreled ambi side plate with appropriate length. Large distal cancellous screws were placed, and further lagging of fracture fragments was performed through the plate. Stable reduction was then maintained after removal of the clamps. Anteroposterior and lateral radiograms revealed anatomical reduction and accurate placement of the appropriate hardware. The wound was then irrigated with copious amount of bacteriostatic-containing sterile saline solution. The fascia was then closed with interrupted 0 Vicryl sutures over the Hemovac drain. The subcutaneous tissue was then closed with interrupted buried simple 2-0 Vicryl sutures. The skin was then closed in routine fashion with excellent apposition of the skin without tension. There were no complications. The patient was awakened from general anesthesia and extubated. Patient was taken to the recovery room in good condition.

INSURANCE CODING, BILLING, AND ACCOUNTS RECEIVABLE

Information has been provided for you to complete the billing and reimbursement cycle for each patient. Provided information includes the following:

- Practice information
- Physician identification numbers
- Fee schedules
- Patient demographics
- Patient medical records
- CMS-1500 claim forms (Place-of-service [POS] codes are found in the introduction to the CPT manual.)
- Ledger forms
- Explanations of payments

DIRECTIONS:

Review the following information as it pertains to each patient encounter and code all billable diagnostic and procedure codes.

- Using the fee schedules provided, complete the CMS-1500 claim form.
- After completing the claim form, complete patient ledgers using the information provided.
- Posting should include all charges, payments, and adjustments and any other actions that should be taken to collect payments.

PRACTICE ACCOUNT NUMBER	**PATIENT REGISTRATION FORM**	DATE

PATIENT ACCOUNT NUMBER	PRACTICE NAME	08-23-xx
17170	MIRACLE CLINIC	☒ NEW ☐ CHANGE

PATIENT INFORMATION (Please write information about the patient here.)

PATIENT'S NAME	SEX	REFERRING DOCTOR		
WORTHINGTON, Mary F.	☐ Male ☒ Female	E.R.		
PATIENT'S ADDRESS 4747 Live Oak Village		REFERRING DOCTOR ADDRESS	CITY	STATE
CITY Anytown	STATE ZIP MO 60600	EMPLOYER'S NAME N/A		TELEPHONE
TELEPHONE 314-555-1786	MARITAL STATUS ☐ Separated ☐ Single ☐ Divorced ☐ Married ☐ Widowed DATE OF BIRTH 10 / 29 / 54	EMPLOYER'S ADDRESS	CITY	STATE
AGE SOCIAL SECURITY NUMBER 434-24-1613	DRIVERS LICENSE NUMBER	EMPLOYMENT STATUS STUDENT STATUS: If 19 Years of Older: ☐ Full-Time ☐ Retired ☐ Part-Time ☐ Not Employed ☐ Full Time ☐ Part Time ☐ Not a Student		

INSURANCE INFORMATION (Please write information about the patient's insurance here.)

PRIMARY INSURANCE COMPANY CHAMPUS	☐ Medical ☐ Dental ☐ Worker's Comp.	SECONDARY INSURANCE COMPANY N/A	☐ Medical ☐ Dental ☐ Worker's Comp.
INSURANCE COMPANY'S ADDRESS P.O. Box 7939		INSURANCE COMPANY'S ADDRESS	
CITY Madison	STATE ZIP WI 53678	CITY	STATE ZIP
GROUP PLAN NUMBER POLICY OR SUBSCRIBER'S NUMBER 474-81-2457 474-81-2457 (N4341613)		GROUP PLAN NUMBER POLICY OR SUBSCRIBER'S NUMBER	

ID CARD INFO   Eff: 06-20-76 Issued: 06-20-9x   EXPIRE: 06-20-9x

POLICYHOLDER INFORMATION Is the secondary policyholder the: ☐ Patient ☐ Primary Policyholder ☐ Other
(Complete the information below if the PATIENT is not the POLICYHOLDER)   (Complete the information below if you checked "Other")

PRIMARY POLICYHOLDER'S NAME WORTHINGTON, Ronald C.	DATE OF BIRTH ___/___/___	SECONDARY POLICYHOLDER'S NAME N/A	DATE OF BIRTH ___/___/___
PRIMARY POLICYHOLDER'S ADDRESS USS Saratoga	TELEPHONE	SECONDARY POLICYHOLDER'S ADDRESS	TELEPHONE
CITY Mayport	STATE ZIP FL 21212	CITY	STATE ZIP
EMPLOYER'S NAME USN (Capt 0-5)	TELEPHONE 314-525-0123	EMPLOYER'S NAME	TELEPHONE
EMPLOYER'S ADDRESS USS Saratoga		EMPLOYER'S ADDRESS	
CITY Mayport	STATE ZIP FL 21212	CITY	STATE ZIP
SOCIAL SECURITY NUMBER RELATIONSHIP TO PATIENT 474-81-2457 ☒ SPOUSE ☐ DEPENDENT ☐ OTHER____		SOCIAL SECURITY NUMBER RELATIONSHIP TO PATIENT ☐ SPOUSE ☐ DEPENDENT ☐ OTHER____	
EMPLOYER PLAN COVERAGE IF CHAMPUS: ☒ Active ☐ Retired ☐ Deceased ☐ YES ☐ No Branch of Service: __US Navy__		EMPLOYER PLAN COVERAGE IF CHAMPUS: ☐ Active ☐ Retired ☐ Deceased ☐ YES ☐ No Branch of Service: _____	

RESPONSIBLE PARTY INFORMATION Responsible party is: ☐ Patient ☐ Primary Policyholder ☐ Secondary Policyholder
(Please complete the information below if the person responsible for paying the fill is not the PATIENT or the POLICYHOLDER.)

RESPONSIBLE PARTY'S NAME	SEX ☐ Male ☐ Female	SOCIAL SECURITY NO. DRIVERS LICENSE NO. LEGAL REPRESENTATIVE ☐ Yes ☐ No
RESPONSIBLE PARTY'S ADDRESS	STATE ZIP	EMPLOYER'S NAME TELEPHONE
TELEPHONE	RELATIONSHIP TO PATIENT ☐ SPOUSE ☐ DEPENDENT ☐ OTHER____	EMPLOYER'S ADDRESS STATE ZIP

I AGREE TO THE ASSIGNMENTS AND FINANCIAL RESPONSIBILITIES SHOWN ON THE BACK OF THIS FORM.
<u>YOU SHOULD READ THOSE TERMS CAREFULLY.</u>

X _____ Date _____
  SIGNED (Patient, or parent if under 18 years of age.)

FIGURE 10-7 Patient registration form for Mary Worthington.

Additional Physician Information

Practice Information			
Miracle Clinic 12 Hope & Getwell Any Town, MO 63010	Ph: (636) 955-8844 Fax: (636) 955-1212	N. Stitches, M.D. I. B. Surgeon, M.D. B. Painless, M.D.	
Tax Lic.: 00998	Medicare Group #	BCBS Group #	Medicaid Group #
EIN: 23-753965	1BX678912345	123456-BC	56897-MO

I.D. Numbers			
Physician	**Personal I.D. #**		
N. Stitches, M.D.	Blue Shield:	234568	
	Medicare:	7891213650	
	Medicaid:	654238-M	
I. B. Surgeon, M.D.	Blue Shield:	121365	
	Medicare:	7894489605	
	Medicaid:	654238-M	
B. Painless, M.D.	Blue Shield:	963258	
	Medicare:	7894521789	
	Medicaid:	951753-M	

Note: The following boxes are part of the superbill on page XX.

Hospital Information
Crystal Memorial Hospital 670 Highway 267 Any Town, MO 63020

Miracle Clinic, P.A.

Tx Lic.: 00998 EIN: 23-753965	12 Hope & Getwell Any Town, MO 63010	Phone: (636) 955-8844 Fax: (636) 955-1212
G A. Good Surgeon, M.D. G I. B. Friendly, M.D.		G N. Stitches, M.D. G B. Painless, M.D.

Account Number:	Patient: Last Name	First Initial	Today's Date ___/___/___

Insurance: ☐ Private   ☐ Medicare   ☐ Medicaid   ☐ HMO
             ☐ PPO   ☐ Tricare   ☐ Other   ☐ Cash

Diagnosis: (1)_____ (2)_____
             (3)_____ (4)_____

X	CPT	Description	DX	AMT	X	CPT	Description	DX	AMT	X	CPT	Description	DX	AMT
Office Visits–New Patient					**Consultations–Office**					**Hospital Services**				
	99201	Problem focus		$35.00		99241	Problem focus		$50.00		99238	Discharge – <30 min		$70.00
	99202	Exp. problem focus		$60.00		99242	Exp. problem focus		$85.00		99239	Discharge – >30 min		$95.00
	99203	Detail		$90.00		99243	Detail		$115.00	**Procedures**				
	99204	Comprehensive		$125.00		99244	Comprehensive		$160.00		10060	I & D abscess		$80.00
	99205	Complex		$160.00		99245	Complex		$210.00		10120	F. B. removal		$65.00
Office Visit–Established Patient					**Hospital Services**						29870	Arthroscopy knee		$1,350.00
	99211	Minimal		$20.00		99221	Int. low complexity		$70.00		29877	Arthroscopy knee		$2,000.00
	99212	Problem focus		$35.00		99222	Int moderate complexity		$105.00		29881	Arthroscopy knee		$2,555.00
	99213	Exp. problem focus		$50.00		99223	Int high complexity		$150.00	**Miscellaneous**				
	99214	Detail		$75.00		99231	Subq E. P. focus		$30.00		36415	Venipuncture		$5.00
	99215	Comprehensive		$115.00		99232	Subq detail		$50.00		45380	Colonoscopy-bx		$1,087.00
Preventative Medicine Services						99233	Subq comp		$75.00		45383	Colonoscopy-surg		$1,415.00
	99381	NP <1 year		$95.00	**Injections**						45385	Colonoscopy-surg		$1,505.00
	99382	NP 1-4 years		$105.00		90724	Flu		$10.00		51725	Cystometro-gram-S		$370.00
	99383	NP 5-11 years		$105.00		90732	Pneumonia		$15.00		51726	Cystometro-gram-C		$550.00
	99392	Est pt <1 year		$85.00		90471	Injection (specify)		$15.00		51772	UPP		$450.00
	99293	Est 1-4 years		$105.00		90772	Antibiotic		$20.00		52000	Cystourethro-scopy		$300.00
Prolonged Services						J1670	Tetanus		$30.00		52005	Cystourethro-scopy		$570.00
	99354	Prolonged care		$180.00		J2510	Penicillin		$15.00		71020	Chest X-ray		$25.00
	99355	Each additional 30 minutes		$95.00		J3301	Kenalog 10 mg		$5.00		93000	EKG		$35.00
											93015	Stress test		$150.00
											99141	Conscious sedation		$100.00

Physician Signature

Return appointment information:

_____Days _____Wks _____Mos

Accept assignment:
☐ Yes ☐ No

Place of service:
☐ Office
☐ Out pt dept
☐ Hospital
☐ Other

Payment
☐ Cash
☐ Check
☐ Charge

$ _____
_____
_____
_____

Today's total fee:

Total due:

**Please remember:
Payment is your responsibility regardless of insurance or other third-party involvement.**

Type of credit card:
_____

Expiration date:
_____

Payment received:

New bal:

Common Accounting Abbreviations Used on Ledgers

Adj	Adjustment	NSF	Not sufficient funds
BCBS	Blue Cross Blue Shield	OV	Office Visit
EOM	End of month	Per ck	Personal check
EOW	End of week	POW	Payment on way
Est Pt	Established patient	PP	Promise to pay
FN	Final Notice	Pym't	Payment
IM inj	Intramuscular injection	Rcv'd	Received
Ins ck	Insurance check	ROA	Received on account
IV	Intravenous injection/infusion	SEP	Separated
MM	Medicare	SK	Skip or skipped
Mcd	Medicaid	U/Emp	Unemployed
MLD	Mailed	w/o	Write-off
NP	New Patient		

Insurance Company Addresses

Aetna Insurance Company P.O. Box 43712 St. Louis, MO 63055	Medicare Part B P.O. Box 98543 St. Louis, MO 63051
BCBS of Missouri P.O. Box 17896 Kansas City, MO 68011	Missouri Medicaid P.O. Box 1546 Jefferson City, MO 68170
GHP Health Plan P.O. Box 50079 St. Louis, MO 63052	United Health Care P.O. Box 6671 St. Louis, MO 63056

•	Above addresses are fictitious. They have been created for use with the exercises.
••	Patient information and fees are for use with the following exercises. Information is not intended to represent actual patient accounts, records, or practice fees.

Correct Coding Initial Bundling Edits							
Arthroscopic procedure bundling edit based on correct code selection:							
27570	29870	29871	29874	29875	29877	29882	29883
29884	36000	64415	64415	64417	64450	64470	69990
90760	90765	90772	90774	90775			
Colonoscopy bundling edits based on correct code selection:							
CPT code: 45383		RVU: 31.6					
45300	45303	45305	15307	45308	45309	45378	45382
45385	45900	45905					
CPT code: 45385		RVU: 27.9					
45300	45303	45305	15307	45308	45309	45378	45382
45383	45900	45905					
Urodynamic studies do not have bundling edits.							

The following pages contain information for coding and billing patient services. In addition, information and forms have been provided to assist you in completing CMS-1500 claim forms and patient ledgers. The final physicians' information on three physicians applies only to patients Luther Alexander through Robert Bell.

Patient 1

Patient 1: Alexander H. Luther	Account # 12345
Patient Information	**Insurance Information**
Name: Luther, Alexander H. Address: 1345 Maple Drive City: Any Town State: MO Zip code: 63022 Telephone #: (636) 555-1515	Primary insurance: Medicare Primary plan number: 222-55-6565-A Group #: N/A Primary policyholder: Luther, Alexander H. Insured DOB: 05-05-19xx
Gender: Male Date of Birth: 05-05-19xx SSN: 222-55-6565 Occupation: Retired Employer: Retired Spouse's name: Luther, Belle M. Spouse's employer: N/A	Relation to patient: Self Second ins info: n/a Secondary plan #: n/a Secondary info: n/a Insured DOB: n/a
Marital status: ☐Single ☒Married ☐Other	Student: ☐Full time ☐Part time

Miracle Clinic
12 Hope & Getwell
Any Town, MO 63010

Patient status:	New: __X__	Est: ____	Consult: ____	Hospital: ____	Other: ____

Account no.: 12345	DOB: 05-05-19xx	Physician: Stitches
Patient name: Luther, Alexander H.	DOS: 03-07-20xx	Insurance: Medicare

Wt: 155	Ht: 5' 11"	BP: 120/80

CC:	Swelling, groin pain
S:	This 67-year-old white male is seen for the first time for swelling and stabbing pain in the left groin area. Patient states he was doing yard work and lifting a heavy object when he experienced the onset of pain. Family history positive for inguinal hernia and hypertension.
O:	Abdomen: mildly tender. Bowel sounds active. Has an inguinal hernia on the left side.
A:	1) Abdominal pain secondary to inguinial hernia 2) Inguinal hernia
CC:	Swelling, groin pain
S:	This 67-year-old white male is seen for the first time for swelling and stabbing pain in the left groin area. Patient states he was doing yard work and lifting a heavy object when he experienced the onset of pain. Family history positive for inguinal hernia and hypertension.
P:	Patient to see Dr. Lawrence Feelgood, a general surgeon, for surgical evaluation of hernia.
	N. Stitches, M.D.

Policy Information		Insurance(s) Information
Policy pays 80% of the allowed amount after deductible Patient has 20% copayment		Deductible met:
*Claim filed 03-07-20xx		
**Received insurance payment check #1235 on 05-26-20xx		
***Patient made payment: Personal check #5678 on 06-26-20xx in the amount of $5.70		

STATEMENT

MIRACLE CLINIC, P.A.
12 Hope & Getwell
Any Town, MO 63010

Ph: (636) 955-8844	Fax: (636) 955-1212
Patient name: Luther, Alexander H.	Account number: 12345
Address: 1345 Maple Drive Any Town, MO 63022 (636) 555-1515	Ph: (636) 555-1515
Primary insurance: Medicare	DOB: 05-05-19xx
Secondary insurance:	

				Balance forward		00

| DATE | REFERENCE | DESCRIPTION | CHARGE | CREDITS | | CURRENT |
				Payments	Adj.	BALANCE

Patient 2

Patient 2: Mary B. Huttson	Account # 12593
Patient Information	**Insurance Information**

Name:	Huttson, Mary B.	Primary insurance:	BC/BS
Address:	1239 Bell Palm	Primary plan number:	12569
City:	Any Town	Group #:	3366
State:	MO	Primary policyholder:	Self
Zip code:	63029	Insured DOB:	09-30-19xx
Telephone #:	(636) 555-7979	Relation to patient:	Self
Gender:	Female	Second ins info:	n/a
Date of Birth:	09-30-19xx	Secondary plan #:	n/a
SSN:	123-45-9876	Secondary info:	n/a
Occupation:	Executive secretary	Insured DOB:	n/a
Employer:	Carlson Plumbing		
Spouse's name:	n/a		
Spouse's employer:	n/a		
Marital status: [X] Single ☐ Married ☐ Other		Student: ☐ Full time ☐ Part time	

Miracle Clinic
12 Hope & Getwell
Any Town, MO 63010

Patient status:	New: ____	Est: ____	Consult: ____	Hospital: <u>O. Pt.</u> Other: ____

Patient name: Mary B. Huttson	DOS: 02-12-20xx	Insurance: BC/BS
Account no.: 12593	DOB: 09-30-19xx	Physician: Painless

BP: 153/98	P: 70	T: 36.9

CC:	Severe cramping abdominal pain
S:	This 30-year-old female presents to outpatient dept complaining of severe cramping abdominal pain associated with bloating, nausea, vomiting, and watery diarrhea. Patient was last seen in the office 3 months ago for f/u of diabetes. Currently on Glucophage and Atenolol for hypertension. Denies fear, chills or other similar symptoms prior to today. Symptoms started around midnight and have been continuous throughout the day. Remarkable for removal of gallbladder 8 years ago.
O:	Tired-appearing white female, awake, alert, and oriented. Feeling weak. ADB: soft, non-tender. Normal bowel sounds. No significant reproducible discomfort. LUNGS: clear. HEART: normal sounds, no murmurs.
CC:	Severe cramping abdominal pain White blood count 8900, hematocrit 41.5, normal differential, electrolyte panel normal, glucose 127, amylase 102, AST 20, ALT 21, Urinalysis (dipstick) normal.
A:	Acute diarrhea, nausea, vomiting caused by viral gastroenteritis Adult-onset diabetes
P:	Hydrate with 1 liter of fluid and IV antiemetics Follow up in the office in 5 days

B. Painless, M.D.

12:30 p.m.	Patient receiving fluids–lying quietly on examination table. States in no distress. Vitals are stable. Still nauseated–no vomiting. Skin color improving. (15-minute assessment)
1:15 p.m.	Patient feeling much better. Improved nausea. One diarrhea stool. Vitals stable. Sipping and retaining water. Patient continues to rest. Will be re-evaluated prior to discharge. (20-minutes patient assessment)
12:30 p.m.	Patient receiving fluids–lying quietly on examination table. States in no distress. Vitals are stable. Still nauseated–no vomiting. Skin color improving. (15-minute assessment)
2:05 p.m.	IV fluids absorbed and discontinued. Condition much improved. Vitals stable. Good skin tone. No vomiting, no diarrhea. Improved strength. Feels okay to go home with husband. Discharged in good condition. Patient to call if symptoms continue or failure to improve. Follow-up in office in 5 days. (20-minute assessment)

B. Painless, M.D.

Policy Information	Insurance(s) Information	
Policy pays 80% of the allowed amount after deductible Patient has 15% copayment		Deductible met:
*Insurance filed 02-14-20xx		
**Received BC/BS check #4567 on 03-24-20xx		
***Patient statement sent 03-25-20xx		
****Patient paid by personal check #2488, 04-05-20xx in the amount of $21.30		

STATEMENT

MIRACLE CLINIC, P.A.
12 Hope & Getwell
Any Town, MO 63010

Ph: (636) 955-8844   Fax: (636) 955-1212

Patient name: Huttson, Mary B.	Account number: 12593
Address: 1239 Bell Palm Any Town, MO 63029 (636) 555-7979	Ph: (636) 555-7979
Primary insurance: BC/BS	DOB: 09-30-19xx
Secondary insurance:	

Balance forward | 00

DATE	REFERENCE	DESCRIPTION	CHARGE	CREDITS Payments	Adj.	CURRENT BALANCE

Patient 3

Patient 3: Mae T. Dovey	Account # 13458
Patient Information	**Insurance Information**
Name: Dovey, Mae T. Address: 1215 Green Drive City: Any Town State: MO Zip code: 63022 Telephone #: (636) 555-1424	Primary insurance: Aetna Primary plan number: 12358 Group #: A7896 Primary policyholder: Mae T. Dovey Insured DOB: 03-05-19xx
Gender: Female Date of Birth: 03-05-19xx SSN: 123-58-5555 Occupation: Shoe maker Employer: Brown Shoe Co. Spouse's name: n/a Spouse's employer: n/a	Relation to patient: Self Second ins info: n/a Secondary plan #: n/a Secondary info: n/a Insured DOB: n/a
Marital status: [X] Single ☐ Married ☐ Other	Student: ☐ Full time ☐ Part time

---

Miracle Clinic
12 Hope & Getwell
Any Town, MO 63010

Patient status: New: ____	Est: _X_	Consult: ____	Hospital: ____	Other: ____

Patient name: Dovey, Mae T.	DOS: 02-12-20xx	Insurance: Aetna
Account no.: 13458	DOB: 03-05-19xx	Physician: Painless

Wt: 110	T: 97.8	BP: 116/78

This 20-year-old white female states she itches all over after a weekend camping trip. Examination shows a raised vesicular rash in the linear distribution on the face, trunk, and extremities. Impression: Contact dermatitis, possible poison oak. Plan: Kenalog 60 mg IM, Hydroxyzine for itch. F/U as needed.

B. Painless, M.D.

Policy Information	Insurance(s) Information
Policy pays 100% of the allowed amount after deductible and co-payment Patient has $20.00 co-payment Medications are allowed at 100% of the billed amount	Deductible: $25.00 Remains:
*Insurance filed 02-14-20xx	
**Patient paid cash 02-12-20xx in the amount of $20.00	
***Received ins payment on 03-31-20xx Check #2789	

STATEMENT

MIRACLE CLINIC, P.A.
12 Hope & Getwell
Any Town, MO 63010

Ph: (636) 955-8844   Fax: (636) 955-1212

Patient name: Dovey, Mae T.	Account number: 13458
Address: 1215 Green Drive Any Town, MO 63022 (636) 555-1515	Ph: (636) 555-1424
Primary insurance: Aetna	DOB: 03-05-19xx
Secondary insurance:	

Balance forward | 00

DATE	REFERENCE	DESCRIPTION	CHARGE	CREDITS		CURRENT BALANCE
				Payments	Adj.	

Patient 4

Patient 4: Mary C. Cathy		Account # 15982	
Patient Information		**Insurance Information**	
Name:	Cathy, Mary C.	Primary insurance:	BCBS
Address:	5960 Happy Lane	Primary plan number:	69853
City:	Any Town	Group #:	B9872
State:	MO	Primary policyholder:	Cathy, Mary C.
Zip code:	63022	Insured DOB:	04-02-19xx
Telephone #:	(636) 555-2772		
Gender:	Female	Relation to patient:	Self
Date of Birth:	04-02-19xx	Second ins info:	n/a
SSN:	585-60-1593	Secondary plan #:	n/a
Occupation:	Registered nurse	Secondary info:	n/a
Employer:	Jefferson Memorial Hospital	Insured DOB:	n/a
Spouse's name:	n/a		
Spouse's employer:	n/a		
Marital status: [X] Single ☐ Married ☐ Other		Student: ☐ Full time ☐ Part time	
Patient status: New: ____ Est: ____ Consult: ____ Hospital: O PT Other: ____			
Patient name: Cathy, Mary C.		DOS: 03-15-20xx	Insurance: BCBS
Account no.: 15982		DOB: 04-12-19xx	Physician: I.B. Surgeon

Crystal Memorial Hospital	670 Hwy 267
Outpatient Department	Any Town, MO 63020

Patient name: Cathy, Mary C.	Account no.: 15982
Date of operation: 04-02-20xx	Room no.:
Surgeon: I.B. Surgeon, M.D.	Assistant:

Preoperative dx:	Occult blood in stool; rectal bleeding	
Postoperative dx:	Polyps diverticulosis (2) of colon	
Operation:	Colonoscopy, flexible, with ablation of tumor(s), polyp(s), or other lesion(s) not amenable to removal by hot biopsy forceps, bipolar cautery or snare	
Anesthesia:	IV conscious sedation Versed 2 mg IV; Fentanyl 50 mcg IV	Drains: None

Procedure:

Pentax video-colonoscopy was passed to the cecum (photo) without difficulty. Patient tolerated the procedure well. On the proximal descending colon an 8 mm polyp was noted and fulgurated with the hot forceps. At 25 cm from the anal verge, a 1.5 cm polyp on a short stalk was snared at mid-stalk and electrocauterized. Except for pandiverticulosis, the remaining mucosa from the anal verge to the cecum was normal. Patient tolerated procedure well and was returned to recovery in satisfactory condition. Instrument and sponge count were correct.

I. B. Surgeon, M.D.

Policy Information	Insurance(s) Information	
Policy pays 80% of the allowed amount after deductible Patient has 20% copayment Secondary procedures are subject to a 50% multiple procedure reduction	Deductible met:	
*Insurance filed 03-16-20xx		
**Received insurance check #7893 on 04-30-20xx		
***Statement sent to patient 05-02-20xx		
****Personal check #8954 received 06-01-20xx in the amount of $410.00		

STATEMENT

MIRACLE CLINIC, P.A.
12 Hope & Getwell
Any Town, MO 63010

Ph: (636) 955-8844   Fax: (636) 955-1212

Patient name: Cathy, Mary C.	Account number: 15982
Address: 5960 Happy Lane Any Town, MO 63022 (636) 555-2772	Ph: (636) 555-1424
Primary insurance: BCBS	DOB: 04-02-19xx
Secondary insurance:	

				Balance forward		00

DATE	REFERENCE	DESCRIPTION	CHARGE	CREDITS Payments	Adj.	CURRENT BALANCE

Patient 5

Patient 5: Robert L. Bell	Account # 15963
Patient Information	**Insurance Information**
Name: Robert L. Bell Address: 1515 Oakwood Place City: Any Town State: MO Zip code: 63022 Telephone #: (636) 555-3258	Primary insurance: BCBS Primary plan number: 455-65-7893 Group #: 2893 Primary policyholder: Robert L. Bell Insured DOB: 01-25-19xx
Gender: Male Date of Birth: 01-25-19xx SSN: 455-65-7893 Occupation: Carpenter Employer: We Build Right Spouse's name: Angela C. Bell Spouse's employer: n/a	Relation to patient: Self Second ins info: n/a Secondary plan #: n/a Secondary info: n/a Insured DOB: n/a
Marital status: ☐ Single ☒ Married ☐ Other	Student: ☐ Full time ☐ Part time

Crystal Memorial Hospital Outpatient Surgical Center	670 Hwy 67 Crystal City, MO 63019-0350
Patient name: Bell, Robert L.	Account no.: 34567891
Date of operation: March 15, 20xx	Room no.:
Surgeon: I.B. Surgeon, M.D.	Assistant: M.R. Helper, M.D.
Preoperative dx: 1) Popliteal cyst. 2) Multiple osteochondral fragments through left knee. 3) Chondromalacia, left patella. 4) Mild degenerative meniscal tear, lateral compartment, left knee.	
Postoperative dx: Same	
Operation: 1) Arthroscopic debridement, left knee. 2) Removal of osteochondral fragments, left knee. 3) Debridement, chondromalacia of the patella.	
Anesthesia: General anesthesia	Drains: None
Procedure:	

The patient was brought to the operating room and placed supine on the operating table. A general endotracheal anesthetic was given. The tourniquet was placed high on the left lower extremity, and the left lower extremity was prepped and draped in a sterile fashion. Through superomedial, inferomedial, and lateral portals, diagnostic arthroscopy was carried out. The suprapatellar pouch showed a significant amount of synovitis, mild to moderate, and there was grade II chondromalacia on the left patella laterally. There were several osteochondral fragments. The fragments were removed. Chondromalacia was eventually debrided, and some other synovium was also taken down.

In the medial compartment, additional osteochondral fragments were identified and removed—both with a shaver and with raspers. At their largest, these measured approximately 4 mm across. The meniscus was probed and without tearing. The anterior cruciate ligament was photographed, probed, and also found to be without laxity or tearing. However, the lateral meniscus showed some degenerative fraying, especially anteriorly into the lateral horn. This was removed using a shaver. Additional osteochondral fragments were then removed in the popliteal fossa. The knee was reexamined and drained and then irrigated out once again and then drained. Then the arthroscope was removed. The knee was injected with 12 mg Celestone and 20 mL of .25% Marcaine.

The portal sites were closed with subcuticular stitches of 4-0 Monocryl. The skin was repaired with Mastisol and ½-inch Steri-Strips applied. Dressing of 4- × 4- inch gauze pads, sterile Webril, and two 6-inch Ace wraps were taken from foot to upper thigh. They were held into position with a Surginet stockinette.

Patient tolerated the procedure well, and there were no complications. The final sponge, needle, and instrument counts were reported as correct.

Policy Information	Insurance(s) Information	
Insurance pays 90% of the allowed amount after deductible Patient has 10% copayment after deductible Secondary procedures are subject to a 50% multiple procedure reduction	Deductible: $100 remaining	
*Insurance billed: March 20, 20xx		
**Received insurance check #5589 April 30, 20xx		
***Statement sent to patient on May 5, 20xx		
****Received personal check #235 on May 30, 20xx in the amount of		

STATEMENT

MIRACLE CLINIC, P.A.
12 Hope & Getwell
Any Town, MO 63010

Ph: (636) 955-8844   Fax: (636) 955-1212

Patient name: Bell, Robert L.	Account number:
Address: 1515 Oakwood Place Any Town, MO 63022	Ph: (636) 555-3258
Primary insurance: BCBS	DOB: 01-25-19xx
Secondary insurance: n/a	

| | | | | Balance forward | | | 00 |

				CREDITS		
DATE	REFERENCE	DESCRIPTION	CHARGE	Payments	Adj.	CURRENT BALANCE

Patient 6

Patient 6: Kristina L. Langford	Account # 13587
Patient Information	**Insurance Information**

Name:	Kristina L. Langford	Primary insurance:	Aetna
Address:	2630 Royal Way	Primary plan number:	408-77-1236
City:	Any Town	Group #:	5656
State:	MO	Primary policyholder:	James K. Langford
Zip code:	63022	Insured DOB:	03-17-19xx
Telephone #:	(636) 555-3489		

Gender:	Female	Relation to patient:	Husband
Date of Birth:	07-06-19xx	Second ins info:	n/a
SSN:	665-15-9874	Secondary plan #:	n/a
Occupation:	Homemaker	Secondary info:	n/a
Employer:		Insured DOB:	n/a
Spouse's name:	James K. Langford		
Spouse's employer:	Do Right Services		

Marital status: ☐ Single ☒ Married ☐ Other   Student: ☐Full time ☐Part time

---

Miracle Clinic
12 Hope & Getwell
Any Town, MO 63010

Patient status: New: ____   Est: _X_   Consult: ____   Hospital: ____   Other: ____

Patient name: Kristina L. Langford	DOB: 07-06-19xx	Insurance: Aetna
Account no.: 13698	Services: Diagnostic procedures	

Date of operation: March 15, 20xx

Surgeon:	I.B. Surgeon, M.D.	Assistant:

Preoperative dx: Stress urinary incontinence

Postoperative dx: Stress urinary incontinence pelvic relaxation

Operation:	Cystometrogram Urethroscopy Urethral pressure profile study (PPS)

Anesthesia: General

Indications: Patient presents for complex cyrtometric and ureteroscopy. She has a history of stress urinary incontinence and pelvic relaxation.

PROCEDURE:

Cystometry was done using complex multichannel cystometric. The patient's first sensation to void was at 14 mL; the second sensation was at 66 mL; and her third sensation was at 365 mL, which is normal bladder capacity. There is no instability noted. She did have a positive stress test, and her valve leak pressure was approximately 155. Her urethra closing pressure was approximately 27, which is normal. Residual urine was zero. Ureteroscopy was then done, with no abnormalities noted. She had positive gaping and positive funneling at the urethrovesical junction. No abnormalities noted of the bladder mucosa.

Policy Information		Insurance(s) Information
Insurance pays 75% of the allowed amount after deductible Patient has 25% copayment Secondary procedures are subject to a 50% multiple procedure reduction		Deductible: $50 due
*Insurance billed: 04-15-20xx		
**Received insurance check #98745 on 04-25-20xx		
***Statement sent to patient on 04-30-20xx		
****Received $25 payment on 05-05-20xx check #3458		

STATEMENT

MIRACLE CLINIC, P.A.
12 Hope & Getwell
Any Town, MO 63010

Ph: (636) 955-8844   Fax: (636) 955-1212

Patient name: Langford, Kristina L.	Account number: 13698
Address: 2630 Royal Way Any Town, MO 63022	Ph: (636) 555-3489
Primary insurance: Aetna	DOB: 03-17-19xx
Secondary insurance: n/a	

Balance forward | 00

DATE	REFERENCE	DESCRIPTION	CHARGE	CREDITS Payments	Adj.	CURRENT BALANCE

REMITTANCE ADVISORY

Patient Name and Account #	DOS	Codes	Billed amount	Allowed amount	Adjust	Ins Payment	Patient Portion
Insurance company: Medicare			Date: May 26, 20xx			Check #1235	
Luther, Alexander H. Acct #12345	03-07-20xx	99xxx	$60.00	$45.00	$15.00	$36.00	$9.00
Insurance company: Blue Cross/Blue Shield							
Huttson, Mary B. Acct #12593	02-12-20xx	99xxx 99xxx	$50.00 $125.00 $175.00	$33.00 $85.00 $118.00	$17.00 $40.00 $57.00	$28.05 $72.25 $100.30	$4.95 $12.75 $17.70
*Payment received March 24, 20xx Check #4567							
Cathy, Mary C. Acct #15982	04-02-20xx	45xxx 45xxx*	$1,505.00 $1,415.00 $2,920.00	$1,450.00 $1,200.00 $2,650.00	$55.00 $815.00 $870.00	$1,160.00 $480.00 $1,640.00	$290.00 $120.00 $410.00
*Comment: Secondary procedures are subject to a 50% multiple procedure reduction. **Payment received 04-30-20xx Check #4888							
Bell, Robert E. Account #34588	03-15-20xx	29xxx*	$2,555.00	$1,785.00	$770.00	$1,515.50	$100.00 $168.50 $268.50
*Comment: Patient has a remaining balance due of $100 on the deductible. **Payment received 04-30-20xx Check #5589							
Insurance company: Aetna							
Dovey, Mae T. Account #13458	02-12-20xx	99xxx 9xxxx Jxxxx	$35.00 $20.00 $25.00 $80.00	$30.00 $18.00 $15.00 $63.00	$5.00 $2.00 $10.00 $17.00	$0.00 $3.00 $15.00 $18.00	$25.00 $20.00
*Payment received 03-31-20xx Check #2789							

On the following pages, six blank CMS-1500 forms have been provided for reference and further practice (Figs. 10-8 through 10-13).

1500

HEALTH INSURANCE CLAIM FORM

APPROVED BY NATIONAL UNIFORM CLAIM COMMITTEE 08/05

FIGURE 10-8 CMS-1500 form.

```
┌─────────┐
│  1500   │
└─────────┘
```

HEALTH INSURANCE CLAIM FORM

APPROVED BY NATIONAL UNIFORM CLAIM COMMITTEE 08/05

☐☐ PICA   PICA ☐☐

1. MEDICARE   MEDICAID   TRICARE   CHAMPVA   GROUP   FECA   OTHER | 1a. INSURED'S I.D. NUMBER   (For Program in Item 1)
   ☐(Medicare #) ☐(Medicaid #) CHAMPUS ☐(Sponsor's SSN) ☐(Member ID#) HEALTH PLAN ☐(SSN or ID) BLK LUNG ☐(SSN) ☐(ID)

2. PATIENT'S NAME (Last Name, First Name, Middle Initial) | 3. PATIENT'S BIRTH DATE MM DD YY   SEX M☐ F☐ | 4. INSURED'S NAME (Last Name, First Name, Middle Initial)

5. PATIENT'S ADDRESS (No., Street) | 6. PATIENT RELATIONSHIP TO INSURED Self☐ Spouse☐ Child☐ Other☐ | 7. INSURED'S ADDRESS (No., Street)

CITY | STATE | 8. PATIENT STATUS Single☐ Married☐ Other☐ | CITY | STATE

ZIP CODE | TELEPHONE (Include Area Code) ( ) | Employed☐ Full-Time Student☐ Part-Time Student☐ | ZIP CODE | TELEPHONE (Include Area Code) ( )

9. OTHER INSURED'S NAME (Last Name, First Name, Middle Initial) | 10. IS PATIENT'S CONDITION RELATED TO: | 11. INSURED'S POLICY GROUP OR FECA NUMBER

a. OTHER INSURED'S POLICY OR GROUP NUMBER | a. EMPLOYMENT? (Current or Previous) YES☐ NO☐ | a. INSURED'S DATE OF BIRTH MM DD YY SEX M☐ F☐

b. OTHER INSURED'S DATE OF BIRTH MM DD YY SEX M☐ F☐ | b. AUTO ACCIDENT? YES☐ NO☐ PLACE (State) | b. EMPLOYER'S NAME OR SCHOOL NAME

c. EMPLOYER'S NAME OR SCHOOL NAME | c. OTHER ACCIDENT? YES☐ NO☐ | c. INSURANCE PLAN NAME OR PROGRAM NAME

d. INSURANCE PLAN NAME OR PROGRAM NAME | 10d. RESERVED FOR LOCAL USE | d. IS THERE ANOTHER HEALTH BENEFIT PLAN? YES☐ NO☐ If yes, return to and complete item 9 a-d.

READ BACK OF FORM BEFORE COMPLETING & SIGNING THIS FORM.
12. PATIENT'S OR AUTHORIZED PERSON'S SIGNATURE I authorize the release of any medical or other information necessary to process this claim. I also request payment of government benefits either to myself or to the party who accepts assignment below.
SIGNED _____ DATE _____
13. INSURED'S OR AUTHORIZED PERSON'S SIGNATURE I authorize payment of medical benefits to the undersigned physician or supplier for services described below.
SIGNED _____

14. DATE OF CURRENT: MM DD YY ILLNESS (First symptom) OR INJURY (Accident) OR PREGNANCY(LMP) | 15. IF PATIENT HAS HAD SAME OR SIMILAR ILLNESS. GIVE FIRST DATE MM DD YY | 16. DATES PATIENT UNABLE TO WORK IN CURRENT OCCUPATION MM DD YY FROM TO MM DD YY

17. NAME OF REFERRING PROVIDER OR OTHER SOURCE | 17a. | 17b. NPI | 18. HOSPITALIZATION DATES RELATED TO CURRENT SERVICES MM DD YY FROM TO MM DD YY

19. RESERVED FOR LOCAL USE | 20. OUTSIDE LAB? YES☐ NO☐ $ CHARGES

21. DIAGNOSIS OR NATURE OF ILLNESS OR INJURY (Relate Items 1, 2, 3 or 4 to Item 24E by Line)
1. |___.___ 3. |___.___
2. |___.___ 4. |___.___
| 22. MEDICAID RESUBMISSION CODE ORIGINAL REF. NO.
23. PRIOR AUTHORIZATION NUMBER

24. A. DATE(S) OF SERVICE From MM DD YY To MM DD YY | B. PLACE OF SERVICE | C. EMG | D. PROCEDURES, SERVICES, OR SUPPLIES (Explain Unusual Circumstances) CPT/HCPCS MODIFIER | E. DIAGNOSIS POINTER | F. $ CHARGES | G. DAYS OR UNITS | H. EPSDT Family Plan | I. ID. QUAL. | J. RENDERING PROVIDER ID. #

1 | | | | | | | | | | NPI
2 | | | | | | | | | | NPI
3 | | | | | | | | | | NPI
4 | | | | | | | | | | NPI
5 | | | | | | | | | | NPI
6 | | | | | | | | | | NPI

25. FEDERAL TAX I.D. NUMBER SSN☐ EIN☐ | 26. PATIENT'S ACCOUNT NO. | 27. ACCEPT ASSIGNMENT? (For govt. claims, see back) YES☐ NO☐ | 28. TOTAL CHARGE $ | 29. AMOUNT PAID $ | 30. BALANCE DUE $

31. SIGNATURE OF PHYSICIAN OR SUPPLIER INCLUDING DEGREES OR CREDENTIALS (I certify that the statements on the reverse apply to this bill and are made a part thereof.)
SIGNED _____ DATE _____
| 32. SERVICE FACILITY LOCATION INFORMATION a. b. | 33. BILLING PROVIDER INFO & PH # ( ) a. b.

NUCC Instruction Manual available at: www.nucc.org | APPROVED OMB-0938-0999 FORM CMS-1500 (08/05)

Right margin vertical text: CARRIER — PATIENT AND INSURED INFORMATION — PHYSICIAN OR SUPPLIER INFORMATION

FIGURE 10-9 CMS-1500 form.

FIGURE 10-10 CMS-1500 form.

1500

HEALTH INSURANCE CLAIM FORM

APPROVED BY NATIONAL UNIFORM CLAIM COMMITTEE 08/05

CARRIER →

☐☐ PICA   PICA ☐☐

1. MEDICARE ☐ (Medicare #)   MEDICAID ☐ (Medicaid #)   TRICARE CHAMPUS ☐ (Sponsor's SSN)   CHAMPVA ☐ (Member ID#)   GROUP HEALTH PLAN ☐ (SSN or ID)   FECA BLK LUNG ☐ (SSN)   OTHER ☐ (ID) | 1a. INSURED'S I.D. NUMBER   (For Program in Item 1)

2. PATIENT'S NAME (Last Name, First Name, Middle Initial) | 3. PATIENT'S BIRTH DATE MM | DD | YY   SEX M ☐ F ☐ | 4. INSURED'S NAME (Last Name, First Name, Middle Initial)

5. PATIENT'S ADDRESS (No., Street) | 6. PATIENT RELATIONSHIP TO INSURED   Self ☐ Spouse ☐ Child ☐ Other ☐ | 7. INSURED'S ADDRESS (No., Street)

CITY   STATE | 8. PATIENT STATUS   Single ☐ Married ☐ Other ☐ | CITY   STATE

ZIP CODE   TELEPHONE (Include Area Code) ( ) | Employed ☐ Full-Time Student ☐ Part-Time Student ☐ | ZIP CODE   TELEPHONE (Include Area Code) ( )

9. OTHER INSURED'S NAME (Last Name, First Name, Middle Initial) | 10. IS PATIENT'S CONDITION RELATED TO: | 11. INSURED'S POLICY GROUP OR FECA NUMBER

a. OTHER INSURED'S POLICY OR GROUP NUMBER | a. EMPLOYMENT? (Current or Previous)   YES ☐ NO ☐ | a. INSURED'S DATE OF BIRTH MM | DD | YY   SEX M ☐ F ☐

b. OTHER INSURED'S DATE OF BIRTH MM | DD | YY   SEX M ☐ F ☐ | b. AUTO ACCIDENT?   PLACE (State)   YES ☐ NO ☐ | b. EMPLOYER'S NAME OR SCHOOL NAME

c. EMPLOYER'S NAME OR SCHOOL NAME | c. OTHER ACCIDENT?   YES ☐ NO ☐ | c. INSURANCE PLAN NAME OR PROGRAM NAME

d. INSURANCE PLAN NAME OR PROGRAM NAME | 10d. RESERVED FOR LOCAL USE | d. IS THERE ANOTHER HEALTH BENEFIT PLAN?   YES ☐ NO ☐ If yes, return to and complete item 9 a-d.

READ BACK OF FORM BEFORE COMPLETING & SIGNING THIS FORM.
12. PATIENT'S OR AUTHORIZED PERSON'S SIGNATURE I authorize the release of any medical or other information necessary to process this claim. I also request payment of government benefits either to myself or to the party who accepts assignment below.

SIGNED _____   DATE _____

13. INSURED'S OR AUTHORIZED PERSON'S SIGNATURE I authorize payment of medical benefits to the undersigned physician or supplier for services described below.

SIGNED _____

PATIENT AND INSURED INFORMATION ↓

14. DATE OF CURRENT: MM | DD | YY ◄ ILLNESS (First symptom) OR INJURY (Accident) OR PREGNANCY(LMP) | 15. IF PATIENT HAS HAD SAME OR SIMILAR ILLNESS. GIVE FIRST DATE MM | DD | YY | 16. DATES PATIENT UNABLE TO WORK IN CURRENT OCCUPATION FROM MM | DD | YY TO MM | DD | YY

17. NAME OF REFERRING PROVIDER OR OTHER SOURCE | 17a. | 17b. NPI | 18. HOSPITALIZATION DATES RELATED TO CURRENT SERVICES FROM MM | DD | YY TO MM | DD | YY

19. RESERVED FOR LOCAL USE | 20. OUTSIDE LAB?   YES ☐ NO ☐ $ CHARGES

21. DIAGNOSIS OR NATURE OF ILLNESS OR INJURY (Relate Items 1, 2, 3 or 4 to Item 24E by Line)

1. ⌞___.___⌟   3. ⌞___.___⌟

2. ⌞___.___⌟   4. ⌞___.___⌟

22. MEDICAID RESUBMISSION CODE   ORIGINAL REF. NO.

23. PRIOR AUTHORIZATION NUMBER

24. A. DATE(S) OF SERVICE From MM DD YY To MM DD YY	B. PLACE OF SERVICE	C. EMG	D. PROCEDURES, SERVICES, OR SUPPLIES (Explain Unusual Circumstances) CPT/HCPCS	MODIFIER	E. DIAGNOSIS POINTER	F. $ CHARGES	G. DAYS OR UNITS	H. EPSDT Family Plan	I. ID. QUAL.	J. RENDERING PROVIDER ID. #
1										NPI
2										NPI
3										NPI
4										NPI
5										NPI
6										NPI

25. FEDERAL TAX I.D. NUMBER   SSN ☐ EIN ☐ | 26. PATIENT'S ACCOUNT NO. | 27. ACCEPT ASSIGNMENT? (For govt. claims, see back) YES ☐ NO ☐ | 28. TOTAL CHARGE $ | 29. AMOUNT PAID $ | 30. BALANCE DUE $

31. SIGNATURE OF PHYSICIAN OR SUPPLIER INCLUDING DEGREES OR CREDENTIALS (I certify that the statements on the reverse apply to this bill and are made a part thereof.)

SIGNED _____   DATE _____

32. SERVICE FACILITY LOCATION INFORMATION   a.   b.

33. BILLING PROVIDER INFO & PH # ( )   a.   b.

PHYSICIAN OR SUPPLIER INFORMATION ↓

NUCC Instruction Manual available at: www.nucc.org   APPROVED OMB-0938-0999 FORM CMS-1500 (08/05)

FIGURE 10-11 CMS-1500 form.

FIGURE 10-12 CMS-1500 form.

FIGURE 10-13 CMS-1500 form.

Glossary

Abuse	Unknowingly defrauding the Medicare program by gaining payment for items or services when there is not legal entitlement to the payment.
Accepting Assignment	The provider of service agrees or is willing to accept as payment the amount allowed/approved by an insurance company as the maximum amount that will be paid for the claim. After the patient has met the annual deductible, the insurance will pay a percentage of the approved/allowed amount and the patient will have a co-payment.
Accounts Payable	Amounts owed by the practice to creditors for property, supplies, equipment, etc.
Accounts Receivable	A/R. The total amount of money owed to the doctor for professional services provided to a patient.
Actual Charge	The amount charged by the practice when providing services.
Adjudicate	A term for processing payment of a claim.
Adjudicator	Person who reviews the claim to determine payments.
Adjunct Codes	Codes used in addition to other services.
Adjustment	The amount corrected on a patient ledger due to an error or the difference in the amount billed by a practice and the amount allowed by the insurance company for payment of a claim.
Adjustments Codes	Codes used by insurance companies to explain actions taken on a remittance notice.
Aging Accounts	Analysis of accounts receivable that indicate delinquency of 60, 90, and 120 days.
Aging Report	Report to track claim status of patient accounts and to identify individual accounts requiring additional work-up for payments and collections.
Allowed Charge	The amount set by the carrier for reimbursement of services.
AMA	American Medical Association.
APGs	Ambulatory patient group. A payment system similar to DRGs but designed for the ambulatory care facility.
Appeal	A request sent to an insurance company or other payer asking that a submitted claim be reconsidered for payment or processing.
Arbitration	Legal method where the patient and physician may agree to resolve any controversy that may occur before an impartial panel.
Assignment	Authorization by a policy holder to allow a third-party payer to pay benefits to a heath care provider.
Assignment of Benefits	Request that money be paid directly to the physician for services rendered on a given claim. In some instances, accepting assignment may result in adjustments or write-offs.
Batching	A deferred or delayed processing basis for imputing data for retrieval at a later date.
Beneficiary	In the Medicare program, one who is eligible to receive Medicare benefits for medical coverage or illness or injury or for death benefits.
Biopsy	Removal of a small amount of tissue to determine the extent of a disease or to determine a diagnosis.
BR	By Report. Based on the codes submitted, the claim may need to have a report sent explaining the charges.
Bundling	Combining lesser services with a major service in order for one charge to include the variety of services.
Capitation	A form of prepayment in which a provider agrees to furnish services to members of a particular insurance program for a fixed fee. Capitations mostly affect monthly payments to primary care physicians in HMO groups.
CF	Conversation Factor. Dollar value multiplier for fee calculation.
Civil Law	Law that enforces private rights and liabilities, as distinguished from criminal law.
CMS	Centers for Medicare and Medicaid Services. The federal agency responsible for maintaining and monitoring the Medicare program, beneficiary services, and Medicaid and state operations.

CMS-1500	A paper claim form submitted to an insurance company to provide billing information regarding patient services.
COB	Coordination of Benefits. A clause that has been written into a health insurance policy stating the primary insurance will take into account benefits payable by a secondary insurance. Prevents overpayment of the charges billed to the patient.
Collection Ratio	The relationship between the amount of money owed and the amount of money collected.
Commercial Payer	Private health insurance company or employer-based group insurance plan that pays claims for eligible participants.
Comorbidity	An ongoing condition that exists with another condition for which the patient is receiving treatment.
Compliance Plan	A structured format stating office policies and procedures to identify and correct inaccurate documentation and billing criteria.
Complication	A disease or condition arising during the course of or as a result of another disease modifying medical treatment requirements.
Component Billing	Billing for each item or service provided to a patient in accordance with insurance carriers' policies.
Conventions	Terms and symbols used to provide instructions for use of diagnostic codes.
Conversion Factor	The dollar amount determined by dividing the actual charge of a service or procedure by a relative value.
Co-payment	The amount the insured has to pay toward the amount allowed by the insurance company for services.
Correct Coding Initiative (CCI)	Bundling edits created by CMS to combine various component items with a major service or procedure.
Covered Entities	Health care providers, health plans, and health care clearing houses.
CPT	*Current Procedural Terminology.* Nomenclature published by the American Medical Association as a means to describe services rendered to a patient using numerical codes.
CPT Code	Procedural description with a five-digit identifying code number.
Cross References	Directions to look in another area for correct code selection.
Customary Charge	The amount representing the charge most frequently used by a physician in a given period of time.
Cycle Billing	Breaking the account receivable amounts into portions for billing at a specific date of the month.
Deductible	The dollar amount that must be paid by the patient before insurance will pay a claim based on coverage plans and benefits.
Defamation	Slander or libel or injury to reputation.
Defendant	Person defending a case. In a malpractice case this is usually the physician.
Demographic Information	Patient identification information. Contains complete patient name, date of birth, Social Security number, and insurance information.
Deposition	Taking of testimony from a witness made under oath although not in an open court. Information is written down or taped to be used in the case of a trial.
Diagnostic Services	Services performed to determine or establish a patient's diagnosis.
DMERC	Durable Medical Equipment Regional Carriers.
DOS	Date of Service.
DRG	Diagnosis-Related Group. Patient classification system to categorize patients who are medically related with respect to diagnosis, treatment, or statistically similar with regard to length of hospital stay.
DRG Rate	A fixed dollar amount payable to hospitals for patient care.
DSM-5	*Diagnostic and Statistical Manual for Mental Disorder, Fifth Edition* (DSM-V). A reference for coding psychiatric disorders or conditions.
Dun/Dunning	A request or message to remind a patient that the account is overdue or delinquent.
E Codes	External Cause of Injury and Disease codes.
E&M Codes	Evaluation & Management codes used to report patient visits, consults, hospital care, and so on.
EDI	Electronic Data Interchange. Computer-to-computer transfer of data between a provider of services and an insurance company or claims processing clearing house.
EIN	National standard Employer Identifier Number (EIN). IRS's federal tax identification number adopted as the national employer identifier (e.g., 42-1212123).
Embezzlement	Willful act of illegally taking an employer's money by an employee.
Encounter Form	Document to record information regarding services provided to a patient used for billing purposes. Also referred to as superbill or fee slip.

Medicare Part A	A national health insurance program for persons over the age of 65 and qualified disabled or blind persons regardless of income, administered by CMS to cover the cost of hospitalizations and nursing facility charges.
Medicare Part B	An elective coverage program offered by CMS for aged and disabled patients to provide benefits for physician and other medical services as part of the Medicare program. This program has a monthly premium that must be paid by the beneficiary to keep the policy in good standing.
Medigap	A specialized insurance policy for Medicare beneficiaries that pays deductibles and co-payment amounts not covered by the Medicare program.
Medi-Medi	Insurance coverage by both Medicare and Medicaid.
Minor Procedures	Services identified by AMA as a starred procedure. For Medicare, these include services with either 0 or 10-days of follow-up care.
Misfeasance	Lawful treatment performed or provided in the wrong way.
Modality	Any physical agent applied to produce therapeutic changes to biologic tissues (e.g., thermal, acoustic, mechanical, etc.).
NEC	Not Elsewhere Classified. A category of codes to be used only when the coder lacks information required to code the term to a more specific category.
Negligence	Omission to do something that should be done under ordinary circumstances. Negligence can involve a wrongful action or an omission of care.
Nonessential Modifiers	Terms listed in parentheses that provide supplemental information but do not affect the code selection.
Nonfeasance	Failure by a physician to anything in regard to a patient's medical condition when the physician has an obligation to act.
NOS	Not Otherwise Specified. This abbreviation is the equivalent of "unspecified."
NPI	National Provider Number (NPI). Number assigned to hospitals, physicians, nursing homes, and other health care providers containing alphanumeric characters plus a check digit (e.g., E3E30KL74-6).
Open Account	Accounts that are subject to charges from time to time.
Open Contract	An account where charges are made from time to time with a 5-year limitation for collection from the date the charge incurred.
Ordering Physician	The physician who orders nonphysician services for the patient such as diagnostic laboratory tests, clinical laboratory tests, pharmaceutical services, or durable medical equipment.
PC	Professional Component. Defines services provided by a physician or other health care professional.
Percentile	The ranking of fees from all providers in a given area to develop a reimbursement base
PHI	Protected Health Information (PHI). Data that could be used to learn a person's health information.
POS	Place of Service. Refers to the physical location where services are provided to a patient (e.g., office, inpatient hospital, etc.).
POS Code	Place-of-Service Codes. Codes used on insurance claim forms to specify the location where services were provided. A complete list is found in the introduction section of the Professional Version of the CPT manual.
Posting	A process of transferring account information from a journal to a ledger.
PPS	Prospective Payment System. A payment method pertaining to hospital insurance based on a fixed dollar amount for a principal diagnosis.
Precertification	A method for preapproving all elective admissions, surgeries, and other services as required by insurance carriers. Approval is essential before receiving payment for services.
Prevailing Charge	The charge most frequently used, in a specific area by physicians, based on specialty. The highest charge in the prevailing range establishes the absolute maximum limitation, or the highest amount a carrier will pay for a service.
PRO	Professional Review Organization. An organization of physicians that reviews services to determine medical necessity.
Professional Courtesy	A discount or fee exception given to a patient at the discretion of the physician.
Profile	A list of CPT codes used by a physician with a corresponding fee that is usually calculated and maintained by a third-party payer.
Providers	Services providers (e.g., physicians, hospitals, pharmacies, nursing homes, durable medical equipment suppliers, dentists, optometrists, and chiropractors).
Qui Tam	Recovery of a penalty brought by an informer in a situation. Generally, a percentage of the recovery is given to the informer for payment.

Endoscopic Procedure	A procedure performed though an existing orifice using a scope to visualize an abnormality or determine the extent of a disease.
EOB	Explanation of Benefits. Form accompanying an insurance remittance with a breakdown and ex of payments for a claim. Also referred to as a remittance advisory (RA).
EOMB	Explanation of Medicare Benefits. Form accompanying an insurance remittance with a breakdov explanation of payments for a claim.
Eponym	Conditions or procedures named after a person or place.
EPSDT	Early and Periodic Screening, Diagnosis, and Treatment. Medicaid preventive medical examinatio
Ethics	Moral principles and standards in the ideal relationship between a physician and patient or betw physicians.
Etiology	The cause of a disease.
Fee Schedule	An established price set by a medical practice for professional services.
Fee Slip	Also referred to as superbill or patient encounter form. A form used to track service information.
FI	Fiscal Intermediary. An insurance company under contract to the government that handles claims Medicare Part A from hospitals, skilled nursing facilities, and home health agencies.
Fraud	An intentional misrepresentation of facts to deceive or mislead another.
Global Period	Specific time frames assigned to a code by an insurance company before additional payment will k made following a surgical procedure (e.g., 10 days, 90 days, etc.).
Global Procedures	Referred to as major surgical procedures that typically have a follow up period of 30, 60, 90, or 12(before you may begin to bill the patient for services related to the original procedure.
HCPCS	Healthcare Common Procedure Coding System. More commonly referred to as "HCPCS" (sometime pronounced *hick pix*). A coding system designed by CMS to report patient services utilizing codes fr(CPT and other alphanumerical codes.
Health Plans	An individual or group plan that provides or pays for the cost of medical care.
Healthcare Providers	Any person or organization that furnishes, bills, or is paid for healthcare in the normal course of busi
Healthcare Clearing House	Companies that translate electronic transactions between the "standard" formats and code sets req under HIPAA and nonstandard formats and code sets.
HIPAA	Health Insurance Portability and Accountability Act. An act passed in 1996 to set standards for electr(health care transactions and to protect the privacy and security of patient health information.
Hospice	An organization (private or public) that provides pain relief, symptom management, and support servi to terminally ill patients and their families.
ICD-9-CM	*International Classification of Diseases, 9th edition, Clinical Modification.* The source of diagnosis codi required by insurance carriers and government agencies.
Indemnity Insurance	Traditional insurance programs referred to as "Fee for Service" programs.
Index	Another term for Volume Two, the alphabetical listing of terms to describe injuries or diseases.
Inquiry	Checking or tracing a claim sent to an insurance company to determine payment or processing status.
Inquiry Letters	Request from an insurance company for additional information required to process a claim for payment
Insurance Adjustment or Write Off	Amount required by an insurance company that must be taken off of a patient's account based on contract agreement and participation.
Judgment	The official decision of the court in regards to an action or suit.
Ledger Card	A record to track patient charges, payments, adjustments and balances due.
Limiting Charge	Typically applies to Medicare reimbursement. This is the absolute maximum fee a physician may charge a Medicare patient when not accepting assignment on the claim. This fee is set by the Centers for Medicare and Medicaid Services (CMS).
Litigation	A lawsuit.
Locum Tenens	A physician who substitutes for another physician who is out of the office for an extended period of time.
Major Procedure	A packaged procedure that includes the operation, local infiltration, digital blocks, and follow-up care for a specific number of days.
Malfeasance	Wrongful treatment of a patient.
Manifestation	Signs or symptoms of a disease.
Medicare	A national health insurance program for persons over the age of 65 and qualified disabled or blind persons regardless of income, administered by CMS.

Ranking Codes	Listing services in their order of importance by dates of service and values. Codes are usually ranked by value from highest to lowest charges.
RBRVS	Resource Based Relative Value Scale. A system of assigning values to CPT codes developed for Medicare to determine reimbursement amounts for services.
Referring Physician	The physician who requests an item or service for the beneficiary for which payment may be made under the Medicare program.
Relative Value Unit (RVU)	A method to calculate fees for services. A unit is translated into a dollar value using a conversion factor or dollar multiplier. The assigned value is generally based on three factors: physician work component, overhead practice expense, and malpractice insurance.
Remittance Advice	Statement sent by an insurance company detailing how submitted claims were processed for payment along with payment amounts.
Review	Process of looking over a claim to assess payment amounts.
Rubric	Three-digit root code for classification of illness, disease, or injury.
RVS	Relative Value Scale. The unit value attached to a code used to determine payment for services.
Skip	A patient who owes a balance on the account who has moved without a forwarding address.
SOF	Signature on File
Specificity	Using ICD-9-CM codes to the highest degree of certainty. Using fourth and fifth digits, as appropriate, while avoiding over use of the unspecified codes.
Statement	An itemized bill sent to the patient describing professional services provided. A request for payment.
Statute of Limitations	The time limit in which a lawsuit may be filed.
Superbill	A multipurpose billing form to track procedure and diagnosis codes during a patient encounter or visit.
Suspended File Report	A listing of claims that have incorrect information such as a posting error or missing information to process the claim.
Tabular	Another name for Volume One of the ICD-9-CM, the numerical listing of disease and injury.
TC	Technical Component. The portion of a test or study that pertains to the use of equipment or technicians.
Therapeutic Services	Services performed for treatment of a specific diagnosis.
Third-Party Payer	A carrier that has an agreement with an individual or organization to provide heath care benefits.
Timely Filing Clause	The amount of time allowed by an insurance company for a claim to be submitted for payment from the date of the service.
TOS	Type of Service. This refers to the services provided to a patient (e.g., Evaluation & Management services, surgery, x-ray, etc.).
Truth in Lending	An agreement between the patient and the physician regarding monthly installments to pay a bill. A truth in lending statement must be signed when payments exceed a 4-month period.
TWIP	Take what insurance pays.
UCR	Usual, Customary, and Reasonable. The reimbursement method that establishes a maximum fee an insurance company will pay for services.
Unbundling Services	Listing services or procedures as separate billable components. While this practice may generate more revenue, it is often an incorrect reporting technique that could result in an insurance company auditing a practice or asking for refunds of paid monies.
Unit Count	A means to report the number of times a service was provided on the same date of service to the same patient (e.g., Removal of 15 lesions).
UPIN	Unique Personal Identification Numbers. A number assigned to each covered provider in the Medicare program to identify the provider who performed the billed service(s).
Utilization Review	The process of assessing medical care services to assure quality, medical necessity, and appropriateness of treatment.
V Codes	Supplemental classification of codes when patient presents for something other than illness or disease.
Withhold Incentive	The percentage of payment held back for a risk account in the HMO program. Withhold arrangements are used to share potential losses or profits with providers of service.
Written Contract	An agreement signed by a patient in which specific payment amounts are made on the account on a monthly basis. These accounts usually have high amounts that will take over 4 months to repay and generally have a 6-year limitation for collection.

Index

Page numbers followed by *f* indicated figures; *t*, tables; *b*, boxes.